Pulmonary Hypertension and Interstitial Lung Disease

Robert P. Baughman • Roberto G. Carbone
Steven D. Nathan
Editors

Pulmonary Hypertension and Interstitial Lung Disease

Second Edition

Springer

Editors
Robert P. Baughman
Department of Medicine
University of Cincinnati Medical Center
Cincinnati, OH, USA

Roberto G. Carbone
Regional Hospital Aosta
and University of Genoa
Genoa, Italy

Steven D. Nathan
Inova Fairfax Advanced Lung Disease and
Transplant Program
Inova Fairfax Hospital
Falls Church, VA, USA

ISBN 978-3-319-49916-1 ISBN 978-3-319-49918-5 (eBook)
DOI 10.1007/978-3-319-49918-5

Library of Congress Control Number: 2017942775

Printed on acid-free paper

This Springer imprint is published by Springer Nature
The registered company is Springer International Publishing AG
The registered company address is: Gewerbestrasse 11, 6330 Cham, Switzerland

Dr. Roberto Carbone wishes to dedicate this book to parents Attilia and Giuseppe Carbone.

Preface

Several years ago, Roberto Carbone began working on a book which would deal exclusively regarding pulmonary hypertension in interstitial lung disease. He asked Drs. Baughman and Bottino to join in this effort as editors and we solicited chapters from experts around the world on this subject. This led to the first edition of *Pulmonary Arterial Hypertension in Interstitial Lung Disease* which was published in 2010. In this edition, Dr. Baughman and Carbone are joined by Dr. Steven Nathan as the third co-editor.

Since that time, several studies have been published regarding the diagnosis and management of pulmonary hypertension in interstitial lung disease. The terminology has changed and pulmonary arterial hypertension is reserved for WHO group 1 patients. Pulmonary hypertension in interstitial lung disease is categorized as either group 3 (e.g. idiopathic pulmonary fibrosis) or group 5 (e.g. sarcoidosis). Thus, we have changed the title of our second edition to *Pulmonary Hypertension in Interstitial Lung Disease*.

In addition to a new title and new co-editor, we have asked our contributors to provide a new version of their respective chapters, not just an update of the prior chapters. For many of the chapters, we sought new authors who have contributed to these respective areas.

The book is divided into two main sections. The first section deals with general principles of diagnosis and management of pulmonary hypertension in interstitial lung disease (PH ILD). Dr. Carbone and colleagues start with a chapter detailing the radiographic imaging seen in various interstitial lung diseases, with insights into how the pattern on high resolution computer tomography (HRCT) scan may help determine the underlying interstitial lung disease. Since patients with significant pulmonary hypertension are poor candidates for surgical biopsy or even bronchoscopic biopsy, many of the PH ILD patients are diagnosed based on HRCT. Dr. Engel describes the findings on heart catheterization which characterize pulmonary hypertension. This includes separating precapillary pulmonary hypertension from pulmonary hypertension due to left ventricular dysfunction. Although pulmonary pathology may not be available as part of the initial assessment of PH ILD, studies of pathology from biopsies and explanted lungs have provided insights into the cause(s) of pulmonary hypertension associated with specific interstitial lung diseases. This is detailed in the chapter by Dr. Nunes and colleagues.

The last two chapters of the general section focus on therapy. Dr. Nathan's group provide a review of the evidence supporting various medical managements for treating pulmonary hypertension in different interstitial lung diseases. In the past few years, some drugs have been shown not only to be ineffective for pulmonary hypertension associated with idiopathic pulmonary fibrosis but also to be potentially harmful. This is not a universal finding, since therapy for pulmonary hypertension with interstitial lung disease associated with scleroderma and sarcoidosis has had positive results. One potential treatment for PH ILD is transplant. Dr. Cordova and colleagues have reviewed this option in the last chapter in the general considerations section.

The second half of the book deals with specific interstitial lung diseases. Dr. Wells' group provide details regarding managing pulmonary hypertension in patients with idiopathic pulmonary fibrosis and other idiopathic interstitial lung diseases. Dr. Baughman and colleagues discuss the evaluation and treatment of sarcoidosis-associated pulmonary hypertension. Dr. Selman's group discuss pulmonary hypertension in patients with hypersensitivity pneumonitis. Dr. Highland and colleagues discuss pulmonary hypertension in interstitial lung disease associated with connective tissue disorders. Dr. Shlobin's group then address several other interstitial lung diseases associated with pulmonary hypertension.

We believe this book will provide a framework for future studies in what is an important aspect of managing both interstitial lung disease and pulmonary hypertension.

The editors wish to thank Stephanie Westendorf for all her help and support for this project.

Cincinnati, OH, USA Robert P. Baughman
Genoa, Italy Roberto G. Carbone
Falls Church, VA, USA Steven D. Nathan

Acknowledgements

Robert Baughman would like to dedicate this book to Elyse Lower, his spouse and most supportive collaborator.

Steve Nathan would like to dedicate this book to his wife Romy and their two sons Jack and Max.

Contents

Contributors

Debabrata Bandyopadhyay, MD, MRCP Department of Thoracic Medicine, Geisinger Medical Center, Danville, PA, USA

Robert P. Baughman, MD Department of Medicine, University of Cincinnati Medical Center, Cincinnati, OH, USA

Simon Bax, BSc, MBBS, MRCP Royal Brompton Hospital, National Heart and Lung Institute, Imperial College London, London, UK

Jean-François Bernaudin Université Paris 13, Sorbonne Paris Cité, Bobigny, France

Histologie et Cytologie, Université Pierre et Marie Curie, Sorbonne Universités Paris, Paris, France

Giovanni Bottino, MD Department of Respiratory Medicine, University of Genoa, Genoa, Italy

Ivette Buendía-Roldán, MSc Instituto Nacional de Enfermedades Respiratorias, Dr. Ismael Cosío Villegas, Tialpan, México DF, Mexico

Roberto G. Carbone, MD, FCCP Regional Hospital Aosta and University of Genoa, Genoa, Italy

Francis Cordova, MD Department of Thoracic Medicine and Surgery, Temple University School of Medicine, Philadelphia, PA, USA

Peter Dorfmüller Service d'Anatomie pathologique et INSERM UMRS 999, LabEx LERMIT, Hôpital Marie Lannelongue, Le Plessis-Robinson, France

Peter J. Engel, MD Ohio Heart and Vascular Center, The Christ Hospital, Cincinnati, OH, USA

Miguel Gaxiola, MD Instituto Nacional de Enfermedades Respiratorias, Dr. Ismael Cosío Villegas, Tialpan, México DF, Mexico

Kristin B. Highland, MD, MSCR Department of Pulmonary and Critical Care Medicine, Respiratory Institute, Cleveland Clinic Foundation, Cleveland, OH, USA

Cynthia Kim, MD Department of Medicine, Division of Pulmonary and Critical Care, David Geffen School of Medicine at University of California, Los Angeles, CA, USA

Marianne Kambouchner Assistance Publique Hôpitaux de Paris, Service d'Anatomie et Cytologie pathologiques, Hôpital Avicenne, Bobigny, France

Christopher S. King, MD Inova Fairfax Advanced Lung Disease and Transplant Program, Inova Fairfax Hospital, Falls Church, VA, USA

Elyse E. Lower, MD Department of Medicine, University of Cincinnati Medical Center, Cincinnati, OH, USA

Assaf Monselise, MD Department of Internal Medicine, University of Tel Aviv, Tel Aviv, Israel

Steven D. Nathan, MD Inova Fairfax Advanced Lung Disease and Transplant Program, Inova Fairfax Hospital, Falls Church, VA, USA

Carmen Navarro, MD Instituto Nacional de Enfermedades Respiratorias, Dr. Ismael Cosío Villegas, Tlalpan, México DF, Mexico

Hilario Nunes, MD, PhD Assistance Publique Hôpitaux de Paris, Service de Pneumologie, Hôpital Avicenne, Bobigny, France

Université Paris 13, Sorbonne Paris Cité, Bobigny, France

Tanmay S. Panchabhai, MD Norton Thoracic Institute, St Joseph's Medical Center, Phoenix, AZ, USA

Laura Price, BSc, MBChB, MRCP, PhD Pulmonary Hypertension Service, Royal Brompton Hospital, National Heart and Lung Institute, Imperial College London, London, UK

Moises Selman, MD Instituto Nacional de Enfermedades Respiratorias, Dr. Ismael Cosío Villegas, Tlalpan, México DF, Mexico

Oksana A. Shlobin, MD Inova Fairfax Advanced Lung Disease and Transplant Program, Inova Fairfax Hospital, Falls Church, VA, USA

Yoshiya Toyoda, MD, PhD Department of Thoracic Medicine and Surgery, Temple University School of Medicine, Philadelphia, PA, USA

Yurdagul Uzunhan Assistance Publique Hôpitaux de Paris, Service de Pneumologie, Hôpital Avicenne, Bobigny, France

Université Paris 13, Sorbonne Paris Cité, Bobigny, France

Dominique Valeyre Assistance Publique Hôpitaux de Paris, Service de Pneumologie, Hôpital Avicenne, Bobigny, France

Université Paris 13, Sorbonne Paris Cité, Bobigny, France

Athol Wells, MBChB, MD, FRACP, FRCP, FRCR Interstitial Lung Disease Unit, Royal Brompton Hospital, National Heart and Lung Institute, Imperial College London, London, UK

John Wort, MA, MBBS, PhD, FRCP, FFICM Pulmonary Hypertension Service, Royal Brompton Hospital, National Heart and Lung Institute, Imperial College London, London, UK

Chapter 1
Radiographic Imaging in Interstitial Lung Disease and Pulmonary Hypertension

Roberto G. Carbone, Assaf Monselise, and Giovanni Bottino

Introduction

Interstitial lung diseases (ILD) is a heterogeneous group of over 200 different diseases of unknown and known cause with common functional characteristics (restrictive physiology and impaired gas exchange) and a common final pathway, eventually leading to irreversible fibrosis [1–5].

In this chapter, the radiographic imaging of the more common conditions of ILD is reviewed, and in particular, Idiopathic Interstitial Pneumonias (IIP), in relation to the presence of pulmonary hypertension, is discussed. A special emphasis is placed on the role of high-resolution computed tomography (HRCT) findings in association with Pulmonary Hypertension (PH) [6–9].

In 2002, the ATS/ERS multidisciplinary panel proposed a classification of IIP that comprises clinical–pathological entities such as Idiopathic Pulmonary Fibrosis.

(IPF), Nonspecific Interstitial Pneumonia (NSIP), Respiratory Bronchiolitis-associated Interstitial Lung Disease (RB-ILD), Cryptogenic Organizing Pneumonia (COP), Acute Interstitial Pneumonia (AIP), Desquamative Interstitial Pneumonia (DIP), and lymphoid interstitial pneumonia (LIP) [1].

R.G. Carbone, MD, FCCP (✉)
Regional Hospital Aosta and University of Genoa, Genoa, Italy
e-mail: carbone.roberto@aol.com

A. Monselise, MD
Department of Internal Medicine, University of Tel Aviv, Tel Aviv, Israel

G. Bottino, MD
Department of Respiratory Medicine, University of Genoa, Genoa, Italy

R.P. Baughman et al. (eds.), *Pulmonary Hypertension and Interstitial Lung Disease*, DOI 10.1007/978-3-319-49918-5_1

IPF is the most common subset IIP occurring most frequently in patients older than 50 years of age, limited to the lower lungs, and associated with a histological pattern termed usual interstitial pneumonia (UIP). Symptoms include dry cough, progressive dyspnea, and finger clubbing that usually precede presentation by 6 months [10–18]. Physiological examination shows crackles over the lower lungs specific for IPF with a high level of accuracy near 100%. In our opinion, only two approaches would allow an earlier diagnosis of IPF: (a) assessment of Velcro crackles by lung auscultation and (b) screening using HRCT [4, 12, 18–20].

Pulmonary Hypertension in Interstitial Lung Disease

PH is defined as a mean pulmonary artery pressure (P pa) ≥ 25 mmHg at rest with a pulmonary capillary wedge pressure ≤15 mmHg and/or a pulmonary vascular resistance ≥3 Wood units [3, 8, 9, 21]. Pulmonary vascular disease is characterized by progressive obliteration and remodeling of the pulmonary arteries, resulting in loss of vascular reserves and the development of precapillary PH. The normal pulmonary circulation is a low resistance, high capacitance circuit with the ability to accommodate the entire cardiac output at low arterial pressure [21]. Assessment of pulmonary vasculature can be made by HRCT. In particular, the measurements of parenchymal vessel diameter, the absolute size of the main PA, and the ratio of the PA diameter (d-PA) to the diameter of the ascending aorta (d-AA) have been shown to correlate with mPAP. Assessment of the d-PA/d-AA ratio has become a widely accepted quick and easy sign for the assessment of PH on HRCT [21]. Two studies have shown that increased PA size may not be reliable for detecting PH in patients with fibrotic lung disease [22, 23]; nevertheless, a correlation between d-PA/d-AA ratio and mPAP was demonstrated in the pulmonary fibrosis group, suggesting this may still be a useful HRCT sign. Segmental artery size has been shown to correlate with mPAP, although not closer than the mean d-PA/d-AA ratio. In HRCT, enlarged main pulmonary artery (>29 mm) or an increased diameter of pulmonary artery as compared with the aorta can be seen in patients with moderate to severe PH [3, 21].

In long-standing severe PH, calcifications of the pulmonary arteries usually affecting the main right or left pulmonary arteries and less commonly the lobar pulmonary arteries may be present. This finding is usually but not invariably associated with irreversible vascular disease.

Recently, a composite index of HRCT and echocardiographic measurements, d-PA/d-AA ratio, and right ventricular systolic pressure (RVSP) have been shown to correlate with mPAP better than either test alone [3]. Moreover, the gold standard using right heart catheterization (RHC) is not always practicable [12, 24]. The World Health Organization (WHO) classification of PH categorizes PH due to chronic lung disease such as ILD under group 3 and it is the second most common cause of PH in the Western world [3]. Currently, available studies suggest that PH is present in up to 70–90% of patients with advanced COPD, showing at most mild PH, and in 50% of patients with IPF. RVSP is estimated >45 mmHg in up to 50% of patients with combined pulmonary fibrosis and emphysema. Even though group 3 PH is usually mild to moderate in severity, it has important clinical and prognostic implications. Notably, the presence of PH in the setting of chronic hypoxic lung disease is associated with worsened exercise capacity, impaired quality of life, and a higher incidence of primary graft dysfunction after lung transplantation. Indeed, the presence of PH is associated with worse survival [3].

There are many reports of PH complicating the course of the more common ILD, such as IPF, connective tissue diseases associated with ILD, and conditions within WHO group 5, such as sarcoidosis. What is surprising though is the relative paucity of data on PH complicating the course of other forms of ILD [25]. In advanced fibrosis, markers of pulmonary vascular disease, including elevated pulmonary vascular resistance, are strongly predictive of early mortality. Noninvasive pulmonary vascular markers are desirable for accurate prognostic assessment [24, 26–28].

Chest X-ray in Interstitial Lung Disease with Pulmonary Hypertension

Radiologic evaluation of dyspneic patients by means of chest X-ray is often a diagnostic challenge since dyspnea may arise from either pulmonary, cardiac, hematological, muscular, or neuropsychiatric diseases [29]. However, most dyspneic patients have pulmonary disease and dyspnea is the main symptom of IPF [1, 7, 10].

While chest-X-ray cannot be considered the primary imaging modality to evaluate patients with IPF, it can be used to roughly assess the extension of the disease and to exclude major complications [3]. In IPF study approximately 10% of patients with histologically proven disease have a normal chest X-ray [3]. In such cases, HRCT will reveal evidence of the disease with a sensitivity of 88% as reported by Orens et al. [30]. Chest-X-ray findings may be consistent with congestive heart failure or could be partly explained by superimposed acute thromboembolic disease. Furthermore, the relative hyperlucency of the right lung base along with the ectasia of the interlobar artery represents the Westermark sign which is highly predictive of pulmonary thromboembolic disease [31].

Although chest X-ray may provide clues of PH, the sensitivity of this procedure is low. Enlarged central pulmonary artery (>15 mm) and elongated retrosternal contact of the right ventricle are typical findings [3].

HRCT in IPF with Pulmonary Hypertension

The role of HRCT finding in ILD is (i) to detect ILD in patients with normal or equivocal chest X-ray, (ii) to focus the differential diagnosis in patients with obvious but nonspecific chest X-ray abnormalities, (iii) to guide the site of lung biopsy, and (iv) to evaluate disease reversibility [1–5]. Ideally, the diagnosis should be supported by surgical lung biopsy (SLB), but this may be not being performed in patients at high risk, such as those with significant pulmonary hypertension.

Recent guidelines have tried to identify those patients in whom the risks of SLB may outweigh the benefits of establishing a definite diagnosis of IPF [1, 2]. On the basis of BTS guidelines [2], when clinical, serological, and instrumental (physiological functional) tests have excluded other common causes of ILD, the diagnosis of IPF is based on HRCT findings combined with procedures as described by the composite physiological index (CPI) levels by Wells [2], making SLB unnecessary. By contrast the lack of a known cause of ILD represents a key factor for SLB in the diagnostic process [1, 2, 8–10]. Also, the presence of a subpleural honeycombing with minimal ground glass, especially in someone over the age of 60 with progressive fibrosis in older patients (>70 years), has a high likelihood of IPF.

In cases where the HRCT shows a predominant reticular pattern of involvement of the lung parenchyma with scattered lobular areas of ground-glass attenuation and upper lobe predominance, chronic hypersensitivity pneumonitis is a common cause, especially in advanced lung disease.

While these findings can also be observed in other ILD, such as chronic hypersensitivity pneumonia [32] and collagen vascular disease [33], the patient does not refer any domestic or professional exposure, and serological tests may result negative. However, while the upper lobe predominance of such a reticular pattern cannot be considered a typical finding of IPF [1, 2, 10, 11], it was indeed described by Hunninghake et al. in 85% of patients with IPF vs. 31% of those with other interstitial pneumonia [34]. In fact, the predominance of reticular densities over the areas of ground-glass attenuation does represent a typical finding of IPF when it is confined to both lung bases and associated with traction bronchiectasies and honeycombing—indeed this may be considered diagnostic for IPF (Fig. 1.1a, b).

In IPF patients, the HRCT findings of pulmonary arterial enlargement may occur even in the absence of PH due to the presence of fibrosis; therefore, it is an unreliable sign of PH in IPF patients [21]. However, PH is common in patients with IPF. Nadrous et al. [35] observed that PH was frequent in advanced IPF and correlated with both low diffusing capacity of the lung for carbon monoxide and low resting arterial oxygen tension. In a retrospective analysis of consecutive pretransplant IPF patients undergoing RHC, Lettieri et al. [36] found that PH was present in approximately one-third of the study population, and that even moderate increases of mean PAP (25 mmHg) correlated with increased mortality. Nathan et al. [37] found that echocardiographic assessment of systolic PAP was not a sufficiently accurate test for the assessment of PH, as nearly a third of patients with normal systolic PAP measured by echocardiography had PH by RHC. As noted earlier, the combination of echo and HRCT may enhance the sensitivity for PH, although the specificity may still be low.

HRCT in NSIP with Pulmonary Hypertension

The most difficult IIP to distinguish from a UIP is NSIP. In contrast to UIP, the dominant feature of NSIP on HRCT imaging is basilar, subpleural, symmetrical, bilateral ground-glass opacity. The latter may be the sole feature in nearly one-third

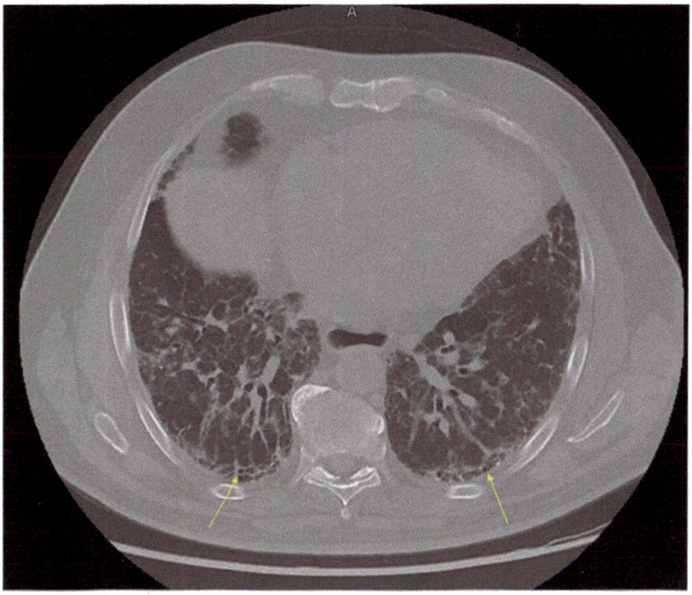

Fig. 1.1 (**a** and **b**) Idiopathic pulmonary fibrosis (IPF) histologically proved usual interstitial pneumonia (UIP). HRCT shows extensive reticular opacities in the lung bases, and subpleural honeycombing with traction bronchiectasis and an increase of interlobular septal thickening especially in the lower lobes (*arrows*)

of patients with NSIP (Fig. 1.2a–c). A peculiar pattern in which the peripheral ground-glass opacity and reticulation spares the immediate subpleural region of lung has been considered suggestive of NSIP (Fig. 1.2d). Irregular linear and reticular opacities are often present in patients with NSIP, and these opacities become increasingly coarse as the fibrotic elements become more pronounced on histopathological specimens. Traction bronchiectasis is often visible and also becomes increasingly prominent as the fibrosis progresses. The radiographic features for NSIP are somewhat tenuous and there was significant disagreement between radiologist on the presence or absence of NSIP vs. surgical lung biopsy (Flaherty).

Data on the prevalence and clinical features of PH in idiopathic NSIP are sparse; in this setting, the level of PH is usually mild to moderate in an echocardiographic study. The mean systolic PAP in this group was 30.2 mmHg. Severe PH has only rarely been described in idiopathic NSIP [37].

HRCT in Respiratory Bronchiolitis and Interstitial Lung Disease (RB-ILD)

Respiratory bronchiolitis (RB) is a histopathologic lesion found in cigarette smokers and is characterized by the presence of pigmented intraluminal macrophages within first- and second-order respiratory bronchioles [20]. It is usually asymptomatic.

a

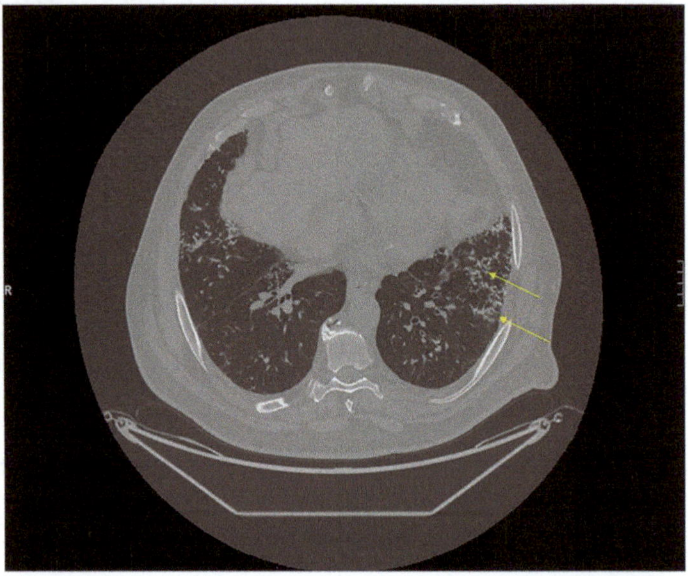

b

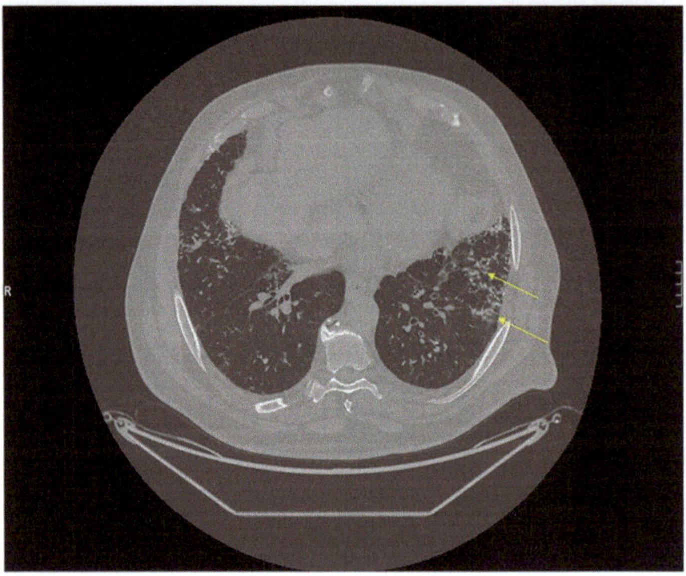

Fig. 1.2 (**a–c**) Nonspecific interstitial pneumonia (NSIP) histologically proven. HRCTs at three levels show reticular opacities and traction bronchiectasis. (**d**) HRCT shows reticular and ground-glass opacities which are symmetrical, predominant in lung bases and at the periphery of the lungs (*arrows*)

RB associated with Interstitial Lung Disease (RB-ILD) and Desquamative Interstitial Pneumonia (DIP) are best regarded as a part of a continuum of smoking-related lung injuries (Fig. 1.3a–c) [38, 39]. Patients with asymptomatic respiratory

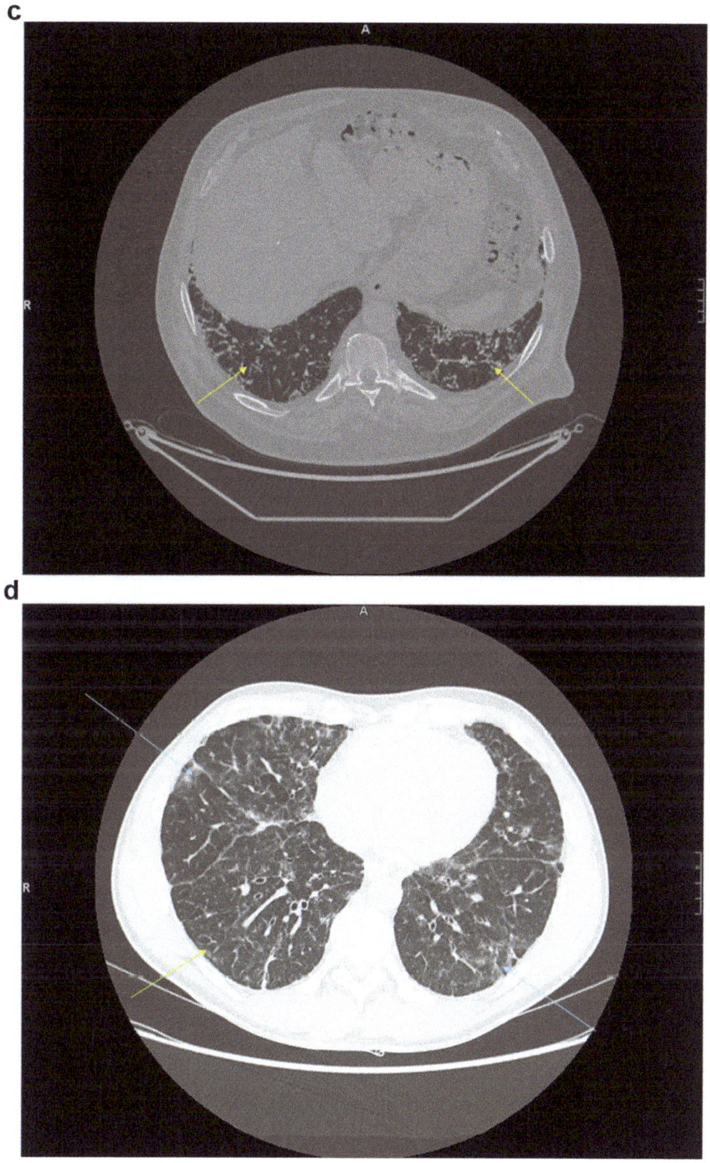

Fig. 1.2 (continued)

bronchiolitis generally show mild centrilobular nodularity and small patches of ground-glass opacity. In RB-ILD, both of these findings particularly that of ground-glass opacity become more extensive. HRCT findings of RB-ILD are at least partially reversible in patients who stop smoking.

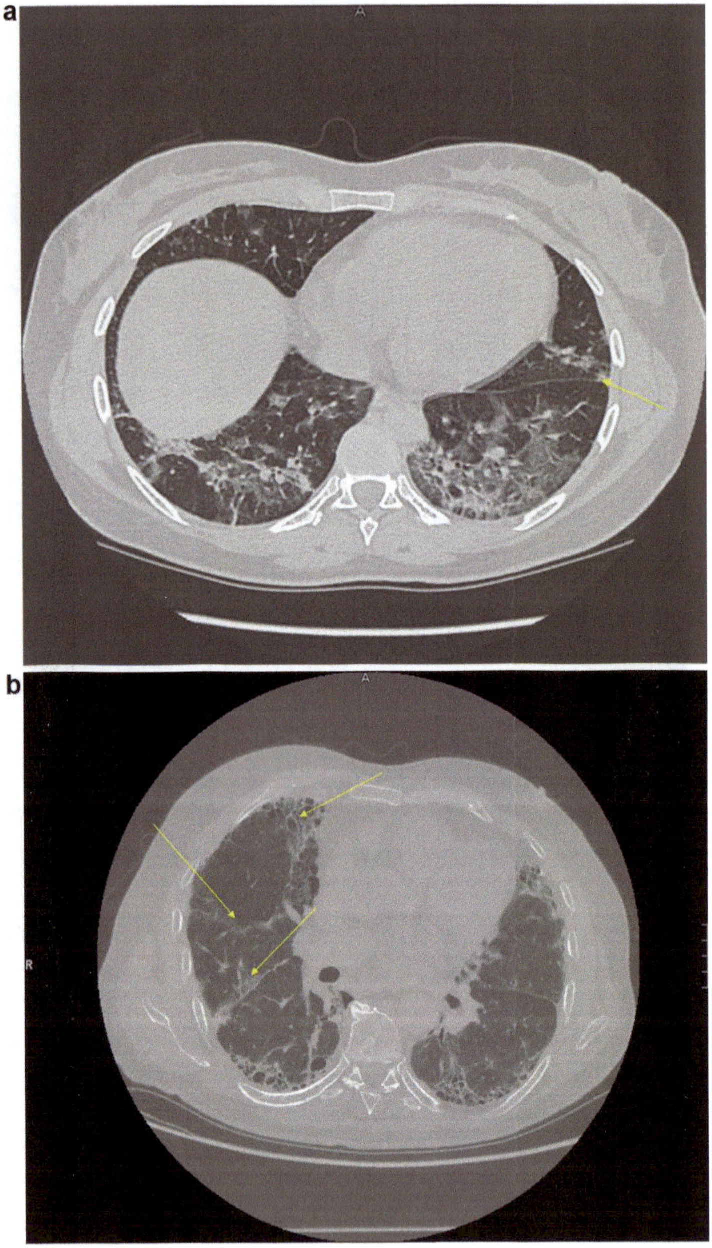

Fig. 1.3 (**a–c**) Desquamative Interstitial Pneumonia (DIP) histologically proven. HRCT show peripheral ground-glass consolidations in the lower lobes and traction bronchiole ecstasies (*arrows*)

c

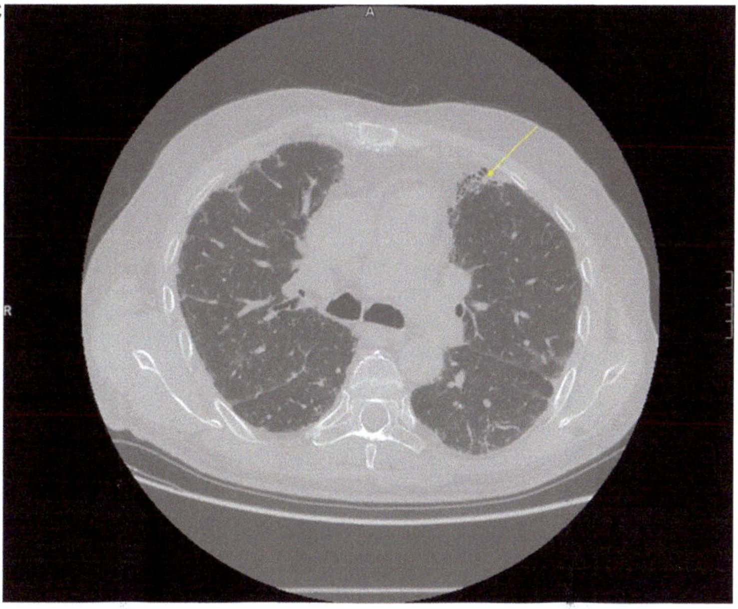

Fig. 1.3 (continued)

HRCT in Cryptogenic Organizing Pneumonia (COP) with Pulmonary Hypertension

COP is also usually radiographically distinct from UIP, most commonly presenting as parenchyma consolidation which is present in 90% of patients. Ground-glass opacity or nodules that frequently regress with treatment. In up to 50% of patients, the consolidation is peripheral or peribronchiolar in distribution, and is more commonly encountered in the lower lobes (Fig. 1.4a and b) [40, 41]. The ATS/ERS Classification [1] recommends the term COP for idiopathic disorders avoiding bronchiolitis obliterans organizing pneumonia (BOOP) because it might cause misleading. However, for the latter now is preferred the definition of organizing pneumonia (OP) and characterized by the presence of a patchy areas of organizing pneumonia [3].

Several variant presentations of COP have been described. In 15% of patients, COP may present as multiple masses, often with poorly circumscribed margins and an air bronchogram.

Patients with COP may also show the "reverse ground-glass halo" sign, or "atoll" sign, on HRCT imaging (Fig. 1.5a–c).

This finding consists of a nodular area of increased attenuation consisting of peripheral consolidation surrounding central ground-glass attenuation. While this finding is not specific for COP, nodules with this morphology are suggestive of COP

a

b

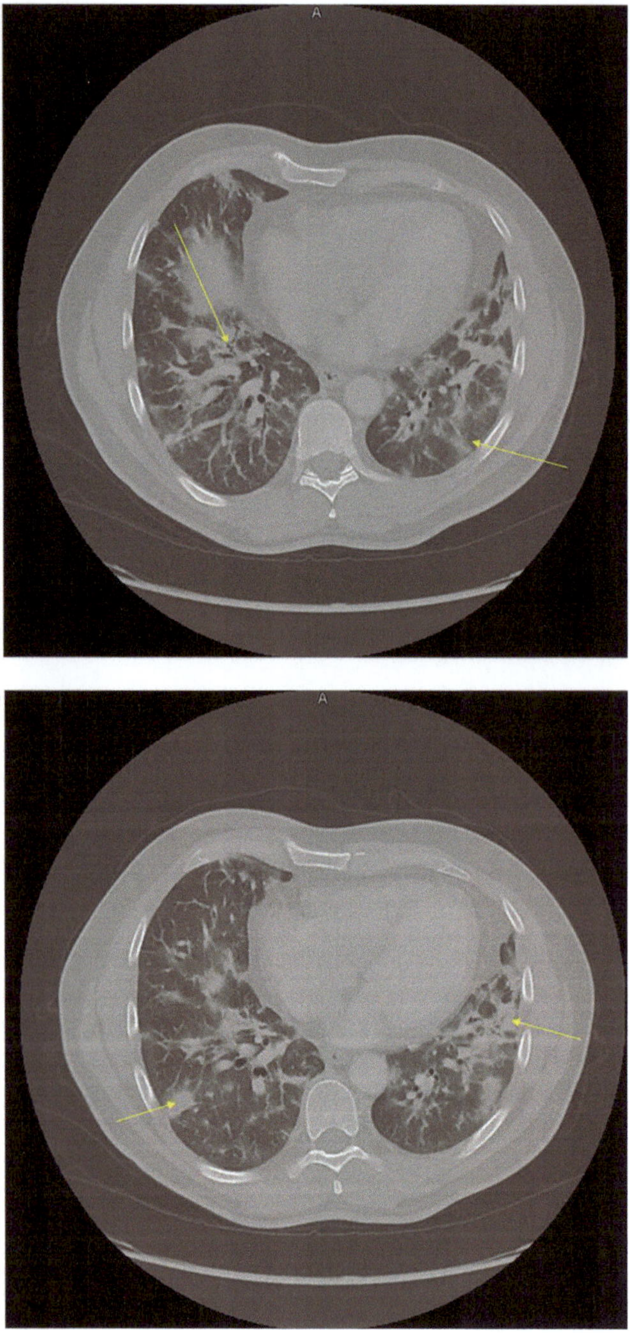

Fig. 1.4 (**a**) Cryptogenic obstructing pneumonia. HRCT shows irregular nodular opacities and peripheral ground-glass consolidation. Some of the small nodules in the lower lobes appear centrilobular in location in combination with bronchiectasis. (**b**) Patchy subpleural area and peribronchial consolidation

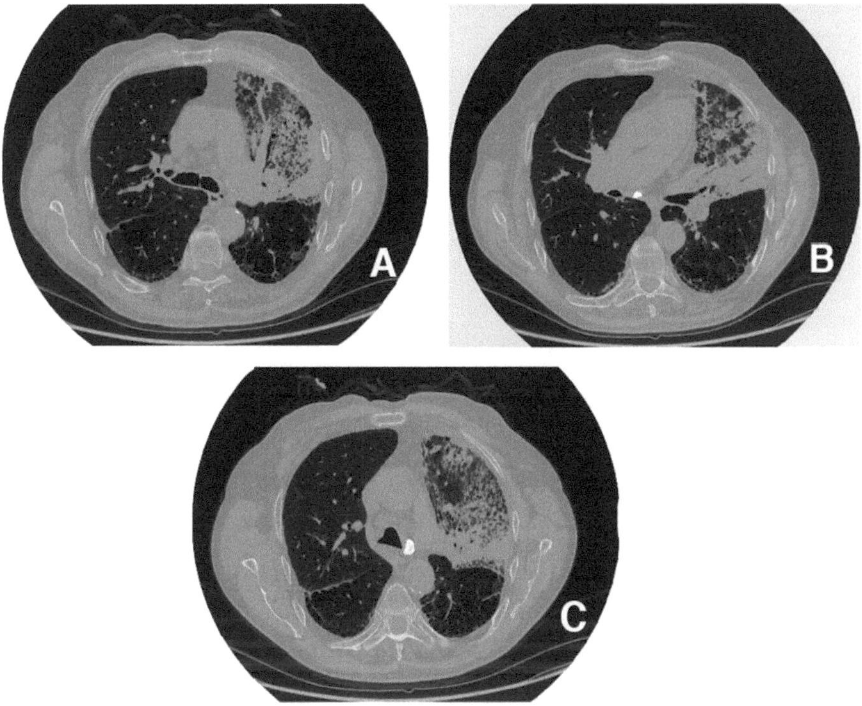

Fig. 1.5 (**a–c**) Patients with COP show the "reverse ground-glass halo" sign, or "atoll" sign, on HRCT imaging

in the appropriate clinical setting. However, a perilobular pattern of linear increased attenuation has been described. PH has only rarely demonstrated in OP and when present PAP is moderate.

HRCT in Acute Interstitial Pneumonia (AIP) with Pulmonary Hypertension

HRCT features can distinguish AIP from UIP. The typical HRCT features of AIP are bilateral, multifocal, or diffuse areas of ground-glass opacity and consolidation, usually without pleural effusion. No zonal distribution is identifiable, although the consolidation is often dependent on location. HRCT findings often reflect the stage of the disease and underlying histopathological process. During the organizing phase of the disease, HRCT findings consistent with evolving fibrosis are often present, including traction bronchiectasis, linear and reticular abnormalities, and architectural distortion. Among survivors, HRCT scans show clearing of most abnormalities, but foci of reticulation, parenchymal distortion, cystic change, or honeycombing may remain (Fig. 1.6a–c) [42–44]. Because AIP usually manifests

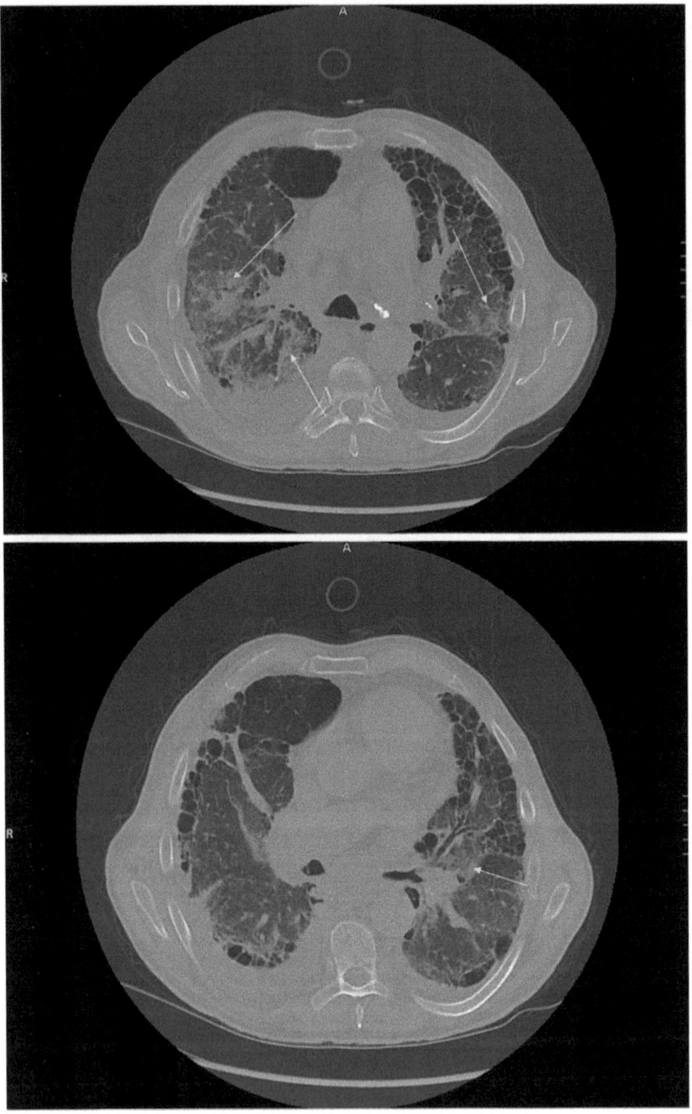

Fig. 1.6 (**a** and **b**) Acute Interstitial Pneumonia (AIP). HRCT show bilateral, multifocal, or diffuse areas of ground-glass opacity and consolidation without pleural effusion (*arrows*). (**c**) Presence of honeycombing with traction bronchiectasis

as acute hypoxemic respiratory failure, it does not enter into the clinical differential diagnosis of the other IIP [45]. By contrast with PH present rarely in OP, in AIP PH shows a severe PAP interesting the 50% of patients because of AIP is considered a severe lung disease with the presence of damage alveolar diffuse and a high mortality risk [46].

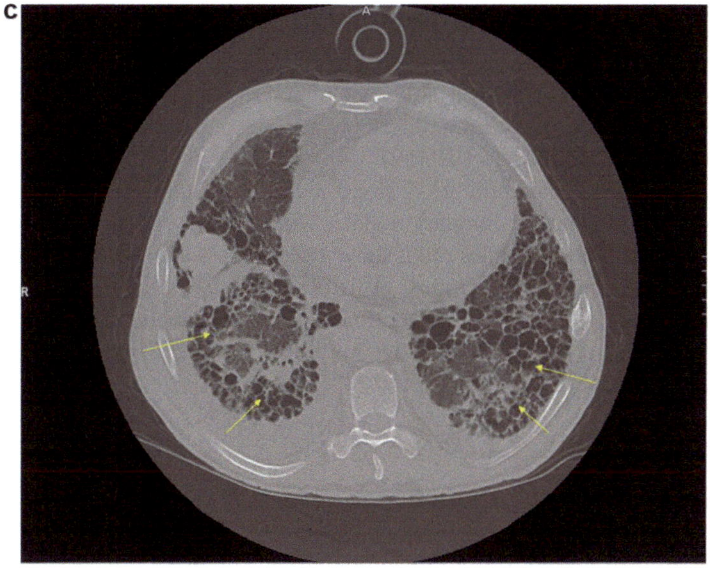

Fig. 1.6 (continued)

HRCT in Desquamative Interstitial Pneumonia (DIP)

HRCT findings show ground-glass opacities present on HRCT images in all cases of DIP. These are due to the spatially homogeneous accumulation of intra-alveolar macrophages and alveolar septal thickening [38]. The abnormality has a lower zone and peripheral distribution in the majority of cases. Irregular linear opacities and a reticular pattern are frequent but are limited in extent and are usually confined to the lung bases. Honeycombing is uncommon, but well-defined cysts may occur within the areas of ground-glass opacity [2, 47, 48]. The cysts are usually round, thin walled, and less than 2 cm in diameter; the ground-glass opacities usually regress with treatment. DIP is associated with a radiological and/or pathological pattern not compatible with UIP and may be the first clinical manifestation of a connective tissue disease.

Therefore, if the diagnosis of IPF is considered it is necessary to systematically look at extra pulmonary signs and biological markers in order to eliminate a connective tissue disease. If signs, symptoms, or biological abnormalities suggesting a connective tissue disease occur during the course of the disease, the diagnosis of IPF should be challenged. Biological markers of an inflammatory syndrome or an extra pulmonary disorder should also be measured.

The investigation of infectious agents, in particular by bronchoalveolar lavage (BAL), may be justified. Examinations that aim to identify a lymph proliferative disorder (protein electrophoresis, immunoelectrophoresis, urinary immunofixation, or cryoglobulinemia) are justified if an ILD other than IPF is suspected.

HRCT in Lymphocytic Interstitial Pneumonia (LIP)

HRCT findings of LIP are variable, but their lymphatic distribution along the peribronchovascular interstitium, interlobular septa, and within the visceral pleura distinguishes this entity from UIP [49].

Lymphoid interstitial infiltration along the centrilobular bronchus, within the center of the secondary pulmonary nodule, will produce centrilobular nodules on the HRCT scan. These nodules often show ground-glass attenuation and are one of the more common manifestations of LIP on HRCT scanning (Fig. 1.7a–c). Sometimes these ground-glass attenuation centrilobular nodules may become confluent and HRCT scans will then show multifocal areas of ground-glass opacity in patients with LIP (Fig. 1.7d).

HRCT and PH in the Complications of ILD

IPF and Superimposed Acute Thromboembolic Disease

IPF and superimposed acute thromboembolic disease is a well-known complication of former accounting for up to 3% of deaths from the disease [36]. While a recent population-based study claims that interstitial lung fibrosis may indeed result from a long-standing clinically occult pulmonary thromboembolism [50], there seems to be no doubt that in some patients the thromboembolic event is superimposed on a preexistent interstitial disease which was not clinically suspected and was first documented by HRCT.

A diagnosis of acute pulmonary thromboembolism can be first suggested by bedside echocardiography and initially ruled out by lung perfusion scintigraphy showing multiple segmental defects in both lungs but scored as a "low probability" scan in view of the chest X-ray findings. Indeed, it is well known that the diagnostic accuracy of this technique may be impaired in presence of diffuse parenchymal lung disease [51]. Thromboembolic disease was then clearly depicted by contrast-enhanced multidetector computed tomography (MDCT) angiography which showed marked ectasia and nonhomogeneous enhancement of the right pulmonary artery, with evidence of an embolus at the emergency of its lower lobar branch as best shown by the coronal reformatted MIP image. As MDCT angiography is currently regarded as the "gold standard" for pulmonary embolism [52], CT findings were not further investigated and the patient was put on an anticoagulant.

MDCT angiography, however, revealed signs of chronic pulmonary arterial hypertension resulting from IPF as both the pulmonary trunk and left pulmonary artery appeared ectasic (>25 mm) but normally patent. As far as the pathophysiology of arterial pulmonary hypertension is concerned, both obstructive and restrictive lung diseases may result in alveolar hypoxia with chronic hypoxic vasoconstriction and vascular remodeling resulting in increased resistances in the pulmonary circulation [53].

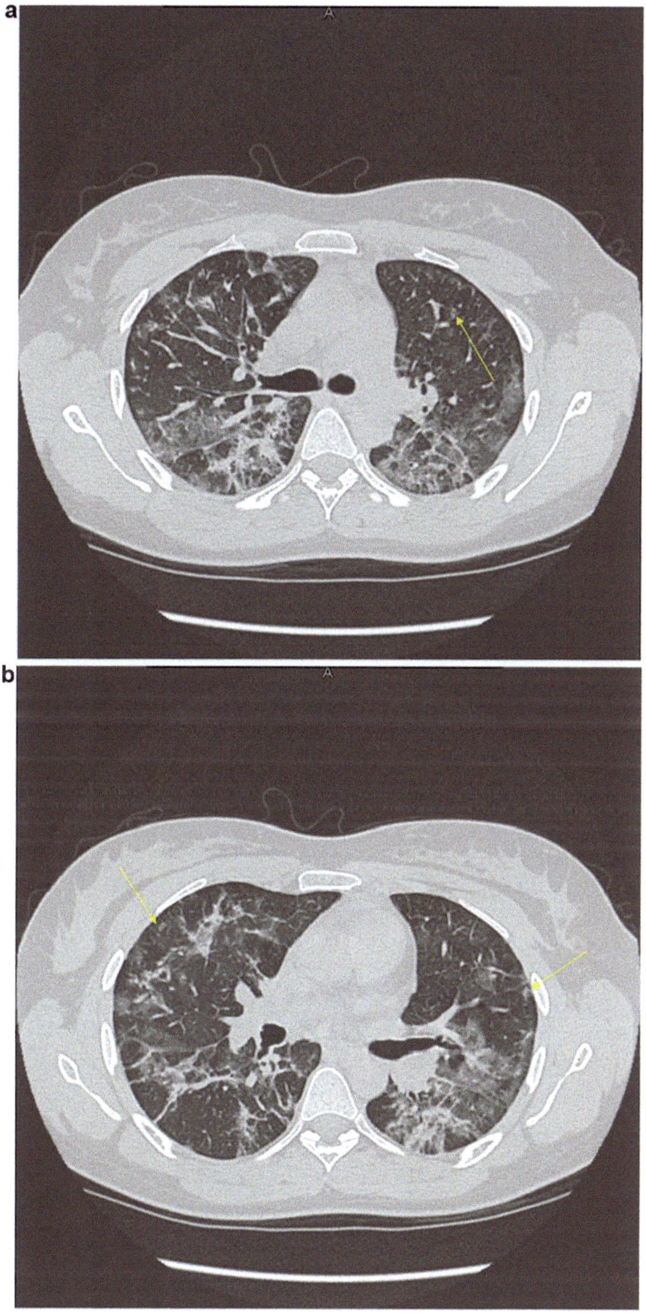

Fig. 1.7 (**a–c**) Lymphocytic Interstitial Pneumonia (LIP) histologically proven. HRCTs show millimeter center-lobular and peripheral lobular nodules (**d**) LIP. A combination of different HRCT patterns: ground-glass, nodular thickening of the peribronchovascular regions and patchy area of ground-glass opacity showed by arrows number 1, 2, 3, respectively

c d

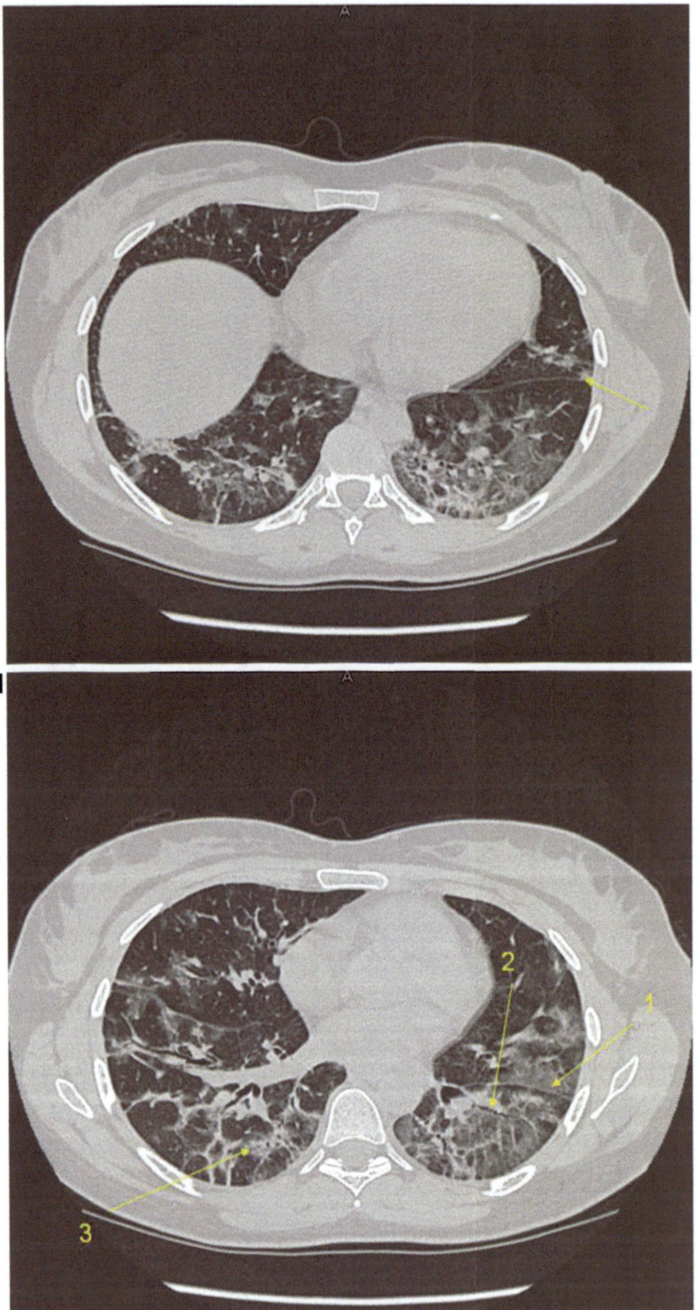

Fig. 1.7 (continued)

HRCT in Acute Exacerbation of IPF and Pulmonary Hypertension

Acute exacerbation is increasingly recognized as an important and relatively common complication of IPF. Diagnostic criteria of acute exacerbation comprise previous or concurrent diagnosis of IPF; unexplained worsening or development of dyspnea within 30 days, HRCT demonstrating new parenchymal opacity on a background of reticular or honeycomb pattern consistent with UIP; exclusion of alternative causes, including infection, left heart failure, or identifiable cause of acute lung injury [54–56]. In this context, Matsushita S, et al. [57] evaluated a change in the size of the main pulmonary (PA) artery in patients with acute exacerbation of interstitial pneumonia (IP). Twenty-nine patients underwent computed tomography at baseline and at the time of acute IP exacerbation for the measurement of the diameters of the main PA and the ascending aorta. The diameter of the main PA was significantly larger at the time of acute IP exacerbation than at baseline, which might reflect the alterations in pulmonary circulation.

HRCT in Combined Pulmonary Fibrosis and Pulmonary Emphysema (CPFE)

The HRCT studies have permitted the identification of the coexistence of pulmonary fibrosis and emphysema (CPFE) [58]. The former centrilobular involves the lower lobes, while the latter involves thc upper lobes of the lung. The most common CPFE is IPF. Patients are smokers and prevalently male, with the physiological functional tests characterized by preserved lung volumes and markedly reduction of the lung transfer of CO. CPFE may be due to pure coincidence, a cohabitation where smokers develop emphysema and for an unknown reason develop an ILD. Both conditions may be related to a common environmental mechanism. HRCT pattern suggestive of NSIP is characterized by basal ground-glass opacities and/or reticular pattern, often with traction bronchiectasis and bronchiole–ectasis without or with minimal honeycombing in morc advanced disease. For this reason, HRCT finding of NSIP is similar to IPF.

The CPFE prognosis is worse than that of IPF especially when significant PH is evaluated and not only for the presence of pulmonary emphysema with a higher level of mortality risk (HR = 4.09) [59].

Any pharmacological treatment for PH in CPFE except for long-term oxygen treatment is not recommended. The high prevalence of PH complicating CPFE has a devastating impact on the natural history of the disease [59] and renders imperative the need for clinical trials.

Cardiogenic Pulmonary Edema

Patients with IPF show an increased prevalence of ischemic heart disease. Kizer et al. [60] found a significantly increased frequency of coronary artery disease detected at angiography in patients with end-stage fibrotic lung disease, including a subset with IPF, compared with patients with other end-stage lung diseases. Mortality and autopsy studies have reported cardiovascular causes of death in between a fifth and a quarter of patients with IPF [61]. Therefore, it is not surprising that cardiogenic pulmonary edema is a common cause of acute deterioration in patients with IPF [62]. The presence of profuse septal thickening on HRCT (an uncommon finding in uncomplicated IPF) with patchy ground-glass opacity and pleural effusions suggests cardiac failure as the cause of deterioration.

Orphan Lung Diseases and Pulmonary Hypertension

Langerhans Cell Histiocytosis (LCH) is a rare bronchiolitis disorder developing exclusively in young smokers [63–65]. HRCT imaging is useful for the diagnosis of this disease showing nodules with centrilobular distribution, cavitated nodules (thick walled cysts), and thin walled cysts which are typical for this disease (Fig. 1.8) [66–70].

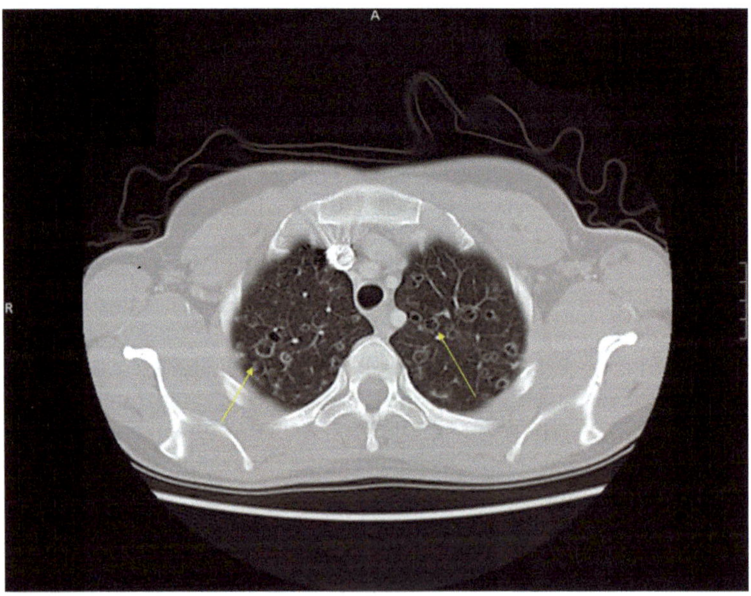

Fig. 1.8 Langerhans cell histiocytosis. HRCT pattern shows nodules with centrilobular distribution, cavitated nodules (thick walled cysts), and thin walled cysts which are typical for this disease. Nodules can be with a general size range of 10–20 mm

Development of severe PH is very common in end-stage disease in patients referred for lung transplantation and appears to be more frequent compared to other end-stage chronic lung diseases [71, 72].

Additionally, PH prevalence is higher than that reported at baseline (38%) increasing to 86% in IPF, with respect to 50–90% at end stage of disease in COPD at the time of lung transplantation [58].

Granulomatosis with polyangiitis (Wegener's) is a rare autoimmune disorder that is characterized by necrotizing granulomatous inflammation and vasculitis affecting predominantly the small vessels [73]. HRCT imaging shows lung nodules and mass that can be cavitated or consolidated: pulmonary infiltrates (alveolitis) and ground-glass opacities (Fig. 1.9a, b) [50, 74]. The presence of PH is correlated with a poor outcome [75]. *Pulmonary amyloidosis nodules* are uncommon in Sjogren's disease (sicca syndrome), a chronic organ-specific autoimmune disease characterized by lymphocytic infiltration of the salivary and lacrimal glands [76]. HRCT identifies multiple pulmonary nodules, some of them in the mediastinum (Fig. 1.10), which show intense uptake on PET–CT scan (Fig. 1.10). The final diagnosis is obtained by a histopathological evaluation of a biopsied nodule, showing peribronchial and perivascular lymphoid nodular hyperplasia, with perivascular and interstitial amyloid deposits seen with Congo red dye (Fig. 1.10) [76]. PH is rare and observed in advanced systemic disease [77]. *Lymphangioleiomyomatosis (LAM)* is a multisystemic disorder affecting prevalently females in their reproductive years with a prevalence of one per 400,000 adult females [78, 79]. LAM is characterized by progressive cystic lung destruction, lymphatic abnormalities, and abdominal tumors and on HRCT imaging the cysts are distributed diffusely and bilaterally throughout normal lung parenchyma (Fig. 1.11) [80]. PH is relatively common in patients with severe pulmonary involvement [78–80].

Behçet disease is a multigenetic inflammatory systemic disorder of unknown etiology. Clinical features include oral and genital ulcers, ocular inflammation, skin lesions, as well as articular, vascular, neurological, pulmonary, gastrointestinal, renal, vascular, and genitourinary manifestations [81]. On HRCT imaging pleural thickening, major fissure thickening, emphysematous changes, bronchiectasis, parenchymal bands, and parenchymal nodules are the most important abnormalities (Fig. 1.12).

Takayasu arteritis (TA) is an inflammatory arteritis affecting large vessels, especially aorta, its main branches, and the pulmonary arteries (119). Arteriography is considered the gold standard for the diagnosis of TA; however, 18 FDG-PET could be an effective imaging modality to estimate the disease activity (Fig. 1.13a, b) [81].

Data on PH for Behcet's and Takayasu's in combination with HRCT findings of various ILD and COPD are reported with the incidence of PH in Table 1.1.

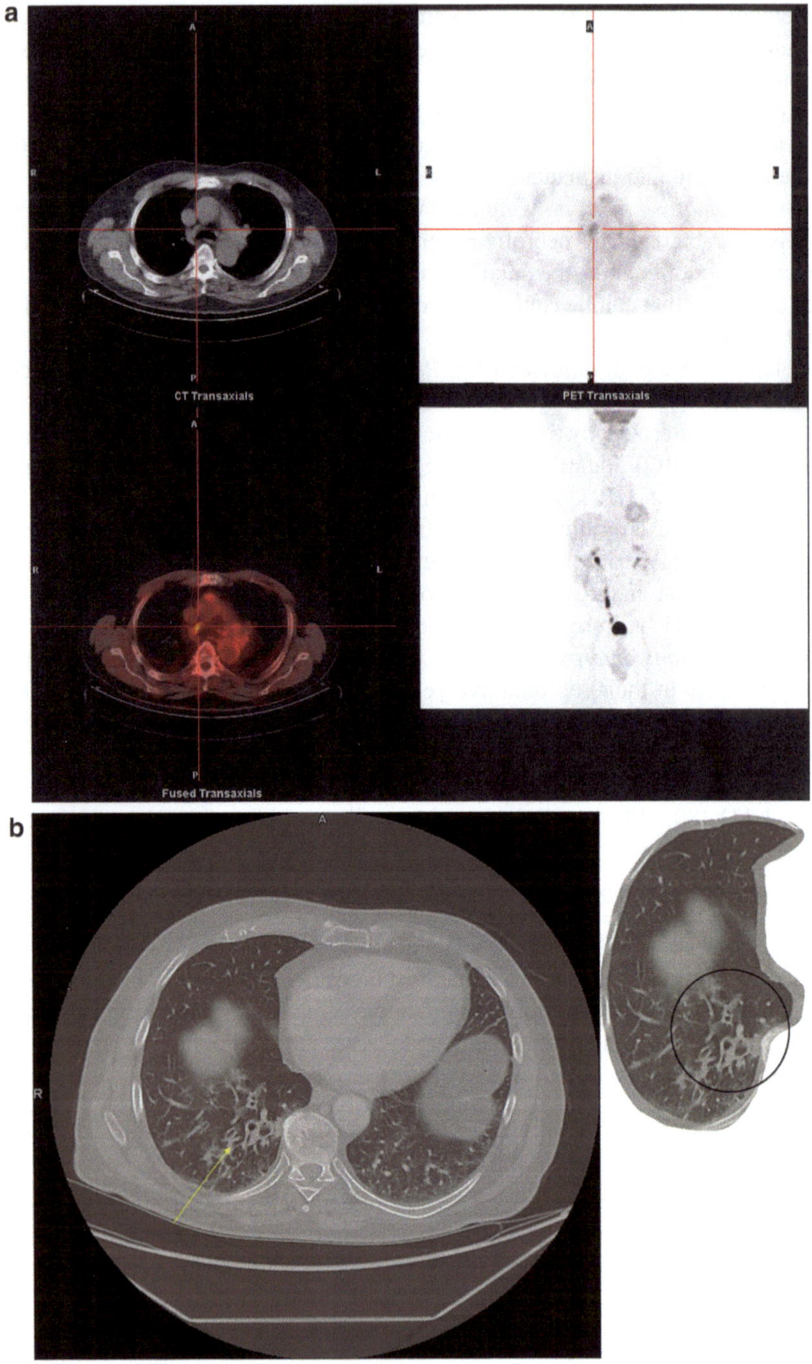

Fig. 1.9 (**a** and **b**) Wegener's granulomatosis. HRCT shows opacities mono or bilateral that can be cavitated (*arrows*) in close correlation with the bronchovascular tissue. In this patient, PET–CT total body scan shows a good regression of disease after 6 months of treatment with steroid and cyclophosphamide

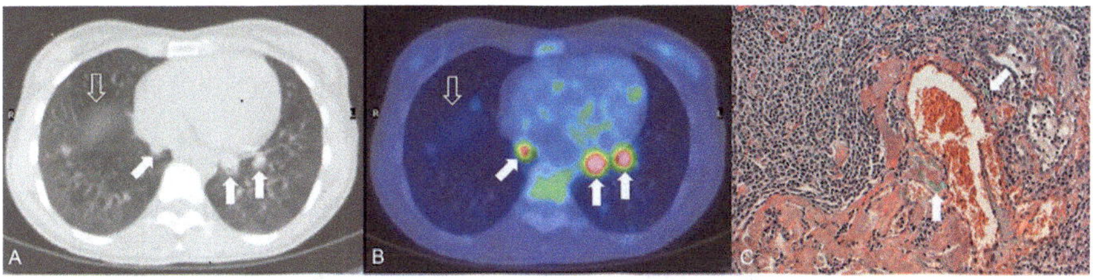

Fig. 1.10 **(a–c)** *Sjogren*'s disease. HRCT shows multiple pulmonary nodules, some of them in the mediastinum, confirmed by PET–CT scan total body. The histological evaluation of biopsied nodules identifies pulmonary amyloidal nodules

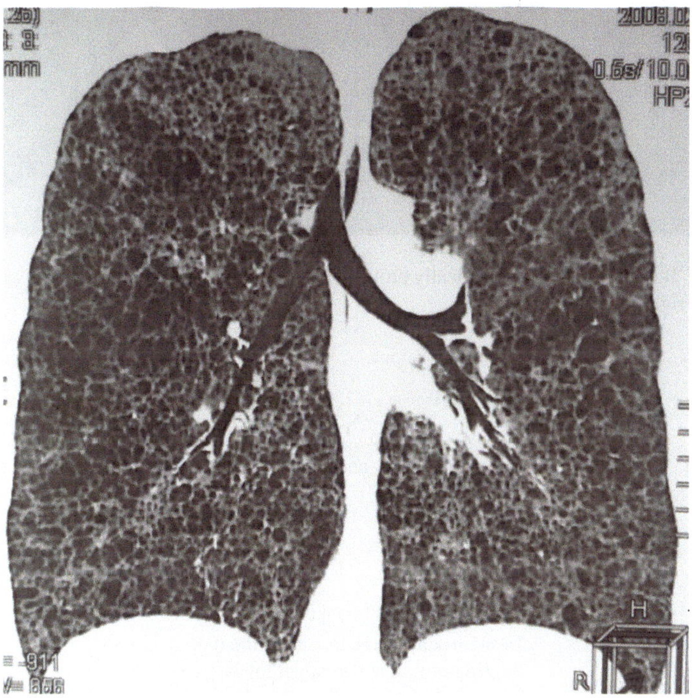

Fig. 1.11 Lymphangioleiomyomatosis. HRCT shows diffuse bilateral with cysts with thick and irregular walls with a reticular aspect (*Courtesy S Harari*)

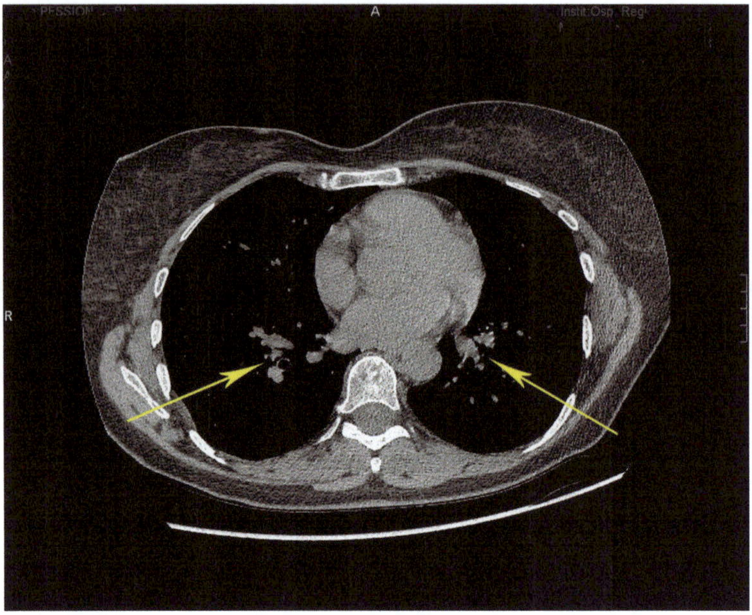

Fig. 1.12 Behçet diseases histologically proven. HRCT shows parenchymal nodules especially in the lower right lobe

Table 1.1 HRCT findings in various ILD, and COPD with reported incidence of pulmonary hypertension

ILD—COPD	HRCT findings	Pulmonary hypertension incidence %
IPF	Reticular pattern honeycombing	36
IPF and emphysema	Basal ground glass opacity without honeycombing bullae upper lobes	55
AIP	Bilateral multifocal ground glass opacity	74
LCH > 35 mmHg	Cavitated nodules	72
LCH > 45 mmHg	Pavitated nodules	45
COP	Parenchyma consolidation ground glass opacity	48
BEHCET's	Pleural and major fissure thickening bronchiectasis	5,11
TAKAYASU's	CT angiography shows abnormality of lung or vessels	50
COPD		36

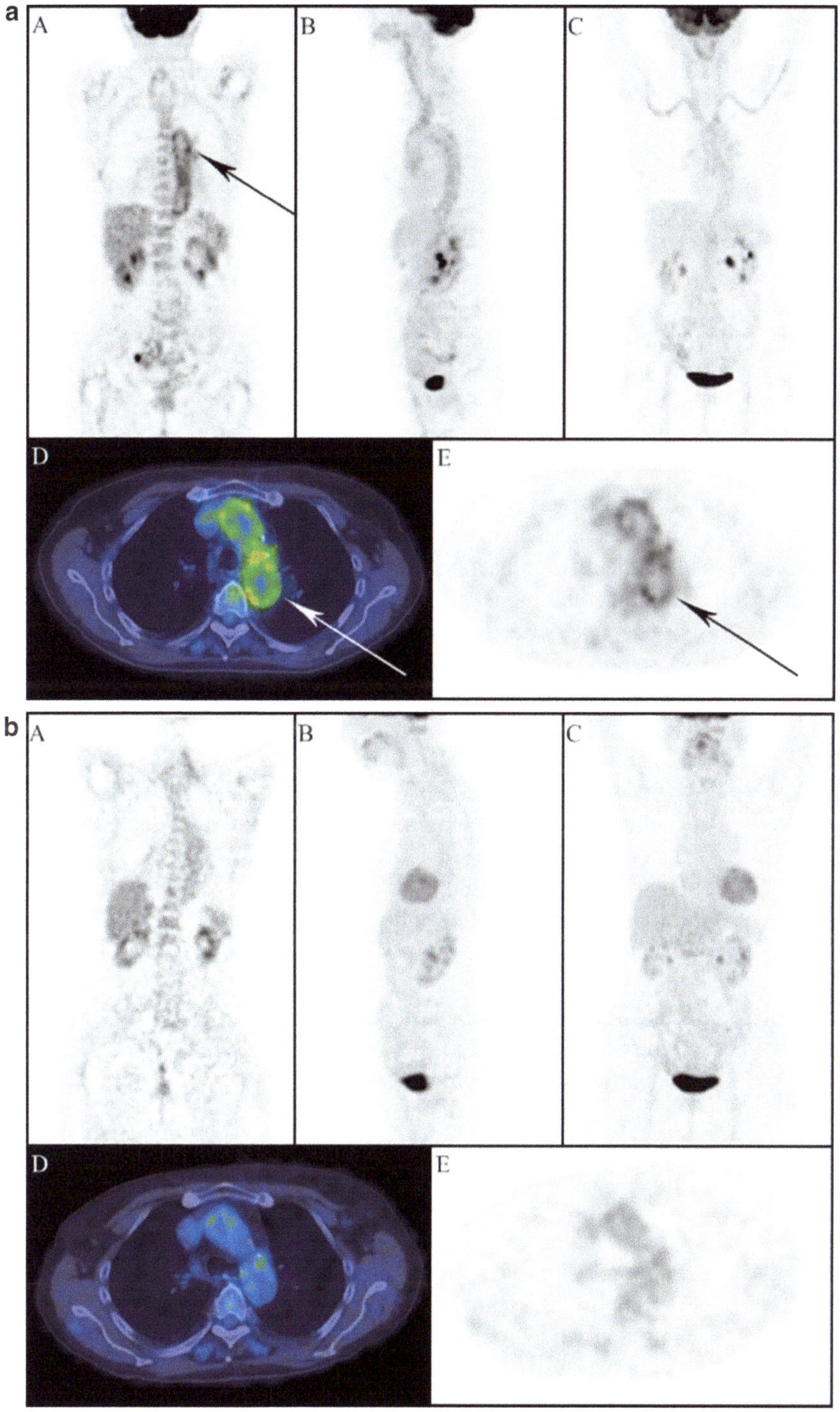

Fig. 1.13 (**a–e**) Takayasu arteritis histologically proven. PET–CT scans may be useful tools for disease monitoring

Acknowledgements The Authors thank Dr. Giulio Salmè, Dr. Karine Versace. Dept. of Radio-Diagnostic Hospital, Director Professor O. Davini. Città della salute e della Scienza di Torino. Dr. Daniele Penna, Dr. Vincenzo Arena, Director of Nuclear Medicine, IRMET, Torino, Dr. Michele Ciro Totaro, Rheumatology Service, Regional Hospital Aosta, Professor Valter Paolini regarding the graphics.

Glossary

AIP	Acute interstitial pneumonia
ANCA	Antineutrophil cytoplasmic antibodies
ATS	American thoracic society
BAL	Bronchoalveolar lavage
BHL	Bilateral Hilar lymphadenopathy
BOOP	Bronchiolitis obliterans organizing pneumonia
BTS	British thoracic society
COP	Cryptogenic organizing pneumonia
COPD	Chronic obstructive pneumonia disease
CPFE	Combined pulmonary fibrosis and pulmonary emphysema
CTD	Connective tissue disease
DIP	Desquamative interstitial pneumonia
ERS	European respiratory society
FDG-PET	18 F-fluoro-2- deoxy-D-glucose Positron emission tomography
HLA	HLA class II alleles (HLA class II can form a complex with antigenic proteins and T-cell receptors to provide the first signal for T-cell activation) have been frequently reported as being involved in the development of sarcoidosis
HRCT	High-resolution computed tomography
IIP	Idiopathic interstitial pneumonias
ILD	Interstitial lung disease
IPF	Idiopathic pulmonary fibrosis
LCH	Langerhans cell histiocytosis
LIP	Lymphoid interstitial pneumonia
MIP	Maximum intensity projection
mPAP	Mean pulmonary arterial pressure
MDCT	Multidetector computed tomography
MRI	Magnetic resonance imaging
NSIP	Nonspecific interstitial pneumonia
OP	Organizing pneumonia
PAH	Pulmonary arterial hypertension
PET–CT	F-18 fluorodeoxyglucose Positron emission computed tomography
PH	Pulmonary hypertension
PVOD	Pulmonary veno-occlusive disease
RB-ILD	Respiratory Bronchiolitis-associated interstitial lung disease

RVSP	Right ventricular systolic pressure
RHC	Right heart catheter
SLB	Surgical lung biopsy
SPECT/CT	Single photon emission computed tomography/computed tomography
WHO	World Health Organization
U.I.	Uptake index
UIP	Usual interstitial pneumonia

References

1. Society AT, Society ER. American Thoracic Society/European Respiratory Society International Multidisciplinary Consensus Classification of the Idiopathic Interstitial Pneumonias. This joint statement of the American Thoracic Society (ATS), and the European Respiratory Society (ERS) was adopted by the ATS board of directors, June 2001 and by the ERS Executive Committee June 2001. Am J Respir Crit Care Med. 2002;165(2):277–304.
2. Wells AU, Hirani N. Interstitial lung disease guideline: the British Thoracic Society of Australia and New Zealand Thoracic Society in collaboration with the and the Irish Thoracic Society. Thorax. 2008;63:v1–v58.
3. Webb RW. The idiopathic interstitial pneumonia. In: Webb RW, Higgins CR. Thoracic imaging. Lippincott, Philadelphia; 2013. pp. 428–50.
4. Hansell DM. Classification of diffuse lung diseases: why and how. Radiology. 2013;268(3):628–40.
5. Cottin V. Interstitial lung diseases. Eur Respir Rev. 2013;22(127):26–32.
6. Carbone RG, Montanaro F, Bottino G. Interstitial Lung Disease; Introduction. In: Baughman RP, Carbone RG, Bottino G, eds. Pulmonary arterial hypertension and interstitial lung diseases. NY Springer; 2009, p 3–12
7. Behr J, Ryu JH. Pulmonary hypertension and interstitial lung disease. Eur Respir J. 2008;31:1357–67.
8. Nathan SD, Carbone RG. Pulmonary hypertension due to fibrotic lung disease: hidden value in a neutral trial. Am J Respir Crit Care Med. 2014;190(2):31–132.
9. Wells AU. The revised ATS/ERS/JRS/ALAT diagnostic criteria for idiopathic pulmonary fibrosis (IPF)—practical implications. Respir Res. 2013;14(Suppl 1):S2.
10. Raghu G, Collard HR, Egan JJ, et al. ATS/ERS/JRS/ALAT Committee on Idiopathic Pulmonary Fibrosis. An official ATS/ERS/JRS/ALAT statement: idiopathic pulmonary fibrosis: evidence-based guidelines for diagnosis and management. Am J Respir Crit Care Med. 2011;183(6):788–824.
11. Cordier JF, Cottin V. Neglected evidence in idiopathic pulmonary fibrosis: from history to earlier diagnosis. Eur Respir J. 2013;42(4):916–23.
12. Meltzer EB, Noble PW. Idiopathic pulmonary fibrosis. Orphanet J Rare Dis. 2008;3:8.
13. American Thoracic Society. Idiopathic pulmonary fibrosis: diagnosis and treatment. International consensus statement. In Am J Respir Crit Care Med. Volume 161. American Thoracic Society (ATS), and the European Respiratory Society (ERS); 2000:646–64.
14. Gross TG, Hunninghake GW. Idiopathic pulmonary fibrosis. N Engl J Med. 2001;345:517–25.
15. The Idiopathic Pulmonary Fibrosis Clinical Research Network. Prednisone, azathioprine, and N-acetylcysteine for pulmonary fibrosis. N Engl J Med. 2012;366:1968–77.
16. Raghu G, Brown KK, Bradford WZ, et al. A placebo-controlled trial of interferon gamma-1b in patients with idiopathic pulmonary fibrosis. N Engl J Med. 2004;350:125–33.
17. Cottin V, Crestani B, Valeyre D, et al. Diagnosis and management of idiopathic pulmonary fibrosis: French practical guidelines. Eur Respir Rev. 2014;23:193–214.

18. Devaraj A. Imaging: how to recognise idiopathic pulmonary fibrosis. Eur Respir Rev. 2014;23:215–9.
19. Lynch DA, Travis WD, Muller NL, et al. Idiopathic interstitial pneumonias: CT features. Radiology. 2005;236(1):10–21.
20. Navaratnam V, et al. The rising incidence of idiopathic pulmonary fibrosis in the UK. Thorax. 2011;66:462–7.
21. Devaraj WAU, Meister MJ, Corte TJ, Hansell DM. The effect of diffuse pulmonary fibrosis on the reliability of CT signs of pulmonary hypertension. Radiology. 2008;249(3):1042–9.
22. Zisman DA, Karlamangla AS, Ross DJ, et al. High-resolution chest CT findings do not predict the presence of pulmonary hypertension in advanced idiopathic pulmonary fibrosis. Chest. 2007;132:773–9.
23. Corte TJ, Wort SJ, Gatzoulis MA, Macdonald P, Hansell DM, Wells AU. Pulmonary vascular resistance predicts early mortality in patients with diffuse fibrotic lung disease and suspected pulmonary hypertension. Thorax. 2009;64:883–8.
24. Nathan SD. Hypersensitivity pneumonitis and pulmonary hypertension: how the breeze affects the squeeze. Eur Respir J. 2014;44:287–8.
25. Enomoto N, Suda T, Kato M, et al. Quantitative analysis of fibroblastic foci in usual interstitial pneumonia. Chest. 2006;130(1):3–5.
26. Corte TJ, Worth SJ, PS MD, et al. Pulmonary function vascular index predicts prognosis in idiopathic interstitial pneumoniar. Respirology. 2012;17:674–80.
27. Lebtahi R, Moreau S, Marchand-Adam S, et al. Increased uptake of 111In-octreotide in idiopathic pulmonary fibrosis. J Nucl Med. 2006;47(8):1281–7.
28. Cardinale L, Volpicelli G, Lamorte A, et al. Revisiting signs, strengths and weaknesses of standard chest radiography in patients of acute dyspnea in the emergency department. J Thorac Dis. 2012;4:398–407.
29. Orens JB, Kazerooni EA, Martinez FJ, et al. The sensitivity of high-resolution CT in detecting idiopathic pulmonary fibrosis proved by open lung biopsy. A prospective study. Chest. 1995;108:109–15.
30. Worsley DF, Alavi A, Aronchick JM, et al. Chest radiographic findings in patients with acute pulmonary embolism: observations from the PIOPED Study. Radiology. 1993;189:133–6.
31. Silva CI, Müller NL, Lynch DA, et al. Chronic hypersensitivity pneumonitis: differentiation from idiopathic pulmonary fibrosis and nonspecific interstitial pneumonia by using thin-section CT. Radiology. 2008;246:288–97.
32. Hwang JH, Misumi S, Sahin H, et al. Computed tomographic features of idiopathic fibrosing interstitial pneumonia: comparison with pulmonary fibrosis related to collagen vascular disease. J Comput Assist Tomogr. 2009;33:410–5.
33. Hunninghake GW, Lynch DA, Galvin JR, et al. Radiologic findings are strongly associated with a pathologic diagnosis of usual interstitial pneumonia. Chest. 2003;124:1215–23.
34. Nadrous HF, Pellikka PA, Krowka MJ, et al. The impact of pulmonary hypertension on survival in patients with idiopathic pulmonary fibrosis. Chest. 2005;128:616S–7S.
35. Lettieri CJ, Nathan SD, Barnett SD, et al. Prevalence and outcomes of pulmonary arterial hypertension in advanced idiopathic pulmonary fibrosis. Chest. 2006;129:746–52.
36. Nathan SD, Shlobin OA, Barnett SD, et al. Right ventricular systolic pressure by echocardiography as a predictor of PH in IPF. Respir Med. 2008;102:1305–10.
37. Hallowell RW, Reed RM, Fraig M, et al. Severe pulmonary hypertension in idiopathic nonspecific interstitial pneumonia. Pulm Circ. 2012;2:101–6.
38. Park JS, Brown KK, Tuder RM, Hale VA, King Jr TE, Lynch DA. Respiratory bronchiolitis-associated interstitial lung disease: radiologic features with clinical and pathologic correlation. J Comput Assist Tomogr. 2002;26:13–20.
39. Lee KS, Kullnig P, Hartman TE, et al. Cryptogenic organizing pneumonia: CT findings in 43 patients. Am J Roentgenol. 1994;162:543–6.

40. Gotway MB, Freemer MM, King Jr TE. Challenges in pulmonary fibrosis ? 1: use of high resolution CT scanning of the lung for the evaluation of patients with idiopathic interstitial pneumonias. Thorax. 2007;62:546–53.
41. Ichikado K, Johkoh T, Ikezoe J, et al. Acute interstitial pneumonia: high-resolution CT findings correlated with pathology. Am J Roentgenol. 1997;168:333–8.
42. Johkoh T, Muller NL, Taniguchi H, et al. Acute interstitial pneumonia: thin-section CT findings in 36 patients. Radiology. 1999;211:859–63.
43. Desai SR, Wells AU, Rubens MB, Evans TW, Hansell DM. Acute respiratory distress syndrome: CT abnormalities at long-term follow-up. Radiology. 1999;210:29–35.
44. Tomiyama N, Muller NL, Johkoh T, et al. Acute respiratory distress syndrome and acute interstitial pneumonia: comparison of thin-section CT findings. J Comput Assist Tomogr. 2001;25:28–33.
45. Tanhiguchi H, Kondoh Y. Idiopathic Interstitial Pneumonia. Respirology. 2016;21:810–20.
46. Hartman TE, Primack SL, Swensen SJ, Hansell D, McGuinness G, Muller NL. Desquamative interstitial pneumonia: thin-section CT findings in 22 patients. Radiology. 1993;187:787–90.
47. Heyneman LE, Ward S, Lynch DA, et al. Respiratory bronchiolitis, respiratory bronchiolitis-associated interstitial disease, and desquamative interstitial pneumonia different entities or part of the spectrum of the same disease spectrum? Am J Roentgenol. 1999;173:1617–22.
48. Johkoh T, Muller NL, Pickford HA, et al. Lymphocytic interstitial pneumonia: thin section CT findings in 22 patients. Radiology. 1999;212:567–72.
49. Strickland NH, Hughes JM, Hart DA, et al. Cause of regional ventilation-perfusion mismatching in patients with idiopathic pulmonary fibrosis: a combined CT and scintigraphic study. Am J Roentgenol. 1993;161:719–25.
50. Polychronopoulos VS, Prakash UB, Golbin JM, et al. Airway involvement in Wegener's granulomatosis. Rheum Dis Clin North Am. 2007;33:755–75.
51. Remy-Jardin M, Pistolesi M, Goodman LR, et al. Management of suspected acute pulmonary embolism in the era of CT angiography: a statement from the Fleischner Society. Radiology. 2007;245:315–29.
52. Rounds S, Cutaia MV. Pulmonary hypertension: pathophysiology and clinical disorders. In: Baum GL, Crapo JD, Celli BR, editors. Textbook of pulmonary diseases. 6th ed. Lippincott Raven, Philadelphia; 1998. p. 1273–93.
53. Collard HR, Moore BB, Flaherty KR, et al. Acute exacerbations of idiopathic pulmonary fibrosis. Am J Respir Crit Care Med. 2007;176:636–43.
54. Fernandez Perez ER, Daniels CE, Schroeder DR, et al. Incidence, prevalence, and clinical course of idiopathic pulmonary fibrosis: a population-based study. Chest. 2010;137:129–37.
55. Kim DS, Park JH, Park BK, Lee JS, Nicholson AG, Colby T. Acute exacerbation of idiopathic pulmonary fibrosis: frequency and clinical features. Eur Respir J. 2006;27:143–50.
56. Matsushita S, Matsuoka S, Yamashiro T, et al. Pulmonary arterial enlargement in patients with acute exacerbation of interstitial pneumonia. Clin Imaging. 2014;38(4):454–7.
57. Papiris SA, Triantafillidou C, Manali ED, et al. Combined pulmonary fibrosis and emphysema. Expert Rev Respir Med. 2013;7(1):19–32.
58. Cottin V, Le Pavec J, Prevot G, et al. Pulmonary hypertension in patients with combined pulmonary fibrosis and emphysema syndrome. Eur Respir J. 2010;35:105–11.
59. Kizer JR, Zisman DA, Blumenthal NP, et al. Association between pulmonary fibrosis and coronary artery disease. Arch Intern Med. 2004;164:551–6.
60. Daniels CE, Yi ES, Ryu JH. Autopsy findings in 42 consecutive patients with idiopathic pulmonary fibrosis. Eur Respir J. 2008;32:170–4.
61. Panos RJ, Mortenson RL, Niccoli SA, King Jr TE. Clinical deterioration in patients with idiopathic pulmonary fibrosis: causes and assessment. Am J Med. 1990;88:396–404.
62. Cordier JF, Johnson SR. Multiple cystic lung diseases. Eur Respir Mon. 2011;54:46–83.
63. Attili AK, Kazerooni EA, Gross BH, et al. Smoking related interstitial lung disease: radiologic-clinical-pathologic correlation. Radiographics. 2008;28:1383–96.

64. Abbott GF, Rosado-de-Christenson MI, Franks TJ, et al. From the archives of the AFIP : pulmonary Langherans cell histiocytosis. Radiographics. 2004;24:821–41.
65. Leatherwood DI, Heitkamp DF, Emerson RE. Best cases from the AFIP: pulmonary Langherans cell histiocytosis. Radiographics. 2007;27:265–8.
66. Moore AD, Godwin JD, Muller NL, et al. Pulmonary histiocytosis X: comparison of radiographic and CT finding. Radiology. 1989;172:249–54.
67. Brauner MW, Grenier P, Mouelhi MM, et al. Pulmonary histiocytosis X: evaluation with high-resolution CT. Radiology. 1989;172:255–8.
68. Brauner MW, Grenier P, Tijani K, et al. Pulmonary Langherans cell histiocytosis evolution of lesions on CT scans. Radiology. 1997;204:497–502.
69. Kim HJ, Lee KS, Johnkoh T, et al. Pulmonary Langherans cell histiocytosis in adults: high-resolution CT-pathology comparisons and evolutional changes at CT. Eur Radiol. 2011;21:1406–15.
70. Fartoukh M, Humbert M, Capron F, et al. Severe pulmonary hypertension in histiocytosis X. Am J Respir Crit Care Med. 2000;161:216–23.
71. Dauriat G, Mal H, Tahbut G, et al. Lung transplantation for pulmonary Langherans' cell histiocytosis : a multicenter analysis. Transplantation. 2006;81:746–50.
72. Nelson D, Specks U. Granulomatosis with polyangiitis (Wegener's). Eur Respir Mon. 2011;54:1–14.
73. Cordier JF, Valeyre D, Guillevin L, et al. Pulmonary Wegener's granulomatosis. A clinical and imaging study of 77 cases. Chest. 1990;97:906–12.
74. Carbone RG, Balleari E, Montanaro F, Monselise A, Ghio R. Exploring correlation between pulmonary hypertension and servival in Wegener Granulomatosis and idiopathic pulmonary fibrosis. Chest. 2008;134 (4_Meeting Abstracts) p137002
75. Carbone R, Cosso C, Cimmino M. Clinical images: pulmonary nodular amyloidosis in Sjögren's syndrome.The J Rheumatol 2015;42(1):134.
76. Launay D, Hachulla E, Hatron P, Jais X, Simonneau G, Humbert M. Pulmonary arterial hypertension: a rare complication of primary Sjogren syndrome: report of 9 new cases and review of the literature. Medicine (Baltimore). 2007;86:299–315.
77. Johnson SF, Cordier JF, Lazor R, et al. European Respiratory Society guidelines for the diagnosis and management of lymphangioleiomyomatosis. Eur Respir J. 2010;35:14–26.
78. Harari S, Torre O, Moss J. Lymphangioleiomyomatosis: what do we know and what are we looking for ? Eur Respir Rev. 2010;35:14–28.
79. Cottin V, Harari S, Jais X, et al. Pulmonary hypertension in lymphangioleiomyomatosis; hemodynamic characteristics in a series of 20 patients. Eur Respir J. 2011;38(Suppl. 55):419 s.
80. Uzun O. Pulmonary involvement in Behçet 's disease and Takayasu's arteritis. Eur Respir Mon. 2011;54:32–45.
81. Lavogiez C, Quéméneur T, Hachulla E, et al. 18FDG PET: a new criterion for disease activity in Takayasu arteritis Rev Med Intern 2006;27(6):478–81.

Chapter 2
Invasive Techniques for Diagnosis of PH

Peter J. Engel

Introduction

During the past two decades, there has been significant progress in the diagnosis and treatment of pulmonary hypertension. As a result of several World Symposia, the definition and classification of PH has been revised and refined. PH is now considered to exist in five diagnostic WHO Groups, with 12 drugs now FDA approved for use only in WHO Group 1, also known as pulmonary arterial hypertension or PAH (see Chap. 6).

Accurate classification of PH is essential to the selection of appropriate therapy, since treatment with PAH-specific drugs may be ineffective or even harmful in patients with WHO Group 2 PH (PH due to left heart disease); conversely, treatment of patients with WHO Group 1 PH with drugs for Group 2 PH will be ineffective at best. It has been hoped that a noninvasive method of could be used for guiding the diagnosis and treatment of PH, but right heart catheterization (RHC) has remained the gold standard for assessing PH. The distinction between precapillary (WHO Groups 1, 3, 4, and 5) and postcapillary (WHO Group 2) PH is vital and depends on not only clinical history and echocardiogram, but most importantly on RHC. In addition, RHC is the only technique that provides crucial information regarding the load imposed on the right ventricle in PAH and the response of the right ventricle to this burden. This chapter will summarize the use of cardiac catheterization in evaluating the patient with suspected PH.

P.J. Engel, MD (✉)
Ohio Heart and Vascular Center, The Christ Hospital,
2123 Auburn Avenue, Suite 137, Cincinnati, OH 45219, USA
e-mail: Puregold76@aol.com

R.P. Baughman et al. (eds.), *Pulmonary Hypertension and Interstitial Lung Disease*, DOI 10.1007/978-3-319-49918-5_2

Methodological Considerations

RHC can generally be performed safely, even in patients with severe pulmonary hypertension. In one multicenter retrospective study of more than 7000 RHC (70% of which were done from the internal jugular approach) performed in patients with severe PH at experienced centers, the rate of serious complications was 1.1% and the procedure-related mortality rate was 0.05% [1].

Certain technological considerations need to be addressed before proceeding to acquisition and interpretation of RHC data. Although the most accurate information regarding ventricular function are obtained with high-fidelity catheters and manipulation of loading conditions (e.g., inferior vena balloon occlusion to reduce right ventricular preload) to construct pressure–volume loops (champion ref), these methods are not feasible in most catheterization laboratories. Fluid-filled catheters therefore remain the standard for invasive assessment of patients with suspected PH. Flow-directed balloon-tipped catheters are used and are inserted in either the femoral or the internal jugular vein and advanced to the right atrium, the right ventricle, the main pulmonary artery, and the wedge position in a smaller pulmonary artery. Since an accurate measurement of the pulmonary artery wedge pressure (PAWP) is of paramount importance (see later), the zero reference level should be chosen to represent the pressure in the center of the left atrium. Failure to do so could result in misclassification and inappropriate treatment of patients with PH. In a study of 196 patients referred to a PH clinic for RHC, various zero reference levels were tested against computed tomography-derived location of the left atrium. It was found that the midthoracic line (measured between the level of the catheterization table and the skin above the sternum) reflected the position of the left atrium most consistently [2], suggesting that this is the most appropriate zero reference level for RHC in patients with suspected PH. Intravenous sedation prior to the procedure is generally unnecessary and may result in respiratory depression, hypoxia, and pulmonary vasoconstriction. Supplementary oxygen is given when needed to maintain systemic O_2 saturations above 90%.

Intravascular volume status prior to RHC is an important consideration. On the one hand, when patients are volume overloaded, pulmonary artery pressure may be considerably higher than in the euvolemic state. On the other hand, when patients with postcapillary PH are vigorously diuresed, PAWP may normalize, leading to hemodynamics more consistent with precapillary PH. Our general practice is to withhold diuretics as tolerated for 4–7 days prior to RHC in patients with clinical risk factors for postcapillary PH. When diuretics have not been withheld and PAWP is found to be unexpectedly low, measurements can be repeated after rapid infusion of 0.5 L of normal saline or ringer's lactate.

Measurements and Definitions

Measurements made at RHC along with normal values are listed in the table. The mean pulmonary artery pressure in normal is 14 ± 3 mmHg, with the upper limit of normal being 20 mmHg. The accepted definition of pulmonary hypertension per se is a mean pulmonary artery pressure (MPAP) greater than or equal to 25 mmHg. It has not yet been determined what the significance is of mean PA pressure between 20 and 25 mmHg, formerly referred to as "borderline PH."

Cardiac output (CO) is a pivotal parameter in determining prognosis and therapy of PH and may be measured by either one of two methods, namely, the thermodilution method or the Fick method. Although these two methods of measuring CO correlate closely with one another, there may be significant differences between the two in any given patient. In one study of 198 patients, many of whom had PAH, studied with RHC, about 36% of patients had greater than 20% difference in CO between the two methods. [3]. Fick CO is measured by dividing O_2 consumption by the arteriovenous O_2 difference. Although the A-VO_2 difference is measured directly during RHC, the O_2 consumption is usually an estimated value derived from tables. This method of CO measurement is termed the indirect Fick method, as opposed to the direct Fick method, which involves direct measurement of oxygen uptake, rarely done in routine cardiac catheterization. For this reason, it was stated in the proceedings of the Fifth World Symposium that thermodilution is the preferred method for CO measurement in PH [4]. The thermodiluton method has been found to be accurate even in the presence of significant tricuspid regurgitation and low cardiac output states [5].

Pulmonary vascular resistance (PVR) is defined as:

$$\text{PVR} = \text{MPAP-PAWP/Cardiac output}$$

The numerator in this equation is also known as the transpulmonary gradient (TPG), which is generally considered to be a reflection of the presence of pulmonary vascular disease when its value exceeds 12–15 mmHg.

Solving this equation for PA pressure.

$$\text{MPAP} = \text{PVR X cardiac output} + \text{PAWP.}$$

Since PAWP is used as a surrogate for left atrial pressure or LVEDP, it can be seen that PA pressure is a variable which is influenced by flow, downstream pressure, and resistance in the vascular bed such that PA pressure rises with increase in left atrial pressure, PA flow (cardiac output), or pulmonary vascular resistance.

Patients with PH generally fall into one of the following hemodynamic profiles:

1. Precapillary PH is defined as MPAP greater than or equal to 25 mmHg accompanied by a PAWP less than or equal to 15 mmHg. Pulmonary vascular resistance (PVR) in these patients is greater than 3 Wood U., and often much higher than this. When precapillary PH is complicated by right ventricular failure, the cardiac index is low (usually less than 2.2 L/min/m^2), the mean right atrial pressure is elevated (greater than 12 mmHg), and the PVR is usually greater than 7 Wood U. Precapillary PH is found in WHO Groups 1 (PAH), 3 (PH due to lung disease), 4 (chronic thromboembolic PH), and 5 (conditions with multifactorial pathogenesis, including sarcoidosis). The distinction between these groups cannot be made from RHC and depends upon results of other tests including pulmonary V/Q scan, pulmonary function testing, and chest CT scan, among others.

2. Postcapillary PH is found only in WHO Group 2 (PH owing to left heart disease, including systolic and diastolic left ventricular dysfunction and left-sided valvular disease) and is defined by a MPAP greater than or equal to 25 mmHg and PAWP >15 mmHg. PVR is usually normal to slightly increased.

3. A subset of patients with PH have a condition variably referred to as "mixed" PH or "combined pre- and postcapillary pulmonary hypertension," usually found in patients with long-standing left ventricular dysfunction. These patients are found at RHC to have MPAP >25 mmHg, PAWP >15, and PVR >3 Wood U.

4. Another group of patients with PH have "high flow" PH. These individuals have MPAP >25 mmHG, PAWP generally less than 15 mmHg, and high cardiac output and PVR <3 Wood U. This combination of findings can be seen in anemia, liver disease, and congenital heart disease with left-to-right shunt such as atrial septal defects. Detection of this condition requires measurement of O_2 saturation of a blood sample from the pulmonary artery (SvO_2), which is important to include routinely during RHC. In cases where SvO_2 is unexpectedly high (e.g., >78%), a formal oxygen saturation run from superior vena cava to pulmonary artery is essential to detect left-to-right intracardiac shunt. SvO_2 is also useful as a method of resolving discrepancies between Fick and thermodilution cardiac output, as SvO_2 is markedly reduced in patients with low cardiac output. Since SvO_2 rises with administration of supplemental oxygen, it is desirable to perform RHC on ambient air.

As noted earlier, the critical factor in distinguishing between precapillary PH and postcapillary PH is the *accurate* measurement of the PAWP, which is used as a surrogate for left ventricular filling pressure. Unfortunately, it is not at all uncommon during RHC that erroneous values for PAWP are obtained. This can result in misclassification of PH, which could result in ineffective and potentially harmful therapy. Apart from appropriate selection of the zero reference level and consideration of volume status, there are several other important factors in assuring that PAWP has been measured accurately:

1. Most or all pressures measured at RHC are measured at end expiration [6]. In a study of 61 patients referred for evaluation of PH and studied with right and left heart catheterization, the use of digitized mean PAWP (commonly reported on routine RHC) tended to underestimate the simultaneously measured end-expiratory left ventricular end-diastolic pressure, which would have resulted in misclassification of 27% of these patients as having precapillary PH (PAH) when the diagnosis was in fact postcapillary PH (PH related to heart failure with preserved ejection fraction) [7]. However, some controversy exists regarding this practice. Le Varge et al. [8] studied 329 patients with RHC and characterized patients as having precapillary or postcapillary "phenotypes" based on clinical and echocardiographic features, and found that 29% of patients who were felt to have the precapillary phenotype would have been misclassified as having postcapillary PH if the diagnosis were based on end-expiratory wedge pressure alone. This experience underscores the need to base PH classification on a comprehensive view of clinical as well as hemodynamic features.

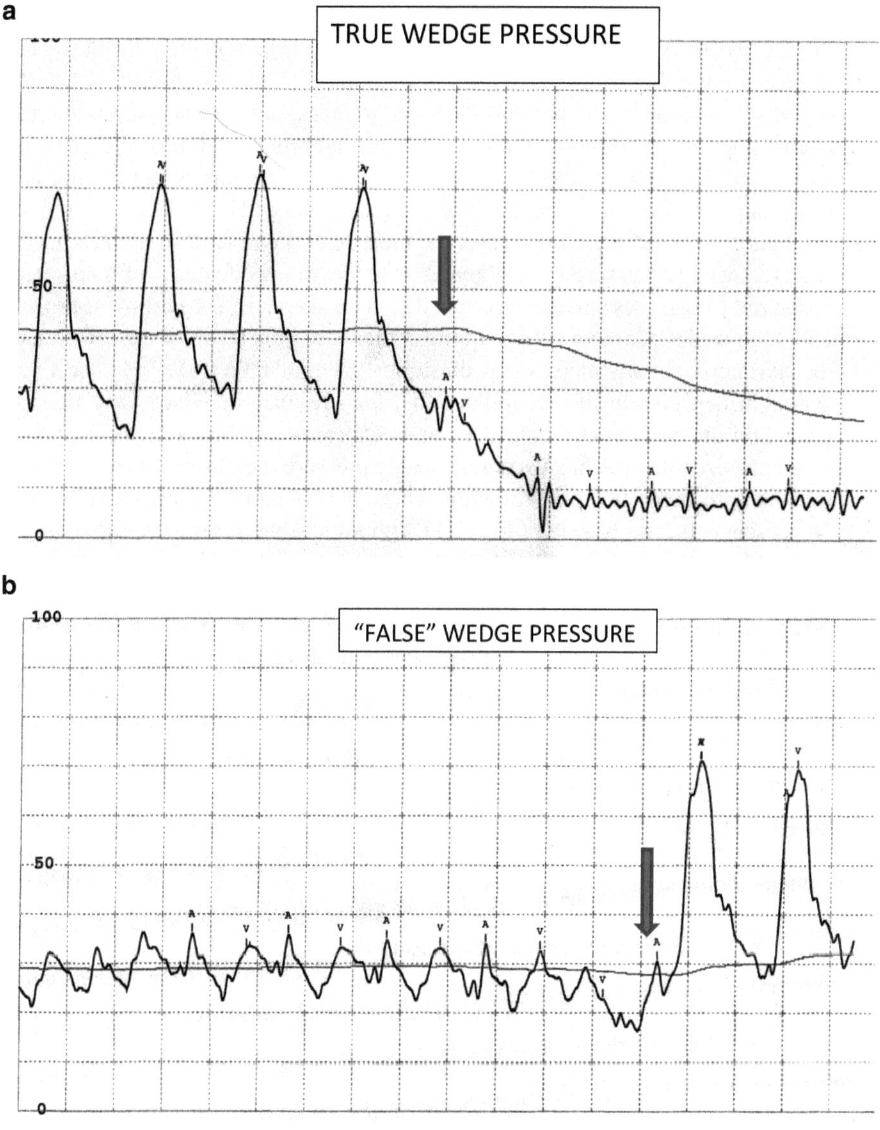

Fig. 2.1

2. In cases of partial occlusion of a small pulmonary artery by the balloon-tipped catheter, there may be continued flow around the catheter tip, resulting in a wedge pressure which may substantially overestimate left atrial pressure. Such partial occlusion tracings often bear little resemblance to "true" wedge pressure measurements, but in some cases may mimic a valid PAWP tracing. Figure 2.1 illustrates such a case. Figure 2.1a shows the pressure tracing with the balloon

inflated, followed by deflation of the balloon with the PA waveform demonstrating severe PH. If the original "wedge" pressure had been accepted, the diagnosis of postcapillary PH would have been made. However, the absence of any gradient between PA diastolic pressure and wedge pressure led to suspicion that the wedge pressure measurement was factitious, and repositioning of the catheter, shown on Fig. 2.1b, resulted in a more acceptable wedge pressure tracing and establishment of the accurate diagnosis of precapillary PH.

3. As demonstrated in the earlier case, the most important factor in identifying an incorrect wedge pressure is heightened awareness of the features of a correctly measured wedge pressure and a certain degree of skepticism regarding unexpectedly high wedge pressure values. In the earlier case, this involved observation of the normalized gradient between diastolic PAP and PAWP (DPG). The DPG should widen greatly in precapillary PH, the presence of which may be suspected on the basis of clinical, ECG, and echocardiographic findings. It should be emphasized that the most accurate wedge pressure measurement is the lowest reading with an atrial waveform with identifiable "a" and "v" waves and "x" and "y" descents (see right side of Fig. 2.1) with noticeable respiratory variation. In cases where the wedge pressure reading is high, confirmation of its accuracy may be obtained by drawing a blood sample from the catheter tip in the wedge position and measuring O_2 saturation of the sample, which should be significantly higher than the SvO_2, usually greater than 90%. In these cases, it is important to remove and discard at least 3 mL of "dead space" blood before obtaining the blood gas sample. When erroneous wedge pressure tracings are suspected it may be useful to deflate the balloon and advance the catheter slightly and reinflate the balloon.
4. When doubt remains regarding the accuracy of the wedge pressure measurement, direct measurement of left ventricular end diastolic pressure with left heart catheterization should be performed. De Oliveira et al. studied 105 patients with PH with right and left heart catheterization and found that PAWP less than or equal to 15 mmHg was a dependable estimate of left ventricular end diastolic pressure. However, 39% of patients with PAWP greater than 15 mmHg actually had left ventricular end diastolic pressure less than 15 mmHg, which would have resulted in misclassification of these patients as having postcapillary PH when the diagnosis was actually PAH [9].

Resting Hemodynamics and Prognosis in PH

Among the measurements made during RHC, the PA pressure itself has the least impact on prognosis and survival. In fact, patients with congenital heart disease and Eisenmenger syndrome often have the highest PA pressures and have the best prognosis when compared to other forms of PAH. Since the most common cause of clinical deterioration and death in PAH (and some other forms of PH) is right ventricular failure, it is not surprising that the parameters on RHC which have the greatest influence in selection of therapy are those which reflect right ventricular function. The REVEAL Registry risk score calculator analyzed data from a registry of over 3000 patients with PAH and focused on 500 patients with incident PAH (diagnosed within 3 months of enrolment). Cardiac index below 2.0 and right atrial pressure greater than 20 mmHg were found to be major factors in determining risk of death. Similar findings were noted in the NIH registry data [10]. In clinical practice, a markedly reduced mixed venous O_2 saturation (e.g., <50%) correlates with low cardiac output and worsened prognosis. Patients with PAH, PVR >7 Wood U., cardiac index <2.0, and right atrial pressure >15 mmHg should be considered candidates for aggressive therapy, often including parenteral prostanoids.

The response of pulmonary hemodynamics to targeted drug therapy for PAH may also be used to help assess prognosis in this disease. Tiede et al. [11] studied 122 patients treated for PAH and compared baseline hemodynamics to those after an average of 4 months of therapy with various guideline-directed PAH drugs. Transplant-free survival at a mean of 4.7 years was significantly better in those patients in whom treatment resulted in short-term increase in CO by >0.22 L/min and decrease in PVR by more than 2 Wood U.

PH "Out of Proportion"

In discussions of PH associated with underlying conditions such as chronic lung disease (CLD) or left heart disease (PH/LHD), the term "out of proportion" has commonly been used to describe individuals in whom the degree of PH is greater than would be expected. This term eluded precise definition and was abandoned as part of the 5th World Symposium on PH. In the case of chronic lung diseases such as chronic obstructive lung disease, interstitial lung disease, or combined pulmonary fibrosis and emphysema, the terms "CLD without PH" (MPAP <25 mmHg), "CLD with PH" (MPAP >25 mmHg), and "CLD with severe PH" (MPAP >35 mmHg or MPAP >25 mmHg and CI <2.0) have been suggested [12]. This schema is based upon the fact that many if not most patients with CLD have mild PH, but a relatively small minority of these patients have MPAP in excess of 35–40 mmHg.

PH has been considered to be "out of proportion" to left heart disease (so-called reactive PH) when TPG is >12 mmHg. However, TPG increases are known to be affected by factors other than vascular remodeling, such as cardiac output, left atrial pressure, and pulmonary artery compliance and distensibility [13]. One large study evaluated 1094 patients with PH/LHD and found that among patients with TPG >12 mmHg, survival was better and pathologic findings of pulmonary vascular remodeling were less advanced in those with a gradient between PA diastolic pressure and PAWP (DPG) of less than 7 mmHg [14]. Based on these considerations, the recommendation was made that the diagnosis of "out of proportion" PH/LHD be abandoned, replaced by classification of PH/LHD into two groups: "isolated postcapillary PH" (MPAP >25 mmHg, PAWP >15 mmHg, TPG >12 mmHg, and DPG <7 mmHg) and "combined postcapillary and precapillary PH"

(MPAP >25 mmHg, PAWP >15 mmHg, TPG >12 mmHg, and DPG >7 mmHg) [15]. Although DPG >7 mmHg may be a valid marker of pulmonary vascular remodeling in PH/LHD and is associated with greater functional impairment [16], two studies have not shown any value of this parameter is assessing prognosis in PH/LHD. Tedford et al. [17] retrospectively studied 5827 patients undergoing hemodynamic evaluation for heart transplant and found no effect of DPG >7 on posttransplant survival. Similarly, Tampakakis et al. [18] retrospectively analyzed hemodynamic data on 1236 patients with nonischemic cardiomyopathy and found that DPG >7 mmHg did not predict worsened survival.

Interventions During RHC

Exercise

Since patients with PH are generally symptomatic with exertion and not at rest, there has been considerable interest in the evaluation of hemodynamics with exercise, particularly as it regards the detection of exercise-induced PH. It has long been known that PAP rises with exercise in normal subjects. The definition of PH included a mean PA pressure >30 mmHg with exercise until the publication of the Fourth World Symposium on Pulmonary Hypertension in 2009. However, this definition was abandoned in the absence of substantive data in the literature on the normal response of intracardiac pressures to exercise.

Although exercise response of PAP has not yet been reintroduced into the definition of PH, there has been some clarification of exercise hemodynamics in normals. Kovacs et al. [19] reviewed the literature on normal individuals studied with RHC. While gender, use of upright vs. supine exercise, use of treadmill vs. cycle ergometry, and upper vs. lower extremity exercise influenced normal values slightly or not at all, the authors found that age played a major role in the hemodynamic response to exercise. Normal resting values at RHC varied little with age, but measurements during light exercise were quite different when younger individuals were compared with individuals older than 50 years (see Table 2.1). The upper limit of normal for mean PAP during light exercise in healthy individuals over 50 was found to be 46 mmHg and frequently exceeded 30 mmHg. Since the rise in CO with a given workload may vary, it is best to describe the response of PA pressure to exercise in relation to CO rather than to workload. In younger healthy subjects, the rise in mean PAP was about 1 mmHg per L/min increase in cardiac output whereas in subjects over 50, the relationship between mean PAP and CO was steeper, amounting to about 2.8 mmHg per L/min rise in CO. In older healthy subjects, exercise resulted in significant rises in PAWP, with some readings in excess of 20 mmHg. In all age groups, the normal response to exercise included a slight decrease in PVR and TPR [20]. This decrease in resistances is explained by vascular recruitment and distensibility of the resistance vessels in the pulmonary circulation, which averages about 2 mm in diameter per mmHg rise in mean PAP [21].

Table 2.1 Normal values in RHC

Normal values	Rest		Exercise		
		Age >50	Light	Heavy	Age >50
Heart rate	76 ± 14		103 ± 14	170 ± 14	
Cardiac output (L/min)	7.3 ± 2.3		15 ± 4	20 ± 4	
Cardiac index (L/min/m^2)	4.1 ± 1.3				
PA systolic (mmHg)	21 ± 4				
PA diastolic (mmHg)	9 ± 3				
PA mean (mmHg)	14 ± 3	15 ± 4	21 ± 4	25 ± 6	29 ± 8[a]
Right atrial mean (mmHg)	3 ± 2				
PAWP (mmHg)	8 ± 3		9 ± 4	15 ± 8	17 ± 6[a]
SvO_2 (%)	68–75				
PVR (Wood U)	1.0 ± 0.5		0.7 ± 0.2	0.6 ± 0.2	0.8 ± 0.2
TPR (U)	2.5 ± 1				
DPG (mmHg)	<7				
TPG (mmHg)	<12				

[a]PA pressure in older individuals was measured with light exercise only

The definition of exercise pulmonary hypertension (including both pulmonary arterial and pulmonary venous hypertension) has become clearer in more recent studies. Herve et al. [22] studied 169 patients with effort dyspnea and normal hemodynamic parameters at rest on right heart catheterization. Patients were exercised utilizing supine bicycle ergometry to exhaustion. Patients with left heart disease (identified by PAWP >20 mmHg with exercise) and those with pulmonary vascular disease could be differentiated with great accuracy from controls without heart or lung disease using the criterion of total pulmonary resistance (TPR = MPAP/CO) rising to >3.0 Wood units with exercise *in addition to* a rise in MPAP to >30 mmHg with exercise. These criteria did not lose their accuracy regardless of age or sex. The distinction between patients with exercise PH and normal also could be made with these criteria regardless of workload, suggesting that the exercise protocol could be stopped at lower workloads, as long as MPAP rises above 30 mmHg at a cardiac output less than 10 L/min.

In the context of the elucidation of normal responses to exercise, the concept of exercise-induced PAH was felt to be an important part of the effort to identify an earlier phase of PAH, with the hope that earlier therapy could prevent its progression. Tolle et al. [23] examined 406 individuals with dyspnea on exertion with invasive hemodynamics and cardiopulmonary exercise testing. Though most of the patients were found to have pulmonary venous hypertension, there was a subgroup of 93 patients in whom resting MPAP was <25 mmHg and exercise resulted in MPAP >30 mmHg, PAWP <20, and PVR >1 Wood U. These patients were felt to have exercise-induced pulmonary arterial hypertension. Although these individuals were felt to have an early stage of PAH, there has been no longitudinal study of these subjects to suggest that they progressed to resting PAH.

Exercise-induced PH has also been observed in other clinical settings. Saggar et al. [24] studied 80 patients with scleroderma with resting and exercise RHC. Of these, 57 had normal resting hemodynamics. Supine lower extremity cycle ergometry was performed in these patients. Of these, nine patients were identified who had "exercise PH," consisting of exercise MPAP >30 mmHg, PAWP <18 mmHg, and TPG >15 mmHg. Despite normal hemodynamics at rest, these patients had higher TPG, PVR, and MPAP at rest than did the rest of the study group. It was postulated that these patients might be suitable for trials of early treatment with PAH-specific drugs. Borlaug et al. [25] studied 55 patients with dyspnea, normal left ventricular ejection fraction, and normal resting hemodynamics. With supine bicycle exercise or arm exercise, 32 patients were found to have HFpEF as defined by PAWP at exercise >25 mmHg; 88% of these were found to have exercise-induced PH (defined as MPAP >30 mmHg), related mainly to elevated PAWP. To date, no randomized controlled studies of treatment with PAH-specific drugs in patients with exercise induced-PH have been published.

Exercise RHC may also serve to clarify the nature of PH in patients with mild PH at rest. We studied 35 patients with dyspnea and mild-moderate PH (MPAP 20–40 mmHg) and normal PAWP at rest. With light arm exercise, 14/35 patients had a rise in PAWP to levels >20 mmHg, indicating the presence of pulmonary venous (postcapillary) hypertension (presented at ISHLT 2009). These patients would have been classified as having precapillary PH (PAH) based on resting hemodynamics. Figure 2.2 illustrates the recordings of right heart pressures at rest and with exercise in one such patient.

Exercise RHC may also aid in assessing the prognosis in an individual with resting hemodynamics consistent with PAH. Chaouat et al. [26] studied 55 patients with incident PAH (median MPAP 51 mmHg) with light exercise (median workload 20 W) prior to initiation of therapy. They found that prognosis in these patients correlated with exercise response, with >50% increase in cardiac index with exercise predicting improved survival after a median follow-up period of 18 months.

Fluid Challenge

Observation of hemodynamic changes in response to volume expansion has been of interest since the description by Bush et al. [27] of a group of patients with occult constrictive pericarditis whose filling pressures rose strikingly with rapid infusion of 1L normal saline solution. It had previously been thought that a rise in PAWP beyond 15 mmHg with rapid saline infusion indicated the presence of pulmonary venous hypertension [28]. However, in a study of 60 individuals without heart disease, the response to fluid challenge was found to be more complex [29]. Healthy subjects were given up to 2 L saline infusion over approximately 20 min while invasive hemodynamics were measured. PAWP was found to rise to 20 ± 3 mmHg and was above 15 mmHg in the great majority of subjects. For any given volume of saline infused, the rate of rise of PAWP was higher in women over the age of 50 years than in younger women and men of all ages. Cardiac index, MPAP, and TPG rose significantly with rapid saline infusion. In a group of 11 patients with HfpEF studied with smaller volumes of normal saline, the rate of rise of PAWP was found to be higher than in normal individuals.

Thus, although the response of PAWP to volume challenge is different in pulmonary venous hypertension than in normals and can yield useful information during RHC, a cutoff value for defining elevated left ventricular filling pressures cannot be identified. In addition, lack of standardization of volume and rate of infusion and

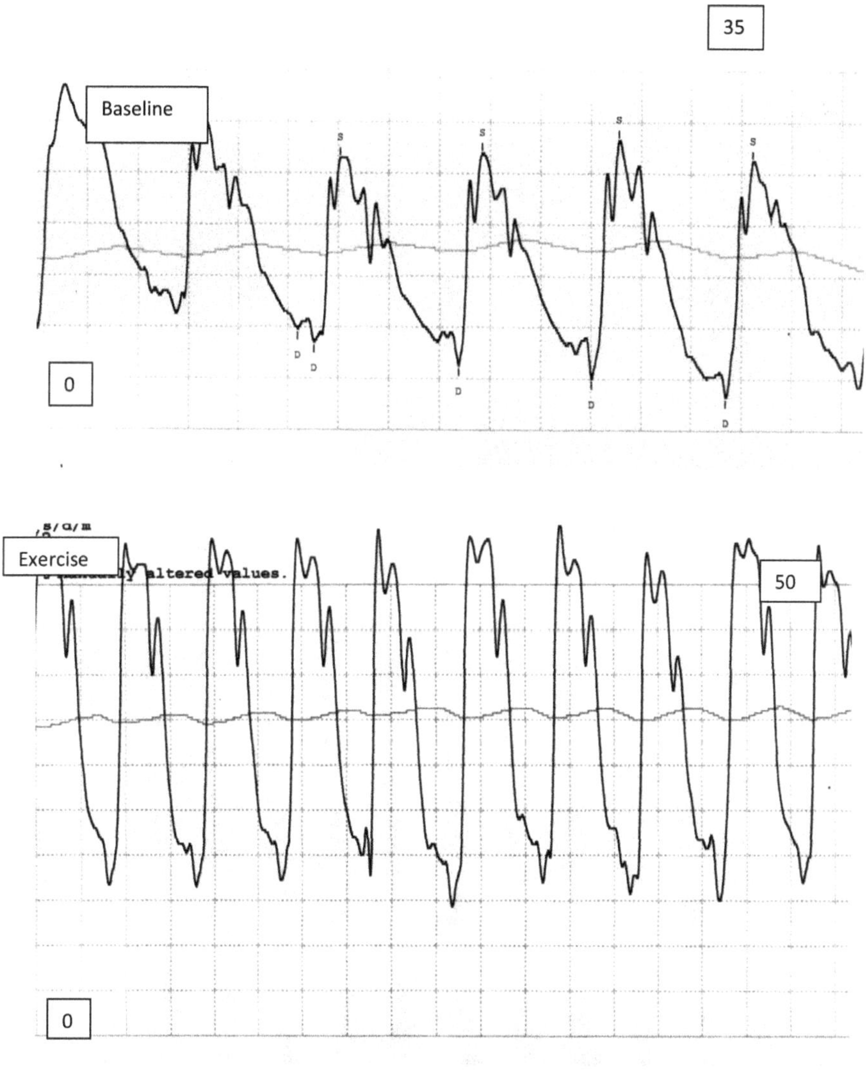

Fig. 2.2

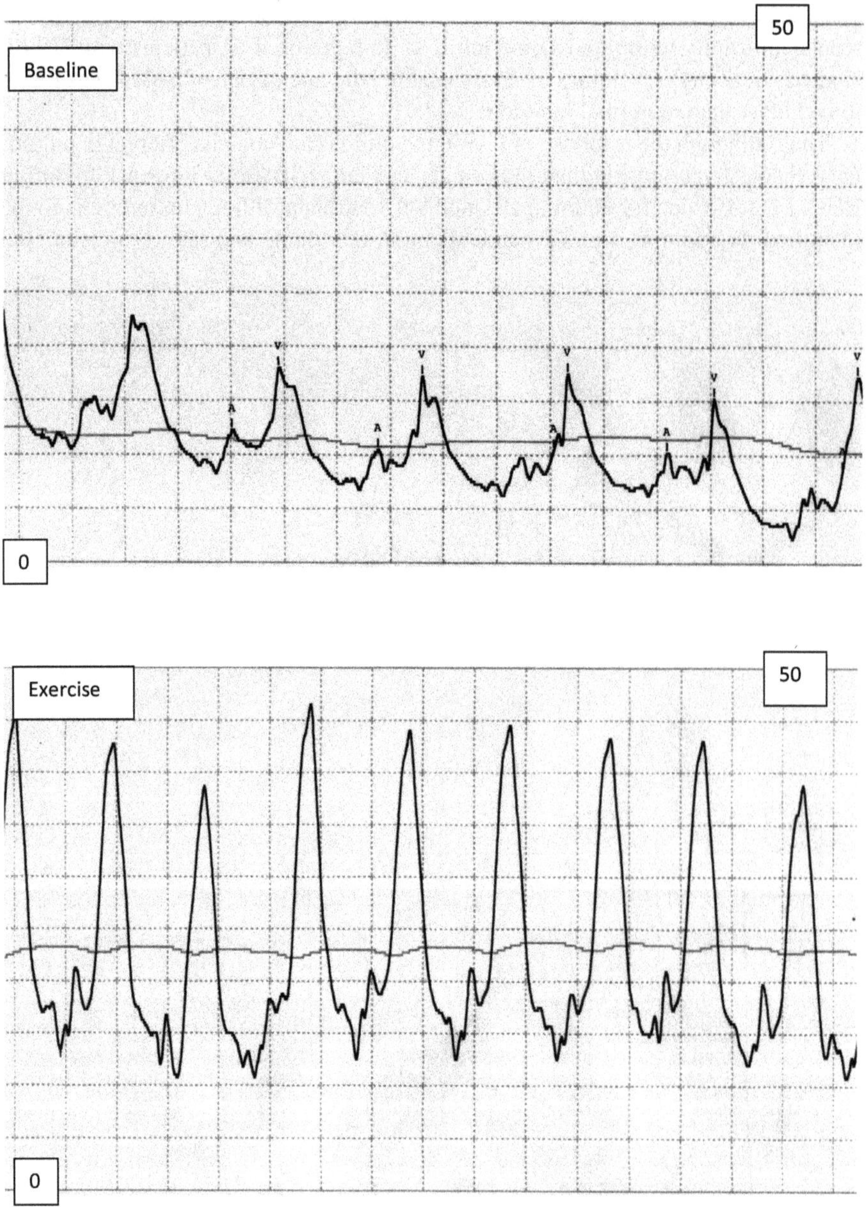

Fig. 2.2 (continued)

volume status at the onset of infusion, as well as gender and age influence on PAWP response prevent fluid challenge from becoming a definitive diagnostic tool in the analysis of the patient with suspected PAH.

Vasodilator Challenge

Since the demonstration more than 20 years ago by Rich et al. [30] that the small subset of patients with PAH who respond to vasodilators during RHC have improved survival when treated with calcium channel blockers, acute administration of vasodilators has become a standard part of the evaluation of patients with PH during RHC. Various agents have been used for this purpose, including inhaled nitric oxide (iNO), intravenous adenosine, and intravenous epoprostenol. The latter agent is not well tolerated when administered acutely in increasing doses. A head-to-head comparison of intravenous adenosine with iNO in 39 patients with PAH showed that iNO was more sensitive than intravenous adenosine in identifying vasoreactive PH and was also better tolerated [31]. Although iNO has become the agent of choice for detection of vasoreactivity in PAH, there is data to support the use of inhaled iloprost as well [32]. A generally accepted definition of vasoreactive PH includes a decrease in MPAP by 10 or more mmHg to a level less than 40 mmHg with no change or an increase in CO.

Vasoreactivity testing is more important in some forms of PH than in others. It is considered essential in initial RHC in patients with idiopathic PAH, in order to identify the subset of patients who can be managed long term with calcium channel blockers; repeat RHC with vasodilator should be considered in these patients to verify persistent vasoreactivity, as a certain proportion of these patients are found to have lost this quality at 12 months after initiation of calcium channel blocker therapy [33]. Vasoreactivity testing is considered of much less importance in patients with PAH related to connective tissue disease, in whom a positive response to iNO is distinctly uncommon. In fact, the only two patients in the literature in whom pulmonary edema occurred with iNO both had scleroderma, one of whom had interstitial lung disease at autopsy [34]. Vasoreactivity testing is generally not performed in patients with PH and interstitial lung disease.

Administration of iNO during RHC may yield information beyond the presence or absence of vasoreactivity. Adverse effects of iNO in patients with left ventricular dysfunction have been described [35]. This response can be used for diagnostic purposes when PH related to diastolic dysfunction (HFpEF) is suspected. Figure 2.3 illustrates one such patient, whose baseline PAWP is borderline at baseline with dramatic rise in PAWP and change in waveform with iNO.

Conclusion

Despite significant advances in evaluation of right ventricular structure and function utilizing noninvasive techniques such as echocardiography and magnetic resonance imaging, RHC remains the gold standard for evaluation of patients with suspected PH. PH is optimally evaluated and treated when the strengths of invasive and noninvasive techniques are allowed to complement one another. RHC is uniquely

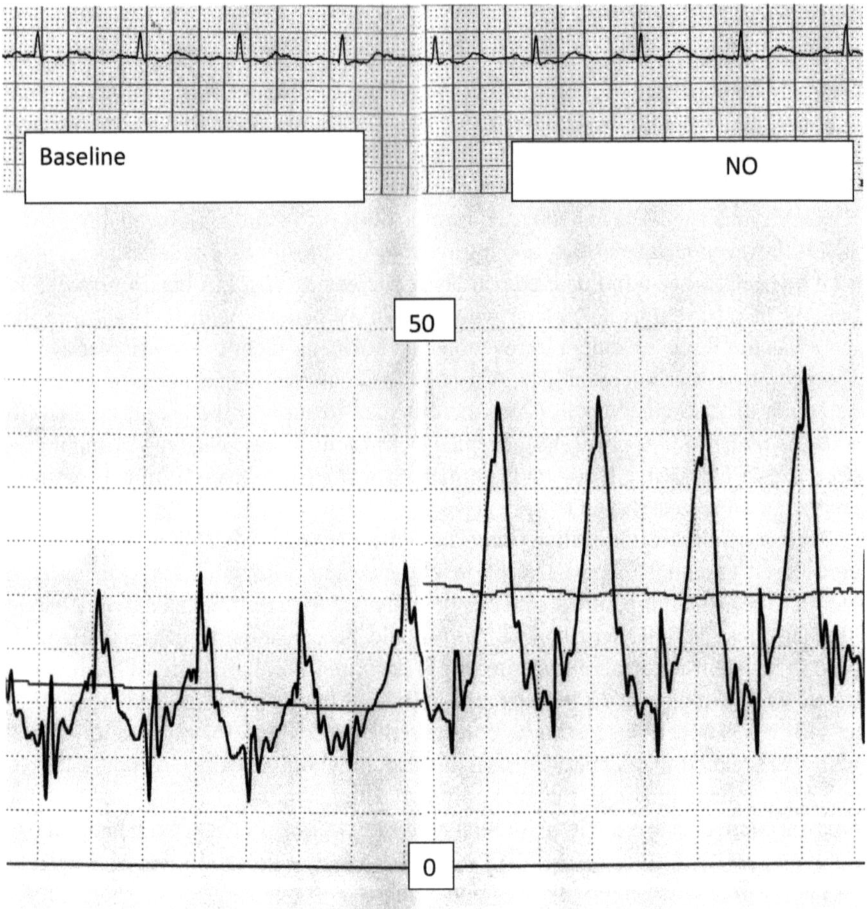

Fig. 2.3

equipped to establish the presence of PAH, distinguish PAH from PH/LHD, determine the severity and nature of the hemodynamic burden, assess prognosis, and guide therapy.

References

1. Hoeper MM, Lee SH, Voswinckel R, Palazzini M, Jais X, Marinelli A, et al. Complications of right heart catheterization procedures in patients with pulmonary hypertension in experienced centers. J Am Coll Cardiol. 2006;48(12):2546–52.
2. Kovacs G, Avian A, Olschewski A, Olschewski H. Zero reference level for right heart catheterisation. Eur Respir J. 2013;42(6):1586–94.

3. Fares WH, Blanchard SK, Stouffer GA, Chang PP, Rosamond WD, Ford HJ, et al. Thermodilution and Fick cardiac outputs differ: impact on pulmonary hypertension evaluation. Can Respir J. 2012;19(4):261–6.
4. Hoeper MM, Bogaard HJ, Condliffe R, Frantz R, Khanna D, Kurzyna M, et al. Definitions and diagnosis of pulmonary hypertension. J Am Coll Cardiol. 2013;62(25 Suppl):D42–50.
5. Hoeper MM, Maier R, Tongers J, Niedermeyer J, Hohlfeld JM, Hamm M, et al. Determination of cardiac output by the Fick method, thermodilution, and acetylene rebreathing in pulmonary hypertension. Am J Respir Crit Care Med. 1999;160(2):535–41.
6. McLaughlin VV, Archer SL, Badesch DB, Barst RJ, Farber HW, Lindner JR, et al. ACCF/AHA 2009 expert consensus document on pulmonary hypertension a report of the American College of Cardiology Foundation Task Force on Expert Consensus Documents and the American Heart Association developed in collaboration with the American College of Chest Physicians; American Thoracic Society, Inc.; and the Pulmonary Hypertension Association. J Am Coll Cardiol. 2009;53(17):1573–619.
7. Ryan JJ, Rich JD, Thiruvoipati T, Swamy R, Kim GH, Rich S. Current practice for determining pulmonary capillary wedge pressure predisposes to serious errors in the classification of patients with pulmonary hypertension. Am Heart J. 2012;163(4):589–94.
8. LeVarge BL, Pomerantsev E, Channick RN. Reliance on end-expiratory wedge pressure leads to misclassification of pulmonary hypertension. Eur Respir J. 2014;44(2):425–34.
9. Oliveira RK, Ferreira EV, Ramos RP, Messina CM, Kapins CE, Silva CM, et al. Usefulness of pulmonary capillary wedge pressure as a correlate of left ventricular filling pressures in pulmonary arterial hypertension. J Heart Lung Transplant. 2014;33(2):157–62.
10. D'Alonzo GE, Barst RJ, Ayres SM, Bergofsky EH, Brundage BH, Detre KM, et al. Survival in patients with primary pulmonary hypertension. Results from a national prospective registry. Ann Intern Med. 1991;115(5):343–9.
11. Tiede H, Sommer N, Milger K, Voswinckel R, Bandorski D, Schermuly RT, et al. Short-term improvement in pulmonary hemodynamics is strongly predictive of long-term survival in patients with pulmonary arterial hypertension. Pulm Circ. 2013;3(3):523–32.
12. Seeger W, Adir Y, Barbera JA, Champion H, Coghlan JG, Cottin V, et al. Pulmonary hypertension in chronic lung diseases. J Am Coll Cardiol. 2013;62(25 Suppl):D109–16.
13. Naeije R, Vachiery JL, Yerly P, Vanderpool R. The transpulmonary pressure gradient for the diagnosis of pulmonary vascular disease. Eur Respir J. 2013;41(1):217–23.
14. Gerges C, Gerges M, Lang MB, Zhang Y, Jakowitsch J, Probst P, et al. Diastolic pulmonary vascular pressure gradient: a predictor of prognosis in "out-of-proportion" pulmonary hypertension. Chest. 2013;143(3):758–66.
15. Vachiery JL, Adir Y, Barbera JA, Champion H, Coghlan JG, Cottin V, et al. Pulmonary hypertension due to left heart diseases. J Am Coll Cardiol. 2013;62(25 Suppl):D100–8.
16. Howard C, Rangajhavala K, Safdar Z. Pulmonary artery diastolic pressure gradient as an indicator of severity of illness in patients with pulmonary hypertension related to left-sided heart disease. Ther Adv Respir Dis. 2015;9(2):35–41.
17. Tedford RJ, Beaty CA, Mathai SC, Kolb TM, Damico R, Hassoun PM, et al. Prognostic value of the pre-transplant diastolic pulmonary artery pressure-to-pulmonary capillary wedge pressure gradient in cardiac transplant recipients with pulmonary hypertension. J Heart Lung Transplant. 2014;33(3):289–97.
18. Tampakakis E, Leary PJ, Selby VN, De Marco T, Cappola TP, Felker GM, et al. The diastolic pulmonary gradient does not predict survival in patients with pulmonary hypertension due to left heart disease. JACC Heart Fail. 2015;3(1):9–16.
19. Kovacs G, Berghold A, Scheidl S, Olschewski H. Pulmonary arterial pressure during rest and exercise in healthy subjects: a systematic review. Eur Respir J. 2009;34(4):888–94.
20. Kovacs G, Olschewski A, Berghold A, Olschewski H. Pulmonary vascular resistances during exercise in normal subjects: a systematic review. Eur Respir J. 2012;39(2):319–28.
21. Naeije R, Vanderpool R, Dhakal BP, Saggar R, Saggar R, Vachiery JL, et al. Exercise-induced pulmonary hypertension: physiological basis and methodological concerns. Am J Respir Crit Care Med. 2013;187(6):576–83.

22. Herve P, Lau EM, Sitbon O, Savale L, Montani D, Godinas L, et al. Criteria for diagnosis of exercise pulmonary hypertension. Eur Respir J. 2015;28
23. Tolle JJ, Waxman AB, Van Horn TL, Pappagianopoulos PP, Systrom DM. Exercise-induced pulmonary arterial hypertension. Circulation. 2008;118(21):2183–9.
24. Saggar R, Khanna D, Furst DE, Shapiro S, Maranian P, Belperio JA, et al. Exercise-induced pulmonary hypertension associated with systemic sclerosis: four distinct entities. Arthritis Rheum. 2010;62(12):3741–50.
25. Borlaug BA, Nishimura RA, Sorajja P, Lam CS, Redfield MM. Exercise hemodynamics enhance diagnosis of early heart failure with preserved ejection fraction. Circ Heart Fail. 2010;3(5):588–95.
26. Chaouat A, Sitbon O, Mercy M, Poncot-Mongars R, Provencher S, Guillaumot A, et al. Prognostic value of exercise pulmonary haemodynamics in pulmonary arterial hypertension. Eur Respir J. 2014;44(3):704–13.
27. Bush CA, Stang JM, Wooley CF, Kilman JW. Occult constrictive pericardial disease. Diagnosis by rapid volume expansion and correction by pericardiectomy. Circulation. 1977;56(6):924–30.
28. Champion HC, Michelakis ED, Hassoun PM. Comprehensive invasive and noninvasive approach to the right ventricle-pulmonary circulation unit: state of the art and clinical and research implications. Circulation. 2009;120(11):992–1007.
29. Fujimoto N, Borlaug BA, Lewis GD, Hastings JL, Shafer KM, Bhella PS, et al. Hemodynamic responses to rapid saline loading: the impact of age, sex, and heart failure. Circulation. 2013;127(1):55–62.
30. Rich S, Kaufmann E, Levy PS. The effect of high doses of calcium-channel blockers on survival in primary pulmonary hypertension. N Engl J Med. 1992;327(2):76–81.
31. Oliveira EC, Ribeiro AL, Amaral CF. Adenosine for vasoreactivity testing in pulmonary hypertension: a head-to-head comparison with inhaled nitric oxide. Respir Med. 2010;104(4):606–11.
32. Jing ZC, Jiang X, Han ZY, Xu XQ, Wang Y, Wu Y, et al. Iloprost for pulmonary vasodilator testing in idiopathic pulmonary arterial hypertension. Eur Respir J. 2009;33(6):1354–60.
33. Sitbon O, Humbert M, Jais X, Ioos V, Hamid AM, Provencher S, et al. Long-term response to calcium channel blockers in idiopathic pulmonary arterial hypertension. Circulation. 2005;111(23):3105–11.
34. Preston IR, Klinger JR, Houtchens J, Nelson D, Mehta S, Hill NS. Pulmonary edema caused by inhaled nitric oxide therapy in two patients with pulmonary hypertension associated with the CREST syndrome. Chest. 2002;121(2):656–9.
35. Loh E, Stamler JS, Hare JM, Loscalzo J, Colucci WS. Cardiovascular effects of inhaled nitric oxide in patients with left ventricular dysfunction. Circulation. 1994;90(6):2780–5.

Chapter 3
Pathology of Vascular Changes in Interstitial Lung Diseases

Hilario Nunes, Peter Dorfmüller, Yurdagul Uzunhan, Dominique Valeyre, Jean-François Bernaudin, and Marianne Kambouchner

Introduction

Interstitial lung diseases (ILDs) embrace a heterogeneous group of disorders with diverse clinical outcomes. ILDs are classically separated into four categories: (i) ILDs of known cause, such as those in relation with occupational or environmental exposures, drugs, connective tissue diseases (CTDs), or vasculitis; (ii) idiopathic interstitial pneumonias (IIPs); (iii) sarcoidosis; and (iv) particular forms of ILDs, such as pulmonary Langerhans cell histiocytosis (PLCH), lymphangioleiomyomatosis (LAM), chronic idiopathic eosinophilic pneumonia [1]. More frequent ILDs are sarcoidosis, CTD-associated ILDs, hypersensitivity pneumonitis, and the chronic fibrosing IIPs, including idiopathic pulmonary fibrosis (IPF) and nonspecific interstitial pneumonia (NSIP).

H. Nunes (✉) • Y. Uzunhan • D. Valeyre
Université Paris 13, Sorbonne Paris Cité, EA2363 "Réponses cellulaires et fonctionnelles à l'hypoxie,", Bobigny, France

Assistance Publique Hôpitaux de Paris, Service de Pneumologie, Hôpital Avicenne, 125 rue de Stalingrad, 93009, Bobigny, France
e-mail: hilario.nunes@avc.aphp.fr

P. Dorfmüller
Service d'Anatomie pathologique et INSERM UMRS 999, LabEx LERMIT, Hôpital Marie Lannelongue, Le Plessis-Robinson, France

J.-F. Bernaudin
Université Paris 13, Sorbonne Paris Cité, EA2363 "Réponses cellulaires et fonctionnelles à l'hypoxie,", Bobigny, France

Histologie et Cytologie, Université Pierre et Marie Curie, Sorbonne Universités Paris, Paris, France

M. Kambouchner
Assistance Publique Hôpitaux de Paris, Service d'Anatomie et Cytologie pathologiques, Hôpital Avicenne, Bobigny, France

R.P. Baughman et al. (eds.), *Pulmonary Hypertension and Interstitial Lung Disease*, DOI 10.1007/978-3-319-49918-5_3

The lung interstitium is the primary site of injury in ILDs, with diverse combinations of inflammation and fibrosis. However, because of anatomic proximity, the disease process is not restricted to the interstitium and also encompasses the airspaces, peripheral airways, and vessels [1]. Accordingly, the pathobiologic mechanisms leading to the parenchymal remodeling and fibrosis in ILDs may also contribute to structural and functional alterations in the pulmonary vasculature. The vascular morphologic changes are extremely protean in ILDs, ranging from nonspecific abnormalities secondary to chronic hypoxic vasoconstriction and/or destruction of the capillary bed to specific involvement, which may affect all types of pulmonary vessels. These changes may be subclinical or result in a variable degree of pulmonary hypertension (PH).

The prevalence and severity of PH vary according to the nature of ILD and disease advancement [2, 3]. In the updated clinical classification of PH, ILDs fall under group 3 ("PH due to lung diseases and/or hypoxia") [4]. Group 5 has been created for "PH with unclear and/or multifactorial mechanisms" in which are included several ILDs, i.e., sarcoidosis, PLCH, LAM, neurofibromatosis, and vasculitis [4]. This distinction from group 3 is justified by the complexity of vascular involvement for these disorders, with some patients exhibiting severe PH insufficiently explained by functional disturbances. PH has a substantial impact on survival of patients with ILDs. In the absence of patent PH, pathologic vascular changes may still have prognostic implications. From a pathogenetic perspective, vascular involvement may also reflect a role in ILDs onset and progression.

This article attempts to describe the pathology of vascular changes observed in ILDs and reviews the most recent literature regarding the pathogenic significance of vascular involvement in this setting. It focuses on the ILDs in which vascular involvement is common and/or clinically relevant, in particular IPF, systemic sclerosis (SSc)-associated ILD, sarcoidosis, and PLCH.

General Considerations

Normal Microanatomy of the Pulmonary Circulation

There are two parallel circulations in the lung, the bronchial and the pulmonary circulation, but to our knowledge, in contrast to the pulmonary circulation, the involvement of the bronchial circulation has not been reported in ILDs. The architecture of the pulmonary vasculature is designed to offer a high compliance and low resistance network of arteries and veins connected to an extensive capillary bed confined within the interalveolar septa [5, 6]. Pulmonary arteries (PAs), capillaries and veins, are connected in series. As a result, arteries and arterioles upstream of the capillaries are referred to as the precapillary vessels and those distal, veinules, and veins, as postcapillary vessels [5, 6].

Despite thinner walls than their systemic analogous, the PAs and veins are similarly constituted of three concentric tunicae. The *intima*, the inner tunica in contact with the blood, consists of a single layer of endothelial cells (ECs), i.e., the endothelium, lying on a basement lamina with subendothelial connective tissue in larger vessels. The *media*, the middle tunica, is composed of various amounts of vascular smooth muscle cells (VSMCs), elastic fibers, and connective tissue, depending on the type of vessel. The *adventitia* is the outer tunica abutting the perivascular tissue. Multiple different cell types contribute to normal vascular function and response to injury. (For an up to date extensive review see [5].)

Normal Pulmonary Arteries

The composition of the arterial wall varies from the proximal artery trunk to the smallest extraalveolar arteries [7].

- The *intima* is mainly composed of the endothelium. Its thickness ranges from 1 to 16% of the total wall thickness. ECs are multifunction highly specialized cells, which in particular secrete factors that maintain the tone of media VSMCs.
- The *media* is constituted of various amounts of VSMCs, elastic fibers, and extracellular matrix providing structural support, vasoreactivity, and elasticity. In comparison to systemic arteries, the media is thin, i.e., 1–3% of the external diameter to 5–10% in less than 100 μm arteries. It varies largely along the arterial tree, and classification of PAs is based on the presence of elastic lamina and the degree of muscularity of the medial layer. Elastic and transitional arteries (>1000 μm external diameter) extend from the hilum to nearly halfway along the bronchial tree. They possess distinctive concentric sheets of elastic fibers, embedded with VSMCs. Muscular PAs (100–1000 μm external diameter), mostly intralobular, accompanying bronchioles are composed of a thin layer of VSMCs sandwiched between well delimited internal and external elastic lamina. Terminal arterioles (<100 μm external diameter) originate from muscular arteries and contain a partial layer of VSMCs that gradually disappear until the arterial wall consists of elastic lamina and endothelium. Into the acinus some arterial branches are partially muscular while others are nonmuscular arteries/arterioles.
- The *adventitia* represents approximately 15% of the external diameter of normal PAs and is larger than 50 μm in diameter [6]. It is a critical regulator of vessel wall function, considered as the principal injury-sensing tissue of the vessel wall [7]. Preacinar arteries are embedded in the loosely organized bronchovascular bundles which in addition encompass airways and lymphatics. In contrast, intraacinar arteries have an intimate relationship with the surrounding alveolar spaces. In case of injury, the heterogeneous population of resident fibroblasts is activated and undergoes a variety of functional changes with consequences on the arterial wall.

Normal Pulmonary Veins

Pulmonary veins duplicate the arterial branching tree but they run independently within the interlobular septa at the periphery of the acinus and lobule. Therefore, the first orders of veins may be defined as preseptal veins. Their microanatomy share similarities to arteries but with thinner walls offering a lower resistance. The media of pulmonary veins is thinner than comparably sized arteries and contains more extracellular matrix collagen and less VSMCs. Intimal thickening may be observed with aging [8].

Hemodynamic Consequences

Histologically, the PAs have thinner walls and far less VSMCs than their systemic analogous. This confers a high distensibility to the pulmonary circulation, which explains its striking ability to accommodate large, i.e., fivefold, increases in cardiac output with only modest increases in pulmonary arterial pressure (PAP) as may occur during exercise. Besides, there is a recruitment phenomenon, with the opening of capillaries that were previously collapsed at rest. Therefore, PH requires ~80% of the vascular bed to be compromised while depending largely of the vascular segments affected [6]. The major site of resistance to pulmonary blood flow resides at the level of small muscular or partially muscular arteries and arterioles. Variations of caliber in these vessels normally regulate pulmonary vascular resistance (PVR) and allow the redistribution of blood flow, which is critical for optimizing ventilation and perfusion matching. Alveolar hypoxia is the major determinant of active changes in PVR. It causes vasoconstriction at the level of precapillary arterioles, which are exposed to the same gas tensions that prevail in the adjacent alveolar spaces [6].

Angiogenesis

Angiogenesis is the physiological or pathological process of new capillary blood vessel sprouting and growth from preexisting vasculature. It is distinct from *vasculogenesis*, the process of de novo formation of blood vessels from the differentiation of precursor cells into ECs that predominantly occurs during embryogenesis. Angiogenesis is the chief architect of tissue injury, repair, and healing responses, which can be beneficial or detrimental depending upon context. Thus, this mechanism may be critical in fibrotic ILDs [9–11]. The homeostatic control of angiogenesis, which attempts to maintain an ideal number of capillaries per unit of lung volume, depends on the simultaneous regulation of stimulatory (angiogenic) and inhibitory (angiostatic) factors.

Vascular Remodeling

It is obvious that the different forms of PH present with either a predominance of arterial remodeling or venous remodeling or a variable contribution of both [12]. In chronic lung diseases, including ILDs, the structural changes that are believed to underlie the development of PH can be roughly separated into two processes: first, remodeling of the resistance PAs and, second, a reduction or rarefaction in the total number of blood vessels in the lung [13, 14]. The major stimuli that are responsible for these changes are chronic alveolar hypoxia, sustained vasoconstriction, chronic inflammation, and excessive shear stress [13, 14]. In chronic lung diseases, vascular changes can be observed even in the absence of overt PH [13, 14].

Arterial Remodeling

Arterial changes can diversely associate [6, 12, 15] (Fig. 3.1)

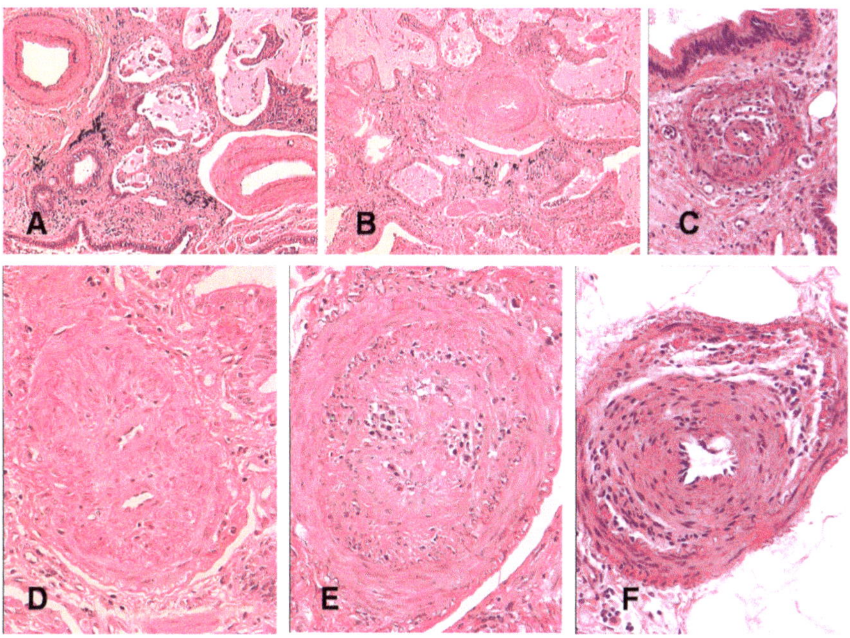

Fig. 3.1 Examples of pulmonary arterial lesions observed in usual interstitial pneumonia (UIP) (**a**, **b**) and nonspecific interstitial pneumonia (NSIP) (**c–f**) (hematoxylin and eosin staining): (**a**, **b**) a concentric medial hypertrophy and paucicellular intimal thickening is observed on sections of pulmonary arteries; note the histopathology background characteristic of UIP (original ×100), (**c**) small artery in a biopsy of NSIP showing a marked intima remodeling with intravascular and perivascular inflammatory infiltrate (original ×200), (**d**–**f**) pulmonary arteries observed in a biopsy of systemic sclerosis-associated NSIP showing plexiform lesions with obliteration of the lumen in **d** and **e** (original ×400)

- *Intimal lesions*: by reducing the luminal area these can be considered as a critical factor in the increase of the PVR in PH. Two forms of intima thickenings may be observed: (i) cellular intimal fibrosis with proliferation/accumulation of fibroblasts and myofibroblasts; (ii) concentric laminar intimal collagen-rich fibrosis; eccentric intimal fibrosis corresponding to organized wall-adherent thrombi or sequelae of vasculitis; (iii) plexiform lesions with proliferation of endothelial cells and fibroblasts (Fig. 3.1d–f).
- *Medial remodeling*: medial hypertrophy and muscularization of arterioles is the earliest most common alteration. It involves muscularized arteries (ranging between 70 and 500 μm in diameter), and precapillary intraacinar vessels (below 70 μm in diameter). Medial thickening has been observed in the lung of normal individuals exposed to cigarette smoke.
- *Adventitial remodeling*: there is growing evidence that the adventitia plays a role in the regulation of pulmonary vascular function, particularly through inflammation and fibroblastic activation. Such mechanisms may be of major importance in ILD-associated PH.

Venous Remodeling

The pulmonary veins may be narrowed by luminal obstruction by intimal fibrosis most commonly eccentric, loose, and paucicellular [16]. Interlobular septal veins may be muscularized and manifest an arterialized pattern. This can be associated with a marked capillary distention into periseptal alveoli and even capillary multiplication (pulmonary capillary hemangiomatosis) (Fig. 3.2) [16]. Occult pulmonary hemorrhage occurs frequently in pulmonary veno-occlusive disease (PVOD), probably due to postcapillary obstruction, with large amounts of hemosiderin found in alveolar macrophages and type 2 pneumocytes as well as deposits in the interstitium [16].

Pathology of Vascular Changes in ILDs

Evaluation of Vascular Changes in ILDs

In ILDs, lung biopsy examination is mostly focused on parenchymal lesions allowing its classification. In contrast with lung tissue studies in PAH, there is still no protocol for the evaluation of vascular lesions in PH associated with disorders of the respiratory system. Accurate assessment necessitates evaluation of all different blood vessels, preacinar and intraacinar arteries, capillaries, intraacinar and postacinar, as well as lymphatics and surrounding tissue. Elastic stains are essential. Pathologists must be aware of the various artifacts mainly due to the absence of inflation at the time of fixation.

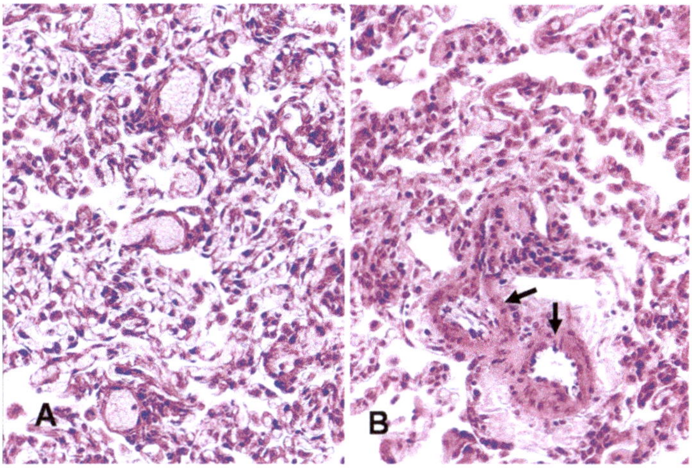

Fig. 3.2 Examples of capillary hemangiomatosis with exuberant proliferation of endothelial cells (**a**, **b**; hematoxylin and eosin staining; original ×400). Note in **b** the medial muscularization of intraacinar arteries

IPF

IPF is the most frequent chronic fibrosing IIP that afflicts primarily the elderly and has a devastating mortality. The prevalence of PH increases with the level of functional impairment, with estimated rates of approximately 5% in IPF patients with mild disease and 32–46% in those referred for lung transplantation [2, 3]. PH is more frequent in cases of combined pulmonary fibrosis and emphysema, which is thought to be a distinct IPF phenotype [17]. PH is indicative of a worse prognosis in IPF. IPF is included in group 3 of the clinical classification of PH [4]. However, PH cannot be explained exclusively by chronic hypoxic vasoconstriction and/or vascular rarefaction, in particular in patients with severe PH.

IPF is associated with the pathologic appearance of usual interstitial pneumonia (UIP), with the primary feature being patchy involvement of lung parenchyma with areas of fibrosis alternating sharply with areas of less affected or normal parenchyma [18]. There is evidence of marked fibrosis, with architectural distortion and sometimes honeycombing, which often is more pronounced in the subpleural and paraseptal parenchyma. The presence of convex subepithelial foci of proliferating fibroblasts and myofibroblasts at the leading edge of fibrosis (so-called fibroblast foci) is characteristic of UIP. When present, Interstitial inflammation is usually mild [18].

Vascular Remodeling and Angiogenesis in IPF

The vascular changes seen in IPF are believed to be related to the effect of chronic alveolar hypoxia with subsequent vascular remodeling and to the reduction of the distal vascular bed by fibrosis. However, these mechanisms cannot account for the broad assortment of structural alterations observed, which can affect all sections of the pulmonary vasculature, including the lung microvasculature [19, 20]. More than five decades ago, Turner-Warwick et al. first reported the presence of aberrant vascularization in IPF, with anastomoses between the systemic (bronchial and/or pleural arteries) and the pulmonary circulation [21]. Over the last years, this issue has been the subject of growing literature and nicely reviewed in several papers [9–11].

Arterial remodeling range from isolated medial hypertrophy and intimal thickening, to complete occlusion of distal PAs and, finally, fibrous atrophy and destruction of affected vessels. Newly formed vessels are also described. Strikingly, vascular remodeling and angiogenesis show a spatially and temporally heterogeneous distribution, paralleling the patchy involvement characteristic of UIP. Overall, there is a reduction in microvessel density, which worsens with the severity of pulmonary fibrosis [22]. However, whereas minimal vascularity is noted in the most fibrotic zones (fibroblastic foci are almost devoid of capillaries), adjacent normal parenchyma is highly vascularized [23, 24]. In honeycombing, the newly formed vessels display an abnormal phenotype, appearing large and dilated, with a lack of elastin layer, which result in reduced vascular compliance [24, 25].

So far, only few studies have correlated vascular changes with pulmonary hemodynamics in IPF [19, 20, 25]. Judge et al. have quantified microvessel density using CD31 immunostaining in the explanted lung from 13 IPF patients [25]. Vascular changes were evidenced in all cases. Neovascularization was significantly increased in areas of cellular fibrosis compared to distant normal lung and significantly decreased in areas of honeycombing. No relationship was found between FVC or DLCO and microvessel density in cellular fibrotic or honeycombing areas, corroborating the fact that lung function is a relatively poor surrogate of vascular involvement in IPF. Conversely, there was a significant inverse link between mPAP and microvessel density in honeycombing areas but not in cellular fibrotic areas [25]. The authors suggested that vascular changes in honeycombing areas, which were reminiscent of PAH, with medial hypertrophy and intimal fibrosis of the muscular PAs and intimal fibrosis of the pulmonary veins, may contribute most significantly to increased PVR, while the neovascularization observed in cellular fibrotic areas may represent an adaptive proliferative change in response to altered PVR rather than a primary event. Alternatively, these findings may indicate that the reduction of the vascular bed by fibrosis plays an important role in the pathogenesis of IPF-associated PH [25].

Two interesting studies have specifically assessed the postcapillary pulmonary system involvement in IPF [19, 20]. Colombat et al. analyzed the lung transplant specimens from 26 IPF patients, with particular attention to vessels in architecturally preserved lung areas using hematoxylin–eosin, iron, and elastin stainings, and correlated vascular changes with pulmonary hemodynamics [20]. Remarkably, the major finding in nonfibrotic zones consisted of occlusion in pulmonary venules and preseptal veins, which was present in 65% of cases and associated with alveolar capillary multiplication and/or muscularization of arterioles in the majority. In these cases with occlusive venopathy, lung parenchyma always exhibited at least moderate diffuse iron deposition in the interstitium and alveolar macrophages. Compared with venous involvement, there were only minor changes in muscular PAs, with no plexiform lesions [20]. Yet, the authors failed to find any significant relationship between venous/venular changes in nonfibrotic zones and mPAP, so that the role of these abnormalities remains speculative [20]. Kim et al. measured alveolar septal capillary density using hematoxylin–eosin, elastin, and CD34 stainings as well as iron deposition in the nonfibrotic zones from surgical lung biopsies (SLB) or explants of 154 IPF patients, and examined their relation with the degree of PH [19]. Both pathologic features were associated with right ventricular systolic pressure at echocardiography, independent of lung function or fibrosis extent [19]. These findings advocate the potential role of postcapillary remodeling in the development of PH.

Angiogenic and Angiostatic Imbalance in IPF

As alluded to earlier, it is now recognized that in IPF both increased capillary density and vascular rarefaction are seen in the same lung at different sites according to the extent of tissue fibrosis [9–11]. It appears likely that the delicate balance between angiogenic and angiostatic factors is disrupted in the fibrotic milieu, with a probable temporal and spatial variation in the expression of these mediators, in keeping with the vascular heterogeneity observed [9–11]. Numerous vascular biologic molecules and signaling pathways have been incriminated in humans with IPF and/or experimental models of pulmonary fibrosis [9–11]. An imbalance in the expression of angiogenic (CXCL5, CXCL8) and angiostatic (CXCL10, CXCL11) chemokines has been demonstrated, with contradictory results [24, 26–30], as well as an imbalance between other angiogenic (vascular endothelial growth factor (VEGF), interleukin (IL)-8), and angiostatic [pigment epithelium-derived factor (PEDF)] factors [23]. Other mechanisms include increased endothelin-1 (ET-1) [31–34], which enhances the neovascularization through induction of VEGF, dysregulation of endostatin [35, 36], a potent inhibitor of angiogenesis, and the angiogenic angiopoictin axis [37]. The most widely investigated mediator is VEGF, the prototypical angiogenic factor. VEGF levels are reduced in the bronchoalveolar lavage (BAL) of IPF patients [38, 39]. Densely fibrotic regions of the IPF lung, especially fibroblastic foci, show a lack of VEGF expression, which is paralleled by augmented expression of PEDF [23, 24, 40]. In contrast, VEGF is overexpressed in the highly vascularized areas of relatively preserved lung [23, 24, 40].

Possible Shared Pathogenic Mechanisms between IPF and PH

The possible shared pathogenic mechanisms between IPF and PH are summarized in Fig. 3.3. This concept of a particular relationship between pulmonary fibrogenesis and vascular remodeling/angiogenesis is in line with the results of two recent studies analyzing gene expression in isolated pulmonary arterioles from IPF patients using laser capture microdissection and microarrays. Patel et al. demonstrated that IPF patients who are free of PH have a similar gene signature to thosc with

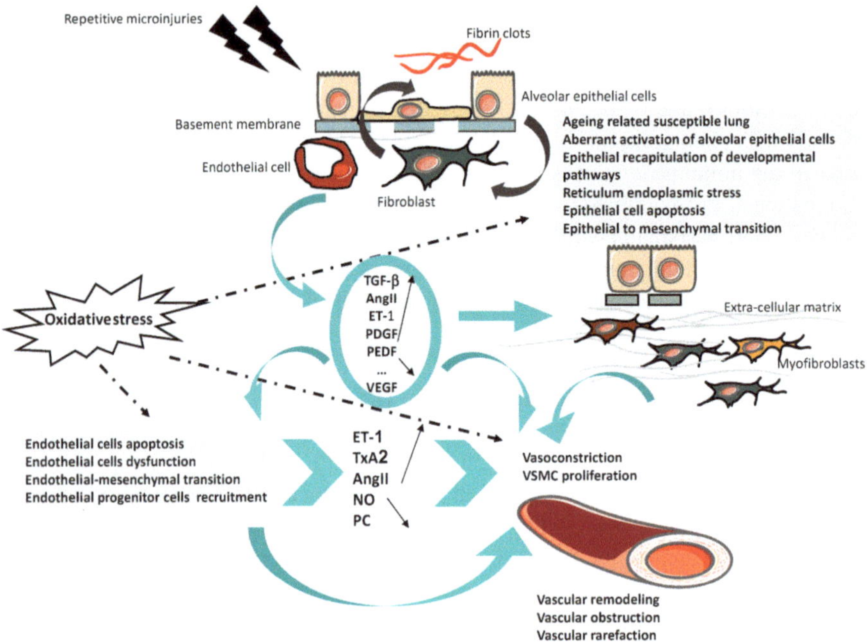

Fig. 3.3 Shared pathogenetic mechanisms between idiopathic pulmonary fibrosis and pulmonary hypertension

coexistent PH, with an exaggerated expression of mediators of SMVCs and ECs proliferation, as compared to controls, suggesting the existence of preclinical pulmonary vascular disease [41]. Interestingly, Hoffmann et al. showed that, even though COPD-associated PH and IPF-associated PH exhibit similar pathologic vascular remodeling, differential gene expression is observed in PA profiles, suggesting that the two conditions are based on distinct mechanisms [42].

IPF is an alveolar epithelial cells (AECs)-driven disorder, with aberrant crosstalk between AECs and fibroblasts [43]. Ageing-related susceptible lung is targeted by repetitive environmental microinjuries, including cigarette smoking, silent microaspiration, and chronic herpes virus infections. Noticeably, Calabrese et al. have suggested that herpes virus infection may be involved in pulmonary vascular remodeling and PH complicating IPF [44]. Also, tobacco is known to be a risk factor for men with PAH [45], as well as in pulmonary veno-occlusive disease [46]. Microinjuries provoke AECs apoptosis and damage of basement membranes, followed by increased vascular permeability and exudation of fibrin [43]. Abnormally activated AECs produce diverse mediators, inducing the formation of fibroblast and myofibroblast foci through the proliferation of resident mesenchymal cells, attraction of circulating bone marrow-derived progenitors of fibroblasts (fibrocytes), and stimulation of epithelial-to-mesenchymal transition [43]. These foci secrete excessive amounts of ECM, resulting in progressive parenchymal remodeling [43].

Several cytokines and growth factors have a critical role in this context, such as transforming growth factor (TGF)-ß, platelet-derived growth factor (PDGF), connective tissue growth factor (CTGF), ET-1, and angiotensin (Ag) II [43]. With a decreased production of VEGF, this environment may also induce ECs apoptosis and/or dysfunction, two key events in vascular remodeling [9–11]. ECs dysfunction leads to decreased production of vasodilators like NO and prostacyclin and increased release of Ag II, thromboxan A2, ET-1, favoring vasoconstriction and VSMCs proliferation [9–11]. Another relevant contributor to PH is the reduction in cross-sectional vascular area due to thrombotic vessels obstruction [47]. Indeed, a procoagulant state is generated [43]. The alveolar fibrin clots due to impaired intra-alveolar fibrinolysis may provide a nidus for fibroblast chemotactic migration and proliferation as well as for neovascularization [43]. In addition to ECs apoptosis or dysfunction, a transdifferentiation of these cells to mesenchymal cells is described and may contribute to both pulmonary vascular remodeling and fibrogenesis [48]. Of interest, this concept of endothelial-to-mesenchymal transition has also recently been shown in PAH [49]. The available evidence also strongly supports the role of enhanced oxidative stress in the pathogenesis of the two processes via myofibroblast accumulation, vasoconstriction, VSMCs proliferation, and ECs alterations [47].

More recently, several studies have been published on the role of circulating endothelial progenitor cells (CECs) and endothelial progenitor cells (EPCs) in the pathogenesis of IPF. It has been suggested that CECs actively participate in the intense remodeling of the pulmonary vasculature in IPF patients. The abundance of CECs and EPCs may indeed reflect the balance between vascular and parenchymal injury/repair with reconstitution of the damaged vascular bed [50, 51]. EPCs represent a subset of bone marrow-derived stem cells with two subtypes. Late EPCs may differentiate into mature ECs and repair injured blood vessels while "early EPCs" (i.e., EPCs that grow into colony forming units on fibronectin following 5–7 days culture) may have angiogenic potential by secreting cytokines such as VEGF and thereby enhance the angiogenic process [52, 53]. Early EPCs levels are reduced in IPF patients. Reduced EPCs numbers have been associated with persistent fibrotic changes in humans following lung injury. Reduced numbers of EPCs may impair normal mechanisms of lung repair. Furthermore, EPCs may act synergically with circulating fibrocytes [54]. These bone marrow-derived mesenchymal progenitor cells involved in IPF are recognized as indicators of a poor prognosis [55]. These cells (fibrocytes and EPCs), recruited by SDF-1/CXCR4 axis in fibrotic areas, have also both been implicated in angiogenic dysregulation observed in IPF [54].

Influence of Angiogenesis/Vascular Remodeling on Pulmonary Fibrogenesis and Vice Versa

It is tempting to speculate that pulmonary fibrogenesis and angiogenesis/vascular remodeling share pathogenic mechanisms and that one process may influence, generate, or perpetuate the other. However, published studies are conflicting. For example, the group of Farkas et al. has elegantly demonstrated in a rat model of pulmonary fibrosis that the local VEGF deficit in fibrotic regions was directly associated with rarefaction of microvascularization, thickening of the PA media, and mPAP elevation through ECs apoptosis. Administration of VEGF ameliorated PH but concomitantly aggravated pulmonary fibrosis via angiogenesis and interplay with TGF-ß. Another study by Richter et al. demonstrated that endostatin was elevated in IPF patients' BALF and plasma and that this antiangiogenic peptide inhibited AECs wound repair, promoting apoptosis and reducing cell viability in vitro [36]. In a study by Almudéver et al., the plasma levels of tetrahydrobiopterin (BHA), the cofactor of NO synthase (NOS), were low in IPF patients while oxidative stress and nitrotyrosine expression was high. In rats, administration of the BH4 precursor sepiapterin attenuated bleomycin-induced pulmonary fibrosis, vascular remodeling, and PH by increasing plasma BH4, decreasing plasma nitrotyrosine, and increasing vascular endothelial NOS [56]. Furthermore, both TGF-ß and ET-1 induced endothelial-to-mesenchymal transition by decreasing BH4 and endothelial NOS expression. In vitro, sepiapterin increased endothelial BH4 and inhibited endothelial-to-mesenchymal transition in human PA ECs [56].

In humans, several agents targeting vascular pathways have been proposed for the treatment of IPF. The results with two dual ET-1 receptor A and B antagonists, Bosentan [57] and Macitentan [58], were negative. Ambrisentan, an ET-1 receptor A antagonist, has proven to be harmful in IPF patients, with a worse progression-free survival and an augmented rate of respiratory hospitalizations [59]. With regard to known complications after vasodilative PAH-specific therapy in PVOD patients, the earlier suggested involvement of pulmonary veins in IPF might be a pivotal negative factor, too [60]. An ex vivo/in vitro study by Milara et al. demonstrated that Sildenafil, a phosphodiesterase 5 inhibitor, had prominent anticontractile and anti-remodeling role in patients with IPF-associated PH [61]. This drug did not show benefit in terms of 6-min walk distance and lung function in patients with advanced IPF [62], but it may be associated with better preservation of exercise capacity as compared with placebo in those with right ventricular systolic dysfunction [63]. Nintedanib, an intracellular inhibitor of multiple receptor tyrosine kinases, including VEGF receptor, has demonstrated to reduce the decline in lung function of IPF patients with mild-to-moderate disease [64].

In summary, IPF is associated with variegated vascular lesions, including profound modifications in lung microcirculation. The pathobiology underlying pulmonary fibrogenesis and angiogenesis/vascular remodeling is closely intertwined but published results regarding their reciprocal influence are controversial. Although it is now clear that the framework of the two processes has temporal and spatial heterogeneity, the significance of such striking heterogeneity in vessels turnover remains elusive. Are vascular changes central to abnormal tissue repair and thereby to progressive fibrogenesis or a peripheral consequence of pulmonary fibrosis? Is angiogenesis an integral part of a protective antifibrotic strategy of the lung in response to the vascular regression observed in severely fibrotic areas to support AECs regeneration? Is this compensatory mechanism trying to limit progressive fibrogenesis actually harmful, leading to the development of PH?

SSc-Associated ILD

SSc is an autoimmune disease, characterized by three pivotal aspects, obliterative and proliferative microvascular involvement, activation of the immune system, and increase of ECM deposition in the skin and internal organs. ILDs and PAH are the two most serious manifestations of disease, responsible for the majority of deaths of SSc patients. SSc-PAH is included in group 1 of the clinical classification of PH, and PH complicating ILD in group 3 [4]. However, a subset of patients, the proportion yet to be determined, have a particular phenotype of SSc lung disease, specifically ILD and associated PH that is disproportionate to the degree of pulmonary fibrosis [2, 3]. This severe PH may be related to concomitant pulmonary vascular disease. The prognosis of patients with a phenotype of both ILD and PH is particularly grim [65, 66].

The most frequent pathologic pattern of ILD involvement is NSIP. A NSIP pattern comprises varying degrees of alveolar wall inflammation or fibrosis, the key feature being the temporal uniformity of lesions, which contrasts to the heterogeneous/patchwork involvement observed in UIP. A UIP pattern is less common in SSc-associated ILD [67].

Vascular changes occur at an early stage in SSc [47, 68]. Autoimmunity plays an important role, as suggested by the presence of a number of autoantibodies in the serum of patients with SSc, including autoantibodies against ECs surface proteins. These cause ECs injury and apoptosis, followed by an inflammatory response; a procoagulant state; and release of profibrotic growth factors such as TGF-β, PDGF, CTGF, and ET-1, which induce intimal proliferation and adventitial fibrosis leading to vessel obliteration. Angiogenesis is deeply dysregulated. The initial inflammation is accompanied by enhanced angiogenic response, as reflected by elevated levels of circulating VEGF. In late stage, there is an overall antiangiogenic environment, with reduced capillary density [47, 68].

Whereas vascular changes have been extensively described in patients with SSc-associated PAH [47, 68–70], there is relatively little knowledge about vascular changes in patients with SSc-associated ILD, in the presence or absence of PH. De Carvalho et al. have systematically compared the vascular and interstitial processes between idiopathic and SSc-associated NSIP. The vessels from lung biopsy specimens were evaluated by semiquantitative analysis for different levels of arterial occlusion: grade I, isolated hypertrophy of the arterial media; grade II, proliferative intimal lesions; grade III, total occlusion of arterial lumen by fibrous tissue; and grade IV, plexiform lesions. Also, the collagen and elastic fibers were quantified in septal interstitium and in preacinar arteries. Unexpectedly, there were no differences in the degree of arterial occlusion between groups or in collagen content of the vascular interstitium. Conversely, the content of septal collagen and elastic fibers, as well as the elastic fibers in the vascular interstitium, was higher in the SSc-associated ILD. This difference in the intensity of elastostic process may indicate the role of autoimmune inflammatory mechanisms affecting the elastic fiber system [71]. The same group demonstrated that alterations in the epithelium and vasculature differ in the pathogenesis of SSc-associated NSIP and idiopathic NSIP [72]. In fact, the lung biopsies from patients with SSc-associated NSIP showed a lower epithelial cell density and a decreased microvascular density (ECs CD34 expression), whereas those with idiopathic NSIP had reduced type II pneumocytes and Clara cells. Furthermore, the vascular activity measured by VCAM expression was much higher in SSc-associated NSIP, suggesting a greater inflammatory component [72]. Vascular density and activity were negatively correlated. DLCO/VA, which is considered as the best functional marker of vascular disease, was more compromised in SSc-NSIP and a direct association was found between vascular density and DLCO/VA [72]. These findings suggest two different profiles of parenchymal–vascular interactions in SSc-NSIP and idiopathic NSIP in response to injury, by repair and remodeling and by repair and regeneration, respectively [72]. Consistently with this reduced microvascular density, patients with SSc-associated ILD have diminished concentrations of VEGF in BAL [73].

Several pathogenic mechanisms may be common between fibrogenesis and angiogenesis/vascular remodeling in SSc, among them endothelial-to-mesenchymal transition. It has been demonstrated that cells coexpressing ECs (CD31 and von Willebrand factor) and mesenchymal markers (α-smooth muscle actin or type I collagen) are present in the endothelium of small PAs from patients with SSc-associated ILD, suggesting that myofibroblasts of endothelial origin may contribute to the production and accumulation of subendothelial fibrotic tissue in the affected vessels that in turn result in their luminal obliteration [74].

Sarcoidosis

Sarcoidosis is a systemic disorder of unknown etiology characterized by the formation of immune granulomas in involved organs, essentially the lungs [75]. PH touches 1–6% of unselected sarcoidosis patients [2, 3]. Although PH can occur in the absence of patent pulmonary involvement, it is much more frequent in advanced lung disease, with a prevalence of 73.8% in patients listed for transplantation [2, 3]. Sarcoidosis is included in group 5 from the clinical classification of PH [4]. In fact, the mechanisms of sarcoidosis-associated PH are diverse: chronic hypoxic vasoconstriction and/or loss of capillary bed following scar tissue accumulation, extrinsic compression of central pulmonary vessels, pulmonary vasculopathy, portopulmonary hypertension, and left heart dysfunction may all play a role [76].

Sarcoid granulomas are formed of clusters of epithelioid and giant cells encircled by a rim of lymphocytes and fibroblasts. A peripheral fibrous ring of varied thickness surrounds the lesions that have a tendency to coalesce, resulting in typical fibrotic nodules [75]. The distribution of sarcoidosis granulomas tends to follow the lymphatics, *i.e.*, peribronchovascular spaces, interlobular septa, and subpleural connective tissue [75].

Vascular Changes in Pulmonary Sarcoidosis

Three seminal studies have assessed comprehensively the incidence and features of pulmonary vascular involvement in sarcoidosis [77–79]. While bronchial blood vessels are rarely affected, granulomatous involvement seems to be very common in the pulmonary circulation [77–79]. Granulomatous angiitis has been described in 53% of transbronchial lung biopsy specimens [77], 69% of open lung biopsies [79], and 100% of autopsy cases [78]. This may occur in any radiographic stage with an equal distribution between upper and lower lobes, and with an extent that is roughly correlated to parenchymal granulomas. Although granulomatous involvement can be seen at all levels, from large branches of PAs to venules, it clearly predominates on the venous side (Fig. 3.4a) and in small vessels [77–79]. Overall, there is evidence of venous involvement only in 65–67% of cases, both venous and arterial involvement in 24–31% and arterial involvement only in 8–11% [77–79]. Granulomas invade the vasculature of elastic PAs in 30% of cases, muscular PAs in 55%, arterioles in 60%, venules in 65%, and interlobular veins in 58%.

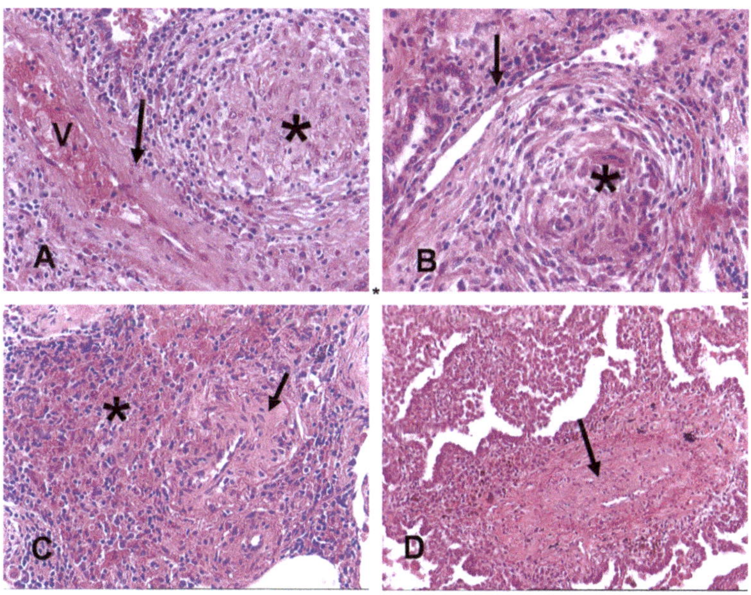

Fig. 3.4 Examples of pulmonary vascular lesions observed in granulomatous interstitial lung diseases: sarcoidosis (**a**, **b**) and Langerhans cell histiocytosis (**c**, **d**) (hematoxylin and eosin staining; original ×400): (**a**) an epithelioid granuloma (*asterisk*) in close contact with the thickened media of a pulmonary vein (V), (**b**) illustrates the close relationship between granulomas (*asterisk*) and the lymphatics (*arrow*) in the vicinity of pulmonary arteries or veins, (**c**, **d**) show pulmonary arteries (*arrows*) lesions with marked medial (**c**) or intimal (**d**) thickening associated with characteristic histiocytic granuloma (Fig. 3.1c; *asterisk*) or perivascular inflammation (Fig. 3.1d)

In both PAs and veins, the distribution of granulomas is segmental and preponderant at the bifurcation of the vessels [77–79]. There is neither fibrinoid necrosis, nor polymorphonuclear leucocyte infiltration. Granulomas have a tropism for the outer wall of arteries and veins, being mainly localized in the adventitia and the outer section of the media, with focal dissociation of elastic fibers and destruction of the external *elastic lamina, as well as around the vasa vasorum* [77–79]. In muscular arteries, granulomas commonly appear along the bronchovascular bundles. Arterioles and venules reveal focal disruption of lamina elastica with occasional obstruction [77–79].

In many cases, both granulomatous vascular involvement and its healed lesions coexist in the same lung at different stages [77–79]. Destruction of vascular architecture can be noted, with loss of media and marked mural and adventitial fibrosis, contributing to luminal narrowing [77–79]. Fibrosis in the venous walls has a tendency to extend into the interlobular space whereas arterial granulomas evolve into fibrosis along the bronchovascular sheaths [77–79].

Nodular lesions, which are formed by the coalescence of numerous granulomas and surrounding lymphocyte inflammation or fibrosis, can incorporate blood vessels and provoke the occlusion of the lumen with subsequent ischemia and eosinophilic necrosis [77–79]. This may represent one of the mechanisms of pulmonary cavitations that are sporadically encountered in sarcoidosis [80]. Noncaseating epithelial cell granulomas, granulomatous angiitis, and necrosis are the pathological hallmarks of necrotizing sarcoid granulomatosis, the taxonomical position of which has long been argued between a truly independent entity and a variant of sarcoidosis [81].

The intimate relationships between granulomas and their supplying lymphatic (Fig. 3.4b) or blood microvascular networks have been investigated by Kambouchner et al. using antipodoplanin, anti-CD34, and anti-CD31 immunostainings in surgical lung biopsies from patients with pulmonary sarcoidosis [82]. While granulomas were closely associated with lymphatics, blood capillaries were rarely seen in the vicinity of lesions, stopping at the boundaries of the fibrous ring bordering granulomas [82]. These observations support the role of airborne particles drained by the lymphatics in the emergence of sarcoidosis granulomas. Conversely, sarcoidosis granulomas can be considered avascular structures, the center of which is therefore subjected to hypoxia. In this hypoxic context, TGF-β, one of the cytokines secreted by sarcoid granulomas, may exert a synergistic action on collagen production by fibroblasts and contribute to the perigranuloma fibrotic progression [82]. This absence of angiogenesis is at variance with the expected findings, in light of the high levels of VEGF in BAL reported in sarcoidosis [83], and in epithelioid cells detected by immunohistochemistry and in situ hybridization [84].

Vascular Changes in Sarcoidosis-Associated PH

Despite extremely frequent vascular involvement in sarcoidosis, clinically significant PH is intringuily rare. In the autopsy series of 40 cases by Takemura et al., all had vascular involvement but only 4 had right heart overload [78]. The reasons why a proportion of sarcoidosis patients will eventually develop this complication remain obscure, with only few publications providing pathologic descriptions of sarcoidosis-associated PH.

Proliferative arteriopathy with plexiform lesions can exist but is exceedingly rare. The complex changes detailed earlier may result in occlusive vasculopathy and, when sufficiently extensive, ultimately lead to PH. Reflecting the venous predilection of vascular granulomatous involvement, a PVOD-like disease is recognized as a cause of sarcoidosis-associated PH [76, 85–87]. The occlusive narrowing of venules and interlobular septal veins by widespread granulomas can mimic PVOD, which has been pathologically authenticated in few cases with active sarcoidosis and PH [85–87]. Besides, Nunes et al. reported an intrinsic venopathy in explanted lungs from 5 patients with fibrotic sarcoidosis and severe PH [76]. This venopathy consisted of marked occlusive intimal fibrosis and recanalization, together with chronic hemosiderosis and iron deposition in elastic lamina in all cases. In opposition, arterial changes were minor with no evidence of plexiform or thrombotic lesions. Scattered granulomas were present in veins in 4 cases whereas arterial granulomas were seen in only 2 cases and neither venous nor arterial granuloma could be found in one patient [76]. These observations suggest the existence of an intrinsic venopathy, which may be an indirect consequence of granulomatous process through the production of various cytokines and growth factors implicated in vascular remodeling. For example, it has been demonstrated that levels of ET-1 in plasma and BAL fluid are elevated in some, albeit not all, sarcoidosis patients [88, 89].

Pulmonary Langerhans Cell Histiocytosis (PLCH)

PLCH is a rare smoking-related disorder that predominantly affects adults aged 20–40 years. It may regress either spontaneously or after smoking cessation [90]. In a minority of patients, PLCH may progress to end-stage lung disease [90]. Although the occurrence of PH is exceptional in patients with early PLCH, it is a common event in the course of advanced lung disease (more than 90% of candidates for lung transplantation) [2, 3]. PLCH is included in group 5 of the clinical classification of PH [4].

While PLCH has traditionally been classified as an ILD, the foremost pathology is that of an inflammatory and destructive bronchiolitis [90]. The pathologic hallmark of PLCH is the presence of stellate nodules composed of large numbers of Langerhans cells (LC) admixed with other inflammatory cells, in particular eosinophils, often organized as loosely formed granulomas in terminal or respiratory bronchioles. Bronchiolocentric lesions may be accompanied by variable lung interstitial inflammation and pigmented alveolar macrophage accumulation in alveolar spaces. More advanced stages are characterized by cystic lung destruction and fibrotic scarring of small airways [90].

There is very little pathologic data on vascular involvement in PLCH. Though generally not marked in early stages, vascular changes seem relatively frequent [91–93]. These are usually observed within regions of prominent involvement with an extension of PLCH inflammation to the walls of small- to medium-sized PAs adjacent to bronchioles in the center of pulmonary lobules (Fig. 3.4c, d) [91–93]. Despite the bronchiolocentric distribution of PLCH lesions, interlobular septal veins may also be affected [91–93].

The development of PH has been ascribed to the presence of intense and widespread vasculopathy. Fartoukh et al. analyzed the lung samples from 12 patients with PLCH-associated PH and found that all of them exhibited changes involving both small- to medium-sized intralobular PAs and interlobular septal veins [94]. Involvement of the intralobular PAs consisted of proliferative arteriopathy with intimal fibrosis and medial hypertrophy, leading to arterial obliteration in 60% of cases [94]. There was no evidence of plexiform or thrombotic lesions. Involvement of the interlobular septal veins consisted of intimal fibrosis, medial hypertrophy, and obliteration in 75% [94]. Aspects of PVOD-like were detected in one-third of the patients, with venular obliteration, hemosiderosis, and capillary dilatation [94]. On the other hand, LC infiltration of a vessel was seen in only one case and vascular abnormalities were noted in areas remote from nodular lesions in half of the patients [94]. In the six patients from whom two subsequent lung specimens (before and after the occurrence of PH) were available, the vasculopathy worsened, whereas parenchymal and bronchiolar lesions remained relatively steady [94]. Consistently, patterns of postcapillary involvement have been identified in two cases of the series by Le Pavec et al. [95]. These observations suggest that intrinsic vasculopathy may be a central process in advanced PLCH.

Remarkably, in contrast to sarcoidosis, PLCH-associated PH has almost not been reported in the absence of long-standing lung disease probably owing to the different distribution of granulomas between the two disorders (primarily bronchiolocentric versus lymphatic). Instead, the venopathy observed in PLCH-associated PH resembles that of fibrotic sarcoidosis and may share similar pathogenesis. Granulomas may have an indirect role through the production of various cytokines and growth factors implicated in vascular remodeling. For example, a number of these mediators can be released by granulomas of PLCH such as PDGF, TGFβ, IL1, and IL6. Cigarette smoke is a known inducer of pulmonary vascular remodeling [96] and may also contribute to the development of PH in PLCH.

References

1. Travis WD et al. An official American Thoracic Society/European Respiratory Society statement: update of the international multidisciplinary classification of the idiopathic interstitial pneumonias. Am J Respir Crit Care Med. 2013;188:733–48.
2. Seeger W et al. Pulmonary hypertension in chronic lung diseases. J Am Coll Cardiol. 2013;62:D109–16.
3. Nathan SD, Hassoun PM. Pulmonary hypertension due to lung disease and/or hypoxia. Clin Chest Med. 2013;34:695–705.
4. Simonneau G et al. Updated clinical classification of pulmonary hypertension. J Am Coll Cardiol. 2013;62:D34–41.

5. Townsley MI. Structure and composition of pulmonary arteries, capillaries, and veins. Compr Physiol. 2012;2:675–709.
6. Tuder RM, Stacher E, Robinson J, Kumar R, Graham BB. Pathology of pulmonary hypertension. Clin Chest Med. 2013;34:639–50.
7. Stevens T et al. Lung vascular cell heterogeneity: endothelium, smooth muscle, and fibroblasts. Proc Am Thorac Soc. 2008;5:783–91.
8. Wagenvoort CA. Morphologic changes in intrapulmonary veins. Hum Pathol. 1970;1:205–13.
9. Farkas L, Kolb M. Pulmonary microcirculation in interstitial lung disease. Proc Am Thorac Soc. 2011;8:516–21.
10. Hanumegowda C, Farkas L, Kolb M. Angiogenesis in pulmonary fibrosis: too much or not enough? Chest. 2012;142:200–7.
11. Renzoni EA. Neovascularization in idiopathic pulmonary fibrosis: too much or too little? Am J Respir Crit Care Med. 2004;169:1179–80.
12. Tuder RM et al. Relevant issues in the pathology and pathobiology of pulmonary hypertension. J Am Coll Cardiol. 2013;62:D4–12.
13. Voelkel NF, Douglas IS, Nicolls M. Angiogenesis in chronic lung disease. Chest. 2007;131:874–9.
14. Hopkins N, McLoughlin P. The structural basis of pulmonary hypertension in chronic lung disease: remodelling, rarefaction or angiogenesis? J Anat. 2002;201:335–48.
15. Tuder RM, Marecki JC, Richter A, Fijalkowska I, Flores S. Pathology of pulmonary hypertension. Clin Chest Med. 2007;28:23–42, vii.
16. Montani D et al. Pulmonary veno-occlusive disease. Eur Respir J. 2016;47:1518–34.
17. Cottin V et al. Combined pulmonary fibrosis and emphysema: a distinct underrecognised entity. Eur Respir J. 2005;26:586–93.
18. Raghu G et al. An official ATS/ERS/JRS/ALAT statement: idiopathic pulmonary fibrosis: evidence-based guidelines for diagnosis and management. Am J Respir Crit Care Med. 2011;183:788–824.
19. Kim K-H et al. Iron deposition and increased alveolar septal capillary density in nonfibrotic lung tissue are associated with pulmonary hypertension in idiopathic pulmonary fibrosis. Respir Res. 2010;11:37.
20. Colombat M et al. Pulmonary vascular lesions in end-stage idiopathic pulmonary fibrosis: Histopathologic study on lung explant specimens and correlations with pulmonary hemodynamics. Hum Pathol. 2007;38:60–5.
21. Turner-Warwick M. Precapillary systemic-pulmonary anastomoses. Thorax. 1963;18: 225–37.
22. Renzoni EA et al. Interstitial vascularity in fibrosing alveolitis. Am J Respir Crit Care Med. 2003;167:438–43.
23. Cosgrove GP et al. Pigment epithelium-derived factor in idiopathic pulmonary fibrosis: a role in aberrant angiogenesis. Am J Respir Crit Care Med. 2004;170:242–51.
24. Ebina M et al. Heterogeneous increase in CD34-positive alveolar capillaries in idiopathic pulmonary fibrosis. Am J Respir Crit Care Med. 2004;169:1203–8.
25. Judge EP, Fabre A, Adamali HI, Egan JJ. Acute exacerbations and pulmonary hypertension in advanced idiopathic pulmonary fibrosis. Eur Respir J. 2012;40:93–100.
26. Keane MP et al. The CXC chemokines, IL-8 and IP-10, regulate angiogenic activity in idiopathic pulmonary fibrosis. J Immunol Baltim Md. 1997;1950(159):1437–43.
27. Keane MP et al. ENA-78 is an important angiogenic factor in idiopathic pulmonary fibrosis. Am J Respir Crit Care Med. 2001;164:2239–42.
28. Burdick MD et al. CXCL11 attenuates bleomycin-induced pulmonary fibrosis via inhibition of vascular remodeling. Am J Respir Crit Care Med. 2005;171:261–8.
29. Keane MP et al. Neutralization of the CXC chemokine, macrophage inflammatory protein-2, attenuates bleomycin-induced pulmonary fibrosis. J Immunol Baltim Md. 1999;1950(162): 5511–8.

30. Russo RC et al. Role of the chemokine receptor CXCR2 in bleomycin-induced pulmonary inflammation and fibrosis. Am J Respir Cell Mol Biol. 2009;40:410–21.
31. Giaid A et al. Expression of endothelin-1 in lungs of patients with cryptogenic fibrosing alveolitis. Lancet Lond Engl. 1993;341:1550–4.
32. Hocher B et al. Pulmonary fibrosis and chronic lung inflammation in ET-1 transgenic mice. Am J Respir Cell Mol Biol. 2000;23:19–26.
33. Saleh D et al. Elevated expression of endothelin-1 and endothelin-converting enzyme-1 in idiopathic pulmonary fibrosis: possible involvement of proinflammatory cytokines. Am J Respir Cell Mol Biol. 1997;16:187–93.
34. Park SH, Saleh D, Giaid A, Michel RP. Increased endothelin-1 in bleomycin-induced pulmonary fibrosis and the effect of an endothelin receptor antagonist. Am J Respir Crit Care Med. 1997;156:600–8.
35. Wan Y-Y et al. Endostatin, an angiogenesis inhibitor, ameliorates bleomycin-induced pulmonary fibrosis in rats. Respir Res. 2013;14:56.
36. Richter AG et al. Soluble endostatin is a novel inhibitor of epithelial repair in idiopathic pulmonary fibrosis. Thorax. 2009;64:156–61.
37. Margaritopoulos GA et al. Investigation of angiogenetic axis Angiopoietin-1 and -2/Tie-2 in fibrotic lung diseases: a bronchoalveolar lavage study. Int J Mol Med. 2010;26:919–23.
38. Koyama S et al. Decreased level of vascular endothelial growth factor in bronchoalveolar lavage fluid of normal smokers and patients with pulmonary fibrosis. Am J Respir Crit Care Med. 2002;166:382–5.
39. Meyer KC, Cardoni A, Xiang ZZ. Vascular endothelial growth factor in bronchoalveolar lavage from normal subjects and patients with diffuse parenchymal lung disease. J Lab Clin Med. 2000;135:332–8.
40. Farkas L et al. VEGF ameliorates pulmonary hypertension through inhibition of endothelial apoptosis in experimental lung fibrosis in rats. J Clin Invest. 2009;119:1298–311.
41. Patel NM et al. Pulmonary arteriole gene expression signature in idiopathic pulmonary fibrosis. Eur Respir J. 2013;41:1324–30.
42. Hoffmann J et al. Distinct differences in gene expression patterns in pulmonary arteries of patients with chronic obstructive pulmonary disease and idiopathic pulmonary fibrosis with pulmonary hypertension. Am J Respir Crit Care Med. 2014;190:98–111.
43. King TE, Pardo A, Selman M. Idiopathic pulmonary fibrosis. Lancet Lond Engl. 2011;378:1949–61.
44. Calabrese F et al. Herpes virus infection is associated with vascular remodeling and pulmonary hypertension in idiopathic pulmonary fibrosis. PLoS One. 2013;8:e55715.
45. Schiess R et al. Tobacco smoke: a risk factor for pulmonary arterial hypertension? A case-control study. Chest. 2010;138:1086–92.
46. Montani D et al. Idiopathic pulmonary arterial hypertension and pulmonary veno-occlusive disease: similarities and differences. Semin Respir Crit Care Med. 2009;30:411–20.
47. Farkas L, Gauldie J, Voelkel NF, Kolb M. Pulmonary hypertension and idiopathic pulmonary fibrosis: a tale of angiogenesis, apoptosis, and growth factors. Am J Respir Cell Mol Biol. 2011;45:1–15.
48. Piera-Velazquez S, Mendoza FA, Jimenez SA. Endothelial to mesenchymal transition (EndoMT) in the pathogenesis of human fibrotic diseases. J Clin Med. 2016;5(4):pii:E45.
49. Ranchoux B et al. Endothelial-to-mesenchymal transition in pulmonary hypertension. Circulation. 2015;131:1006–18.
50. Yamada M et al. Increased circulating endothelial progenitor cells in patients with bacterial pneumonia: evidence that bone marrow derived cells contribute to lung repair. Thorax. 2005;60:410–3.
51. Burnham EL et al. Increased circulating endothelial progenitor cells are associated with survival in acute lung injury. Am J Respir Crit Care Med. 2005;172:854–60.
52. Fadini GP, Losordo D, Dimmeler S. Critical reevaluation of endothelial progenitor cell phenotypes for therapeutic and diagnostic use. Circ Res. 2012;110:624–37.

53. Malli F et al. Endothelial progenitor cells in the pathogenesis of idiopathic pulmonary fibrosis: an evolving concept. PLoS One. 2013;8:e53658.
54. Smadja DM et al. Cooperation between human fibrocytes and endothelial colony-forming cells increases angiogenesis via the CXCR4 pathway. Thromb Haemost. 2014;112:1002–13.
55. Moeller A et al. Circulating fibrocytes are an indicator of poor prognosis in idiopathic pulmonary fibrosis. Am J Respir Crit Care Med. 2009;179:588–94.
56. Almudéver P et al. Role of tetrahydrobiopterin in pulmonary vascular remodelling associated with pulmonary fibrosis. Thorax. 2013;68:938–48.
57. King TE et al. BUILD-3: a randomized, controlled trial of bosentan in idiopathic pulmonary fibrosis. Am J Respir Crit Care Med. 2011;184:92–9.
58. Raghu G et al. Macitentan for the treatment of idiopathic pulmonary fibrosis: the randomised controlled MUSIC trial. Eur Respir J. 2013;42:1622–32.
59. Raghu G et al. Treatment of idiopathic pulmonary fibrosis with ambrisentan: a parallel, randomized trial. Ann Intern Med. 2013;158:641–9.
60. Huertas A et al. Pulmonary veno-occlusive disease: advances in clinical management and treatments. Expert Rev Respir Med. 2011;5:217–29. quiz 230–231
61. Milara J et al. Vascular effects of sildenafil in patients with pulmonary fibrosis and pulmonary hypertension: an ex vivo/in vitro study. Eur Respir J. 2016;47:1737–49.
62. Idiopathic Pulmonary Fibrosis Clinical Research Network et al. A controlled trial of sildenafil in advanced idiopathic pulmonary fibrosis. N Engl J Med. 2010;363:620–8.
63. Han MK et al. Sildenafil preserves exercise capacity in patients with idiopathic pulmonary fibrosis and right-sided ventricular dysfunction. Chest. 2013;143:1699–708.
64. Richeldi L et al. Efficacy and safety of nintedanib in idiopathic pulmonary fibrosis. N Engl J Med. 2014;370:2071–82.
65. Launay D et al. Clinical characteristics and survival in systemic sclerosis-related pulmonary hypertension associated with interstitial lung disease. Chest. 2011;140:1016–24.
66. Le Pavec J et al. Systemic sclerosis-related pulmonary hypertension associated with interstitial lung disease: impact of pulmonary arterial hypertension therapies. Arthritis Rheum. 2011;63:2456–64.
67. Wells AU, Denton CP. Interstitial lung disease in connective tissue disease—mechanisms and management. Nat Rev Rheumatol. 2014;10:728–39.
68. Le Pavec J, Humbert M, Mouthon L, Hassoun PM. Systemic sclerosis-associated pulmonary arterial hypertension. Am J Respir Crit Care Med. 2010;181:1285–93.
69. Dorfmüller P et al. Fibrous remodeling of the pulmonary venous system in pulmonary arterial hypertension associated with connective tissue diseases. Hum Pathol. 2007;38:893–902.
70. Overbeek MJ et al. Pulmonary arterial hypertension in limited cutaneous systemic sclerosis: a distinctive vasculopathy. Eur Respir J. 2009;34:371–9.
71. de Carvalho EF et al. Arterial and interstitial remodelling processes in non-specific interstitial pneumonia: systemic sclerosis versus idiopathic. Histopathology. 2008;53:195–204.
72. Franco de Carvalho E, Parra ER, de Souza R, Muxfeldt A'b Saber A, Capelozzi VL. Parenchymal and vascular interactions in the pathogenesis of nonspecific interstitial pneumonia in systemic sclerosis and idiopathic interstitial pneumonia. Respir Int Rev Thorac Dis. 2008;76:146–53.
73. De Santis M et al. A vascular endothelial growth factor deficiency characterises scleroderma lung disease. Ann Rheum Dis. 2012;71:1461–5.
74. Mendoza FA, Piera-Velazquez S, Farber JL, Feghali-Bostwick C, Jiménez SA. Endothelial cells expressing endothelial and mesenchymal cell gene products in lung tissue from patients with systemic sclerosis-associated interstitial lung disease. Arthritis Rheumatol. 2016;68:210–7.
75. Valeyre D et al. Sarcoidosis. Lancet Lond Engl. 2014;383:1155–67.
76. Nunes H et al. Pulmonary hypertension associated with sarcoidosis: mechanisms, haemodynamics and prognosis. Thorax. 2006;61:68–74.
77. Takemura T et al. Pulmonary vascular involvement in sarcoidosis: granulomatous angiitis and microangiopathy in transbronchial lung biopsies. Virchows Arch A Pathol Anat Histopathol. 1991;418:361–8.

78. Takemura T, Matsui Y, Saiki S, Mikami R. Pulmonary vascular involvement in sarcoidosis: a report of 40 autopsy cases. Hum Pathol. 1992;23:1216–23.
79. Rosen Y, Moon S, Huang CT, Gourin A, Lyons HA. Granulomatous pulmonary angiitis in sarcoidosis. Arch Pathol Lab Med. 1977;101:170–4.
80. Hours S et al. Pulmonary cavitary sarcoidosis: clinico-radiologic characteristics and natural history of a rare form of sarcoidosis. Medicine (Baltimore). 2008;87:142–51.
81. Rosen Y. Four decades of necrotizing sarcoid granulomatosis: what do we know now? Arch Pathol Lab Med. 2015;139:252–62.
82. Kambouchner M et al. Lymphatic and blood microvasculature organisation in pulmonary sarcoid granulomas. Eur Respir J. 2011;37:835–40.
83. Vasakova M et al. Bronchoalveolar lavage fluid cellular characteristics, functional parameters and cytokine and chemokine levels in interstitial lung diseases. Scand J Immunol. 2009;69:268–74.
84. Tolnay E, Kuhnen C, Voss B, Wiethege T, Müller KM. Expression and localization of vascular endothelial growth factor and its receptor flt in pulmonary sarcoidosis. Virchows Arch Int J Pathol. 1998;432:61–5.
85. Hoffstein V, Ranganathan N, Mullen JB. Sarcoidosis simulating pulmonary veno-occlusive disease. Am Rev Respir Dis. 1986;134:809–11.
86. Portier F et al. Sarcoidosis simulating a pulmonary veno-occlusive disease. Rev Mal Respir. 1991;8:101–2.
87. Jones RM et al. Sarcoidosis-related pulmonary veno-occlusive disease presenting with recurrent haemoptysis. Eur Respir J. 2009;34:517–20.
88. Reichenberger F et al. Different expression of endothelin in the bronchoalveolar lavage in patients with pulmonary diseases. Lung. 2001;179:163–74.
89. Terashita K et al. Increased endothelin-1 levels of BAL fluid in patients with pulmonary sarcoidosis. Respirol Carlton Vic. 2006;11:145–51.
90. Tazi A. Adult pulmonary Langerhans' cell histiocytosis. Eur Respir J. 2006;27:1272–85.
91. Basset F et al. Pulmonary histiocytosis X. Am Rev Respir Dis. 1978;118:811–20.
92. Friedman PJ, Liebow AA, Sokoloff J. Eosinophilic granuloma of lung. Clinical aspects of primary histiocytosis in the adult. Medicine (Baltimore). 1981;60:385–96.
93. Travis WD et al. Pulmonary Langerhans cell granulomatosis (histiocytosis X). A clinicopathologic study of 48 cases. Am J Surg Pathol. 1993;17:971–86.
94. Fartoukh M et al. Severe pulmonary hypertension in histiocytosis X. Am J Respir Crit Care Med. 2000;161:216–23.
95. Le Pavec J et al. Pulmonary Langerhans cell histiocytosis-associated pulmonary hypertension: clinical characteristics and impact of pulmonary arterial hypertension therapies. Chest. 2012;142:1150–7.
96. Henno P et al. Tobacco-associated pulmonary vascular dysfunction in smokers: role of the ET-1 pathway. Am J Physiol Lung Cell Mol Physiol. 2011;300:L831–9.

Chapter 4
Treatment of Pulmonary Hypertension in Interstitial Lung Disease

Christopher S. King and Steven D. Nathan

Introduction

The interstitial lung diseases (ILD) are a heterogeneous group of disorders characterized by diffuse pulmonary parenchymal infiltrates. The prognosis of ILD varies among the specific etiologies, but frequently results in substantial morbidity and mortality. For example, idiopathic pulmonary fibrosis (IPF), the commonest form of the idiopathic interstitial pneumonias, has a median survival of only 2.5–5 years [1, 2]. The pharmacologic therapy of ILD varies with the underlying cause, but generally focuses on attenuating inflammation and resultant fibrosis through the use of corticosteroids, alternative immunosuppressant agents, and antifibrotics for IPF. Although frequently prescribed, the data supporting the utility of pharmacologic therapy in ILD is limited. Recent landmark trials of pirfenidone and nintedanib in IPF, while representing a major advance in the treatment of IPF, illustrate this point [3, 4]. The mean change in forced vital capacity (FVC) over 52 weeks was −235 mL for pirfenidone versus −428 mL for placebo while the adjusted annual rate of change with nintedanib was −114.7 mL versus −239.9 mL for placebo [3, 4]. It appears that even with the availability of these agents, the relentless downhill course of IPF will continue, as will the search for further therapeutic targets.

The treatment of pulmonary hypertension (PH) is an attractive potential target for therapy in ILD. PH has been reported to complicate the course of many ILDs including IPF, sarcoidosis, pulmonary Langerhans cell histiocytosis (PLCH), connective tissue disease-associated ILD (CTD-ILD), and chronic hypersensitivity pneumonitis [5, 6]. The development of PH is associated with decreased exercise tolerance as measured by six-minute walk testing (6MWT) and cardiopulmonary exercise testing, increased oxygenation desaturation on exertion, and reduced

C.S. King, MD • S.D. Nathan, MD (✉)
Inova Fairfax Advanced Lung Disease and Transplant Program, Inova Fairfax Hospital, 3300 Gallows Road, Falls Church, VA 22042, USA
e-mail: christopher.king@inova.org; steven.nathan@inova.org

R.P. Baughman et al. (eds.), *Pulmonary Hypertension and Interstitial Lung Disease*, DOI 10.1007/978-3-319-49918-5_4

survival [7–10]. A number of studies have examined the response to pulmonary vasodilator agents in PH complicating ILD (PH-ILD). However, no study has conclusively demonstrated benefit from the use of vasodilator therapy in PH-ILD. In the following chapter, we will examine the arguments both for and against pharmacologic treatment of PH-ILD, review the results of prior studies, and discuss potential pitfalls in trial design that may explain the negative results of studies thus far. We will then provide a guideline for the treatment of PH-ILD based on the authors' clinical experience.

Rationale to Treat

Reasonable arguments can be made both for and against the treatment of PH-ILD. Proponents of treatment point to the paucity of effective treatments for fibrotic lung disease, coupled with the availability of numerous pulmonary vasodilator therapies with demonstrated efficacy in World Health Organization (WHO) Group 1 PH, as compelling reasons to pursue therapy [11]. This argument can be countered by the fact that, as of yet, no randomized, controlled trial (RCT) has conclusively demonstrated clinical benefit from the treatment of PH-ILD with pulmonary vasodilators.

The development of PH-ILD is associated with significantly reduced exercise tolerance and increased dyspnea in comparison to ILD patients with similar pulmonary function and demographics [12]. PH-ILD also substantially impacts mortality. Lettieri, et al. found that patients with IPF and right heart catheterization (RHC) documented PH, had a 1-year mortality of 28% versus 5.5% in those without PH [9]. In a study by Nadrous and colleagues, patients with IPF with right ventricular systolic pressures greater than 50 mmHg on transthoracic echocardiography (TTE) were demonstrated to have a 1-year mortality > 50% [13]. PH has also been associated with increased mortality in sarcoidosis and systemic sclerosis [14, 15]. Given the association of the development of PH with adverse outcomes, it seems plausible that the treatment of PH may improve symptomatology and survival. This hypothesis only holds true if PH-ILD is a "maladaptive" phenomenon that becomes the primary driving force for outcomes, rather than a surrogate marker for severity of disease (Fig. 4.1). If PH develops as a consequence of obliteration of the pulmonary vasculature due to progressive fibrosis, this likely represents an "adaptive" phenomenon unlikely to respond to vasodilator therapy. There may be a subset of patients with PH-ILD that develop PH that is "disproportionate" to the fibrotic burden of their disease. In the case of "disproportionate" PH (DPH), the pathophysiology underlying the development of PH is likely distinct from those with proportionate disease and may be amenable to therapy. This concept with be explored further later in the chapter.

There is frequently concern that pulmonary vasodilator therapy in PH-ILD has the potential to cause adverse outcomes. Theoretically, pulmonary vasodilators may "un-do" hypoxemic pulmonary vasoconstriction in the areas with the most severe

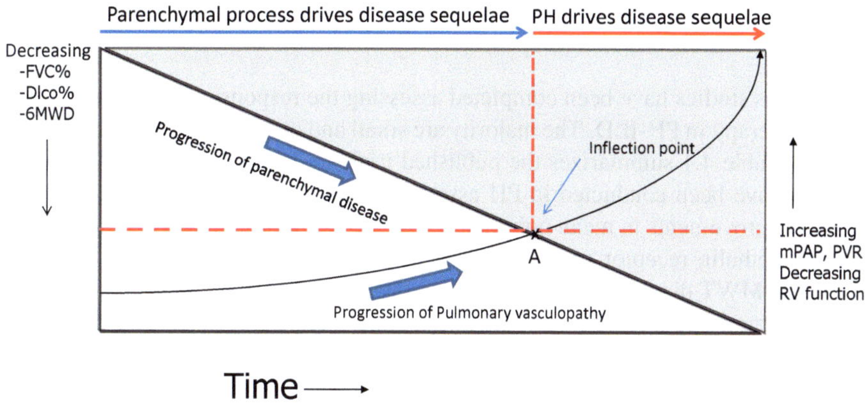

Fig. 4.1 Development of disproportionate pulmonary hypertension. Graphical depiction of the concept of disproportionate pulmonary hypertension. The curve depicts the temporal clinical course of a patient with interstitial lung disease (the *x*-axis). Over time, the mean pulmonary artery pressure (mPAP) and pulmonary vascular resistance (PVR) increase as the forced vital capacity (FVC), diffusing capacity of the lung from carbon monoxide (DLco), and six-minute walk test distance (6MWD) decrease. At inflection point A, outcomes and functional limitation are driven more by pulmonary hypertension than parenchymal lung disease. This is the point where "disproportionate pulmonary hypertension" has developed

parenchymal disease, leading to ventilation–perfusion (V/Q) mismatch and hypoxemia. In a small, open-label trial by Ghofrani, et al., worsened V/Q mismatch and oxygenation was seen in patients with PH-ILD treated with intravenous epoprostenol; however, those treated with oral sildenafil actually demonstrated improved V/Q matching and gas exchange [16]. Similar favorable effects on systemic oxygenation were seen in a small study of inhaled iloprost and a large RCT of sildenafil in IPF [17, 18]. Worsening of V/Q mismatch and systemic oxygenation does not necessarily equate to lack of efficacy. If pulmonary vasodilator therapy improves pulmonary hemodynamics leading to an increased cardiac output and increased tissue oxygen delivery, then patients may feel better and have improved exercise tolerance despite decreased oxygen saturations. This concept is supported in a recent study by Hoeper and colleagues evaluating the response to riociguat in PH-ILD. Subjects in this trial experienced decreased arterial oxygen saturation, but increased mean cardiac output, decreased pulmonary vascular resistance (PVR), and improved mixed venous oxygen saturation [19]. Another potential concern with vasodilator therapy in interstitial lung disease is the possibility of causing pulmonary edema due to pulmonary veno-occlusive disease. Indeed, the distribution of the fibrosis may result in patchy areas of pulmonary veno-occlusive like lesions. Distinguishing patients who have a preponderance of such lesions might be important in excluding patients who are predisposed to a deleterious response to pulmonary vasoactive therapy. It is gratifying however that reports of overt pulmonary edema due to PH-ILD therapy are rare [20].

Results of Prior Studies

Numerous studies have been completed assessing the response to pulmonary vasodilator therapy in PH-ILD. The majority are small and unblinded with inherent limitations. Table 4.1 summarizes the published trials to date [16–19, 21–47]. Several studies have been conducted in PH associated with sarcoidosis. Two small RCTs found improvements in mean pulmonary artery pressure (mPAP) and PVR with the dual endothelin receptor antagonist (ERA) bosentan, but no significant improvement in 6MWT distance [40, 43]. An open-label trial of ambrisentan in sarcoidosis demonstrated improvements in WHO functional class in patients who completed the full 24-week trial, but the study had a dropout rate of >50% with a high incidence of reported side effects [42]. Le Pavec and colleagues published a retrospective series of 14 patients with PLCH and PH treated with various vasodilator therapies. In the 12 patients with follow-up data available, 67% had an improvement in functional class and 45% improved their 6MWT distance by ≥10% [36]. A small open-label trial of bosentan in systemic sclerosis ILD and PH suggested benefit in 6MWT distance and WHO functional class; however, a larger RCT of bosentan in 163 patients with systemic sclerosis ILD failed to demonstrate a significant improvement in 6MWT distance [37, 38]. It should be noted however that patients in this study did not necessarily have PH.

The majority of reasonably powered RCTs of PH-ILD have been conducted in IPF patients. The results with ERAs in this population have been disappointing thus far. The BUILD-1 study examined the effects of bosentan in 158 patients with IPF. Bosentan failed to demonstrate superiority over placebo in increasing 6MWT distance at 12 months. However, a trend toward delay in time to death or disease progression was observed with bosentan (HR = 0.613; 95% CI, 0.126–0.789, $p = 0.119$) [24]. The follow-up BUILD-3 study again compared bosentan to placebo in a larger RCT of 616 patients. No improvement was seen in the primary endpoint of time to disease progression or death or in secondary endpoints including health-related quality of life or dyspnea [25]. A smaller RCT of bosentan in 60 patients with idiopathic pulmonary fibrosis and RHC-confirmed PH failed to demonstrate improvements in pulmonary hemodynamics, symptoms, or functional capacity [34]. The MUSIC trial of macitentan therapy in IPF also failed to demonstrate an improvement in the primary endpoint of change in FVC [27]. The ARTEMIS-IPF study of ambrisentan was terminated early for lack of efficacy and the potential for harm with the suggestion of increased respiratory hospitalizations and risk of disease progression [26]. It should be noted that the earlier trials of ERA therapy in IPF were evaluating purely the antifibrotic effects of the drugs rather than specifically targeting PH-ILD in this population. ARTEMIS-PH, a study evaluating the effects of ambrisentan in IPF patients with PH confirmed via RHC, was terminated early by the sponsor after a subgroup analysis of patients with PH in the ARTEMIS-IPF failed to demonstrate a positive signal [48]. Most recently, the RISE-IIP trial of riociguat in patients with idiopathic interstitial pneumonia was terminated early for suggestion of increased risk of death and serious adverse events in the treatment arm in comparison to the placebo group [46].

Table 4.1 Studies of pulmonary vasodilator therapy in interstitial lung disease

Lung disease	Investigator	Year	Study design	Pts	Therapy	Results	Comments
IPF	Collard et al. [21]	2007	Open-label	14	Sildenafil	57% improved 6MWT by ≥20%	Median follow-up of 91 days
IPF	Zisman et al. [18]	2010	RCT	180	Sildenafil	Failed to improve 6MWT by ≥20%	Improved oxygen saturation and QOL
IPF	Jackson et al. [22]	2010	RCT	29	Sildenafil	No difference in 6MWT or Borg score	
IPF	Gunther et al. [23]	2007	Open-label	12	Bosentan	No worsening of gas exchange	
IPF	Krowka et al. [44]	2007	RCT	51	Iloprost	No difference in 6MWT, NYHA FC, dyspnea score	
IPF	King et al. [24]	2008	RCT	158	Bosentan	Failed to improve 6MWT	Trend to delayed death or disease progression
IPF	King et al. [25]	2011	RCT	610	Bosentan	No effect on time to IPF worsening or death	
IPF	Raghu et al. [26]	2013	RCT	492	Ambrisentan	Terminated early for lack of efficacy in time to clinical worsening	In 32 patients with PH, no change in time to disease progression
IPF	Raghu et al. [27]	2013	RCT	178	Macitentan	Failed to alter primary endpoint of change in FVC	Not focused on patients with PH
CTD-ILD	Mittoo et al. [28]	2010	Retrospective	13	Bosentan Sildenafil	No decline in 6MWT or FVC over mean follow-up of 34 months	No treatment-related toxicity

(continued)

Table 4.1 (continued)

Lung disease	Investigator	Year	Study design	Pts	Therapy	Results	Comments
ILD	Olschewski et al. [17]	1999	Open-label	8	Nitric oxide, Epoprostenol IV and inhaled	Inhaled prostanoids resulted in improved pulmonary gas exchange	
ILD	Ghofrani et al. [16]	2002	Open-label	16	Sildenafil or epoprostenol	Sildenafil improved V/Q matching and oxygenation	Prostacyclin worsened V/Q matching
ILD	Minai et al. [29]	2008	Retrospective	19	Epoprostenol ($n = 10$) Bosentan ($n = 9$)	15/19 improved 6MWT distance >50 m	
ILD	Chapman et al. [30]	2009	Retrospective	5	Sildenafil	Improved 6MWT	Decreased mPAP 2–12 months
ILD	Corte et al. [31]	2010	Retrospective	15	Sildenafil	Improved 6MWT and lower BNP	
ILD	Badesch et al. [32]	2011	Open-label	21	Ambrisentan	6MWT distance worsened; BNP improved	Study included mixed PH population
ILD	Hoeper et al. [19]	2013	Open-label	22	Riociguat	Improved CO and PVR but not mPAP	Arterial saturation decreased but mixed-venous increased
ILD	Zimmerman et al. [33]	2014	Open-label, observational	10	Sildenafil ($n = 5$) Tadalafil ($n = 5$)	Increased CO and decreased PVR	No change in 6MWT or BNP
ILD	Corte et al. [34]	2014	RCT	60	Bosentan	No effect on hemodynamics, symptoms, or functional capacity	RHC confirmed PH
ILD	Saggar et al. [35]	2014	Open-label	15	Treprostinil	Improved hemodynamics without hypoxemia	All had mPAP $\geq$ 35 mmHg

Lung disease	Investigator	Year	Study design	Pts	Therapy	Results	Comments
ILD	Brewis et al. [45]	2015	Retrospective	118	PDE-5i	Unchanged 6MWT, decreased bnp	
ILD	RISE-IIP [46]	2016	RCT	147	Riociguat	Terminated early for harm	
PLCH	Le Pavec et al. [36]	2012	Retrospective	14	ERA ($n = 8$)	WHO functional class improved in 67%; mPAP and PVR improved	No worsening of oxygenation
					PDE-5 ($n = 3$)		
					Inhaled prostanoid ($n = 1$)		
					ERA + PDE-5 ($n = 2$)		
SSc-ILD	Ahmadi-Simab et al. [37]	2006	Open-label, prospective	8	Bosentan	Improved 6MWT and WHO FC	
SSc-ILD	Seibold et al. [38]	2010	RCT	163	Bosentan	No improvement in 6MWT	
SSc-ILD	Furuya et al. [39]	2011	Open-label	9	Bosentan	No effect on decline in lung function	

6MWT six-minute walk test, *BNP* brain natriuretic peptide, *CO* cardiac output, *CTD-ILD* connective tissue disease-associated interstitial lung disease, *ERA* endothelin receptor antagonist, *FC* functional class, *FVC* forced vital capacity, *ILD* interstitial lung disease, *IPF* idiopathic pulmonary fibrosis, *mPAP* mean pulmonary artery pressure, *QOL* quality of life, *PDE-5i* phosphodiesterase 5 inhibitor, *PF* pulmonary fibrosis, *PH* pulmonary hypertension, *PLCH* pulmonary Langerhans cell histiocytosis, *PVR* pulmonary vascular resistance, *RCT* randomized, controlled trial, *RHC* right heart catheterization, *SSc-ILD* systemic sclerosis interstitial lung disease, *V/Q* ventilation/perfusion, *WHO* World Health Organization

The most encouraging study of vasodilator therapy in PH-ILD to date is the STEP-IPF study. This RCT compared sildenafil with placebo in a population of patients with advanced IPF. The study enrolled only patients with single breath diffusing capacity (DLCO) < 35% predicted [18]. Based on experience from previous studies, approximately 50% of the patients in this study would have PH [49]. Although the study failed to demonstrate a difference in the primary endpoint of a ≥20% increase in 6MWT distance, sildenafil improved a number of secondary endpoints including quality-of-life measures, arterial oxygen saturation, and DLCO [18]. There was also a trend toward a mortality benefit at 24 weeks in the treatment arm ($p = 0.07$) [18]. A subgroup analysis of data from STEP-IPF performed by Han and colleagues found that in patients with right ventricular systolic dysfunction on TTE, sildenafil resulted in a preservation of exercise capacity as measured by the 6MWT [50]. Clearly, the current medical literature on vasodilator therapy in PH-ILD has significant limitations; however, the studies to date provide proof of concept of PH-ILD as a potential therapeutic target.

Selecting the Appropriate Population to Treat

As summarized earlier, studies of vasodilator therapy for PH-ILD to date have shown glimmers of potential but have failed to conclusively demonstrate benefit. Improper patient selection for therapy may be a reason for this. Longitudinal study of IPF patients demonstrates that the majority of patients with IPF will develop PH as their lung disease progresses [51]. It has also been shown that lung volume measurements alone cannot predict the development of PH in advanced lung disease, suggesting that factors other than progressive fibrosis cause PH in some advanced lung disease patients [49]. In summary, PH frequently develops over time with progressive respiratory failure and worsening parenchymal disease; however, there is also a distinct population of patients who develop PH with lesser degrees of parenchymal involvement. This implies that discrete pathophysiologic mechanisms aside from pulmonary parenchymal destruction may contribute to the development of PH-ILD. In affected patients, exhausted circulatory reserve from PH may drive exercise limitation and mortality, rather than the ventilatory and gas exchange limitations that invariably accompany fibrotic lung disease. It is in this population of PH-ILD patients that treatment with pulmonary vasodilator theoretically has the greatest potential for benefit.

The concept of DPH can be loosely defined as elevations in pulmonary pressures associated with parenchymal lung disease that are greater than would be expected for the degree of parenchymal lung destruction. Exact definitions for DPH remain elusive and the term DPH has been discouraged in the most recent PH guidelines given the lack of a consensus definition [52]. The guidelines suggest instead the term "ILD with severe PH" for an mPAP ≥35 mmHg or an mPAP ≥25 mmHg with an associated cardiac index (CI) of less than 2.0 L/min [52]. The appropriateness of a single threshold value for defining DPH is not well validated. The traditional definition of

PH as an mPAP ≥25 mmHg is frequently applied to PH-ILD, but lesser mPAP thresholds are also associated with adverse outcomes [53]. Perhaps the mPAP at which PH becomes "disproportionate" is variable and dynamic with higher pressure thresholds for more severe restrictive disease. More likely, it is not a numerical threshold that should define "disproportionate" PH, but rather the physiologic consequences of the increased afterload. It may be that DPH occurs when PH leads to right heart decompensation. This concept is supported by the subgroup analysis of the STEP-IPF trial, in which treatment with sildenafil preserved exercise capacity in patients with IPF and evidence of right ventricular systolic dysfunction on TTE [50]. Despite this hypothesis, the precise patient population who might benefit from the treatment of PH-ILD remains unknown. Based on the limited available data, a trial of closely monitored therapy might be reasonable in PH-ILD patients, where PH appears to be a key factor driving exercise limitation, especially if there is evidence of right ventricular dysfunction or a depressed CI. Carefully designed RCTs focused on the enrollment of patients with DPH will be required to delineate the appropriate threshold for initiation of vasodilator therapy in PH-ILD.

Treatment of Pulmonary Hypertension in Interstitial Lung Disease

The treatment of PH-ILD can be divided into three major categories: primary, adjunctive, and PH-specific therapies. Primary therapy is focused on the underlying ILD. Delaying progression of the underlying lung disease will aid in maintaining functional status and oxygenation as well as curtailing the factors perpetuating the PH. It should be noted that with the exception of steroids for stage 2 and 3 sarcoidosis and select patients with CTD-ILD, systemic therapy has not been demonstrated to improve hemodynamics in PH-ILD [54, 55]. Whether new antifibrotic therapies for IPF will alter the natural history of PH-ILD in this condition remains to be determined. Given the high mortality associated with the development of PH-ILD, lung transplantation may afford a survival benefit. Appropriate candidates should be referred for lung transplantation evaluation and potential listing at the time of diagnosis.

Adjunctive therapies are focused on mitigating comorbid conditions and consequences of lung disease. Resting and exertional hypoxemia should be sought and corrected with supplemental oxygen. Active smokers should be counseled on tobacco use with aggressive smoking cessation interventions implemented when appropriate. Sleep-disordered breathing should be investigated and appropriately treated with weight loss and continuous positive airway pressure (CPAP) ventilation. Notably, CPAP has been demonstrated to reduce pulmonary pressures in patients with OSA [56]. Heart failure with preserved ejection fraction (HFpEF) and coronary artery disease are common comorbidities in patients with ILD [57]. Appropriate medical therapy and cardiology referral should be instituted for these conditions when present.

Table 4.2 Factors suggestive of pulmonary hypertension in interstitial lung disease

• Dyspnea "out of proportion" to pulmonary function test results
• New desaturations despite stable lung volumes
• D_{LCO} <35% predicted
• FVC/D_{LCO} ratio >1.5
• Ratio of main pulmonary artery to aorta diameter >1 on CT
• Desaturation <88% on room air on 6MWT
• Distance <200 meters on 6MWT
• Pulse rate recovery <13 beats/min following 6MWT
• Elevated pro-BNP

6MWT six-minute walk test, *CT* computed tomography, D_{LCO} diffusing capacity of the lung for carbon monoxide, *FVC* forced vital capacity, *pro-BNP* prohormone of brain natriuretic peptide

Fibrotic lung disease is a risk factor for venous thromboembolism which should be sought and treated in the appropriate clinical context [57]. Interestingly, coumadin was found to be harmful in a study as a primary therapy for IPF; nonetheless, anticoagulation should not be withheld in IPF or other fibrotic disease patients in the context of documented thromboembolic events [58]. Finally, advanced lung disease is frequently complicated by deconditioning. Clinicians should consider patient referral for pulmonary rehabilitation, which has been demonstrated to improve quality of life and exercise tolerance in this population [59].

The role for PH-specific therapies in PH-ILD remains poorly defined. To date, no pulmonary vasodilator therapy has been approved for the treatment of PH-ILD. Despite this, it is reasonable to screen for PH in patients with ILD and persistent dyspnea which may be accompanied by one or more of the following: a markedly reduced DLCO (<35% predicted), reduced significantly compromised 6MWT distance (<200–300 m), desaturation <88%, or an impaired pulse rate recovery after 6MWT [5]. Table 4.2 provides a list of findings suggestive of PH-ILD. Screening is typically performed by TTE, although this test can be technically challenging and suffers from imperfect accuracy in advanced lung disease [60]. Confirmatory RHC should be performed if there is the clinical suspicion for PH warranting this [5]. There are many factors that can contribute to the clinicians' level of suspicion for PH. These can be used in a Bayesian fashion to decide if the suspicion is high enough to warrant RHC. Before recommending a RHC, it is important to have an appreciation for how the results of this test might potentially alter the patient's management. This encompasses not only the decision to institute vasoactive therapy but also includes obtaining potentially important prognostic information as well the discovery of other treatable conditions. Specifically, RHC may reveal evidence of volume overload or heart failure with preserved ejection fraction (HFpEF), which may warrant diuretic and other therapies. The decision to pursue a

Table 4.3 Treatment of pulmonary hypertension in interstitial lung disease

Primary therapies (Interventions to improve the interstitial lung disease)	
• Antifibrotic therapy for IPF (pirfenidone, nintedanib) • Immunosuppression for CTD-ILD • Steroids, alternative agents for sarcoidosis	*Key points* • Does not improve pulmonary hemodynamics directly in most ILD
Adjunctive therapies	
• Oxygen • Smoking cessation • Treatment of sleep-disordered breathing • Pulmonary Rehabilitation	*Key points* • Helps maintain functional status and oxygenation • May curtail factors exacerbating PH
Pulmonary hypertension specific therapies	
• Diuretics • Pulmonary Vasodilators	*Key points* • Pulmonary vasodilator therapy has not been conclusively demonstrated to improve outcomes in PH-ILD • Should only initiate vasodilator therapy for PH-ILD in a clinical trial or at a center with expertise in the treatment of PH

ILD interstitial lung disease, *PH* pulmonary hypertension

trial of vasodilator therapy should be guided by the clinician's sense as to what the primary driver of the patient's symptomatology is. If PH-ILD is deemed to be the primary factor responsible for limited exercise tolerance, it may be reasonable to institute a trial of therapy with a pulmonary vasodilator. In doing so, a baseline 6MWT should be performed to establish an objective means of assessing response to therapy. Patients should be closely monitored for worsening hypoxemia and the development of pulmonary edema. If vasodilator therapy is initiated outside the setting of a clinical trial, it should be done only at experienced centers with expertise in treating PH. Current data is too limited to make specific recommendations regarding individual agents or dosing regimens. Based on existing data in IPF patients, the use of agents targeting the nitric oxide pathway such as sildenafil is likely preferable to the ERA class of agents. Given the paucity of data supporting the use of vasodilator therapy in PH-ILD, every effort should be made to enroll patients into available clinical trials. Table 4.3 provides a summary of recommended the recommended treatment for pulmonary hypertension in interstitial lung disease.

Treatment of Pulmonary Hypertension in Sarcoidosis

Many clinicians believe sarcoid-associated PH (SAPH) is a distinct clinical entity which warrants a separate discussion from other forms of PH-ILD. Numerous etiologies can lead to the development of SAPH including fibrosis-associated obliteration of the vascular bed, pulmonary vascular compression by mediastinal lymphadenopathy, granulomatous arteritis, pulmonary veno-occlusive disease, hypoxia-induced pulmonary vasoconstriction, portopulmonary hypertension secondary to sarcoid liver disease, and left ventricular dysfunction [61]. Given the myriad of possible etiologies resulting in SAPH, RHC is mandatory to delineate the cause and severity of PH (Fig. 4.2).

Similar to other forms of PH-ILD, the optimal management of SAPH remains controversial. There is fairly universal agreement that appropriate adjunctive therapies including oxygen supplementation, smoking cessation, vaccinations, and treatment of sleep-disordered breathing should be instituted. The role of corticosteroids as a primary treatment of SAPH is debated, with reports of both benefit and harm

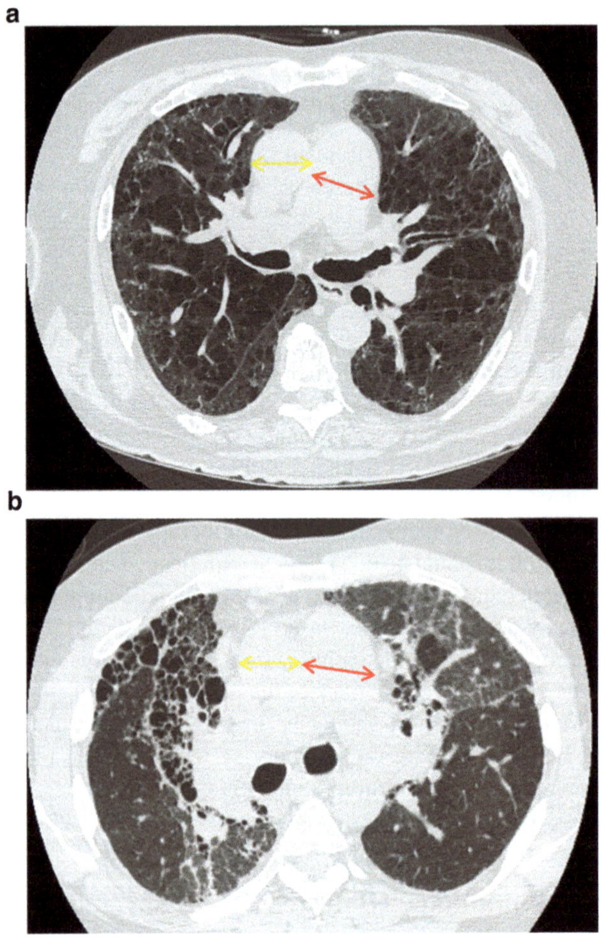

Fig. 4.2 CT imaging of pulmonary hypertension in interstitial lung disease. Both CTs show an enlarged pulmonary artery (*red arrow*) as compared to the ascending aorta (*yellow arrow*). The patient in CT (**a**) has combined pulmonary fibrosis and emphysema, while CT (**b**) is from a patient with sarcoidosis

[62]. It has been suggested that specific subgroups, including those with active inflammation or compression of the proximal pulmonary arteries by adenopathy, may derive benefit, while those with marked fibrosis are unlikely to improve [62]. Numerous studies of pulmonary vasodilator therapy for SAPH have been undertaken; however, their small size and surrogate primary endpoints limit the ability to draw conclusions as to the efficacy of treatment with these agents. Several case series have reported on the efficacy of PDE-5 inhibitors in SAPH [63–65]. In the largest of these retrospective reports, Keir and colleagues found that treatment with sildenafil in 29 SAPH patients led to improved functional class and echocardiographic parameters [64]. Two case series have reported on the efficacy of prostanoid therapy in SAPH [47, 66]. A series of 15 patients treated with inhaled iloprost found a significant improvement in quality of life and improved hemodynamics in 6/15 (40%) of the patients [47]. The most studied class of pulmonary vasodilators in SAPH are the ERAs. A prospective, open-label trial evaluated ambrisentan in 21 patients with SAPH over 24 weeks. No difference in 6MWT distance or symptoms was found, and less than half the patients were able to tolerate therapy for the study duration [42]. In the only RCT of vasodilator therapy for SAPH completed to date, 35 patients were treated with bosentan for 16 weeks. Treated patients demonstrated a reduction in mPAP and PVR, but bosentan therapy failed to improve the 6MWT distance [43]. Table 4.4 provides a summary of prospective studies of pulmonary vasodilator therapy in sarcoid-associated pulmonary hypertension.

The available data suggests that pulmonary vasodilator therapy can improve the hemodynamic profile of patients with SAPH. Whether these hemodynamic improvement translate into sustained improvements in functional capacity and patient outcomes remains to be seen. At this time, there are no approved therapies for the treatment of SAPH. If treatment of SAPH with vasodilator therapy is undertaken, it

Table 4.4 Prospective studies of pulmonary vasodilator therapies in sarcoidosis

Investigator	Year	Study design	Pts	Therapy	Results	Comments
Baughman et al. [40]	2006	RCT	35	Bosentan	Decreased mPAP and PVR	No change in 6MWT
Baughman et al. [47]	2009	Prospective, open-label	15	Iloprost	Decreased mPap in ~1/3	
Judson et al. [42]	2011	Prospective, open-label	21	Ambrisentan	In those completing study, improved WHO functional class	High dropout rate
Baughman et al. [43]	2006	RCT	35	Bosentan	Improved PVR and mPAP	No change in 6MWT

6MWT six-minute walk test, *mPAP* mean pulmonary artery pressure, *PVR* pulmonary vascular resistance, *RCT* randomized, controlled trial, *WHO* World Health Organization

should be done so in the context of a clinical trial or at an expert center with experience in the management of this complex disorder.

Future Directions

Further clinical trials assessing the response to pulmonary vasodilator therapy are required. Careful attention to study design is essential in determining the optimal population for the treatment of PH-ILD. Clinical trialists will need to select an appropriate hemodynamic threshold for pulmonary pressures and the maximal amount of permissible parenchymal disease in order to isolate a population of patients with DPH most likely to respond to vasodilator therapy. Selection of appropriate endpoints for such studies is of paramount importance as well. Consideration could be given to composite endpoints which can capture disease worsening from a number of aspects rather than individual endpoints such as 6MWT distance, hospitalizations, and mortality. The authors recommend the referenced review article to readers interested in a more thorough discussion of issues surrounding clinical trial design in PH-ILD [48].

Conclusion

PH-ILD is associated with significant morbidity and mortality. Given the limited treatment options available for ILD, the treatment of PH in this population is an enticing therapeutic target. Clinicians should maintain a high index of suspicion for PH-ILD, particularly in patients with a markedly reduced DLCO, pronounced oxygen desaturation, or severe exercise limitation. Provision of supplemental oxygen and appropriate evaluation for and treatment of comorbid conditions such as sleep-disordered breathing, HFpEF, coronary artery disease, and venous thromboembolism are of paramount importance. Numerous studies exist evaluating the use of pulmonary vasodilator therapy in PH-ILD, but no clear benefits have been conclusively demonstrated in RCTs. In order to study an enriched population, the concept of DPH will require clearer understanding and definition. Targeting this patient population in future RCTs is necessary to address the complex issue of the role of pulmonary vasoactive agents.

References

1. Travis WD, Costabel U, Hansell DM, King TE Jr, Lynch DA, Nicholson AG, et al. An official American Thoracic Society/European Respiratory Society statement: update of the international multidisciplinary classification of the idiopathic interstitial pneumonias. Am J Respir Crit Care Med. 2013;188(6):733–48.

2. Nathan SD, Shlobin OA, Weir N, Ahmad S, Kaldjob JM, Battle E, et al. Long-term course and prognosis of idiopathic pulmonary fibrosis in the new millennium. Chest. 2011;140(1):221–9.
3. King TE Jr, Bradford WZ, Castro-Bernardini S, Fagan EA, Glaspole I, Glassberg MK, et al. A phase 3 trial of pirfenidone in patients with idiopathic pulmonary fibrosis. N Engl J Med. 2014;370(22):2083–92.
4. Richeldi L, du Bois RM, Raghu G, Azuma A, Brown KK, Costabel U, et al. Efficacy and safety of nintedanib in idiopathic pulmonary fibrosis. N Engl J Med. 2014;370(22):2071–82.
5. Nathan SD, Hassoun PM. Pulmonary hypertension due to lung disease and/or hypoxia. Clin Chest Med. 2013;34(4):695–705.
6. Oliveira RK, Pereira CA, Ramos RP, Ferreira EV, Messina CM, Kuranishi LT, et al. A haemodynamic study of pulmonary hypertension in chronic hypersensitivity pneumonitis. Eur Respir J. 2014;44(2):415–24.
7. Armstrong HF, Schulze PC, Bacchetta M, Thirapatarapong W, Bartels MN. Impact of pulmonary hypertension on exercise performance in patients with interstitial lung disease undergoing evaluation for lung transplantation. Respirology. 2014;19(5):675–82.
8. King TE Jr, Tooze JA, Schwarz MI, Brown KR, Cherniack RM. Predicting survival in idiopathic pulmonary fibrosis: scoring system and survival model. Am J Respir Crit Care Med. 2001;164(7):1171–81.
9. Lettieri CJ, Nathan SD, Barnett SD, Ahmad S, Shorr AF. Prevalence and outcomes of pulmonary arterial hypertension in advanced idiopathic pulmonary fibrosis. Chest. 2006;129(3):746–52.
10. Shorr AF, Wainright JL, Cors CS, Lettieri CJ, Nathan SD. Pulmonary hypertension in patients with pulmonary fibrosis awaiting lung transplant. Eur Respir J. 2007;30(4):715–21.
11. Simonneau G, Gatzoulis MA, Adatia I, Celermajer D, Denton C, Ghofrani A, et al. Updated clinical classification of pulmonary hypertension. J Am Coll Cardiol. 2013;62(25 suppl):D34–41.
12. Glaser S, Noga O, Koch B, Opitz CF, Schmidt B, Temmesfeld B, et al. Impact of pulmonary hypertension on gas exchange and exercise capacity in patients with pulmonary fibrosis. Respir Med. 2009;103(2):317–24.
13. Nadrous HF, Pellikka PA, Krowka MJ, Swanson KL, Chaowalit N, Decker PA, et al. Pulmonary hypertension in patients with idiopathic pulmonary fibrosis. Chest. 2005;128(4):2393–9.
14. Shorr AF, Davies DB, Nathan SD. Outcomes for patients with sarcoidosis awaiting lung transplantation. Chest. 2002;122(1):233–8.
15. Trad S, Amoura Z, Beigelman C, Haroche J, Costedoat N, le Boutin TH, et al. Pulmonary arterial hypertension is a major mortality factor in diffuse systemic sclerosis, independent of interstitial lung disease. Arthritis Rheum. 2006;54(1):184–91.
16. Ghofrani HA, Wiedemann R, Rose F, Schermuly RT, Olschewski H, Weissmann N, et al. Sildenafil for treatment of lung fibrosis and pulmonary hypertension: a randomised controlled trial. Lancet. 2002;360(9337):895–900.
17. Olschewski H, Ghofrani HA, Walmrath D, Schermuly R, Temmesfeld-Wollbruck B, Grimminger F, et al. Inhaled prostacyclin and iloprost in severe pulmonary hypertension secondary to lung fibrosis. Am J Respir Crit Care Med. 1999;160(2):600–7.
18. Idiopathic Pulmonary Fibrosis Clinical Research Network, Zisman DA, Schwarz M, Anstrom KJ, Collard HR, Flaherty KR, Hunninghake GW. A controlled trial of sildenafil in advanced idiopathic pulmonary fibrosis. N Engl J Med. 2010;363(7):620–8.
19. Hoeper MM, Halank M, Wilkens H, Günther A, Weimann G, Gebert I, et al. Riociguat for interstitial lung disease and pulmonary hypertension: a pilot trial. Eur Respir J. 2013;41(4):853–60.
20. Cottin V. Treatment of pulmonary hypertension in interstitial lung disease: do not throw out the baby with the bath water. Eur Respir J. 2013;41(4):781–3.
21. Collard HR, Anstrom KJ, Schwarz MI, Zisman DA. Sildenafil improves walk distance in idiopathic pulmonary fibrosis. Chest. 2007;131(3):897–9.
22. Jackson RM, Glassberg MK, Ramos CF, Bejarano PA, Butrous G, Gomez-Marin O. Sildenafil therapy and exercise tolerance in idiopathic pulmonary fibrosis. Lung. 2010;188(2):115–23.

23. Gunther A, Enke B, Markart P, Hammerl P, Morr H, Behr J, et al. Safety and tolerability of bosentan in idiopathic pulmonary fibrosis: an open label study. Eur Respir J. 2007;29(4):713–9.
24. King TE Jr, Behr J, Brown KK, du Bois RM, Lancaster L, de Andrade JA, et al. BUILD-1: a randomized placebo-controlled trial of bosentan in idiopathic pulmonary fibrosis. Am J Respir Crit Care Med. 2008;177(1):75–81.
25. King TE Jr, Brown KK, Raghu G, du Bois RM, Lynch DA, Martinez F, et al. BUILD-3: a randomized, controlled trial of bosentan in idiopathic pulmonary fibrosis. Am J Respir Crit Care Med. 2011;184(1):92–9.
26. Raghu G, Behr J, Brown KK, Egan JJ, Kawut SM, Flaherty KR, et al. Treatment of idiopathic pulmonary fibrosis with ambrisentan: a parallel, randomized trial. Ann Intern Med. 2013;158(9):641–9.
27. Raghu G, Million-Rousseau R, Morganti A, Perchenet L, Behr J, Group MS. Macitentan for the treatment of idiopathic pulmonary fibrosis: the randomised controlled MUSIC trial. Eur Respir J. 2013;42(6):1622–32.
28. Mittoo S, Jacob T, Craig A, Bshouty Z. Treatment of pulmonary hypertension in patients with connective tissue disease and interstitial lung disease. Can Respir J. 2010;17(6):282–6.
29. Heresi GA, Minai OA. Bosentan in systemic sclerosis. Drugs Today. 2008;44(6):415–28.
30. Chapman TH, Wilde M, Sheth A, Madden BP. Sildenafil therapy in secondary pulmonary hypertension: is there benefit in prolonged use? Vascul Pharmacol. 2009;51(2–3):90–5.
31. Corte TJ, Gatzoulis MA, Parfitt L, Harries C, Wells AU, Wort SJ. The use of sildenafil to treat pulmonary hypertension associated with interstitial lung disease. Respirology. 2010;15(8):1226–32.
32. Badesch DB, Feldman J, Keogh A, Mathier MA, Oudiz RJ, Shapiro S, et al. ARIES-3: ambrisentan therapy in a diverse population of patients with pulmonary hypertension. Cardiovasc Ther. 2012;30(2):93–9.
33. Zimmermann GS, von Wulffen W, Huppmann P, Meis T, Ihle F, Geiseler J, et al. Haemodynamic changes in pulmonary hypertension in patients with interstitial lung disease treated with PDE-5 inhibitors. Respirology. 2014;19(5):700–6.
34. Corte TJ, Keir GJ, Dimopoulos K, Howard L, Corris PA, Parfitt L, et al. Bosentan in pulmonary hypertension associated with fibrotic idiopathic interstitial pneumonia. Am J Respir Crit Care Med. 2014;190(2):208–17.
35. Saggar R, Khanna D, Vaidya A, Derhovanessian A, Maranian P, Duffy E, et al. Changes in right heart haemodynamics and echocardiographic function in an advanced phenotype of pulmonary hypertension and right heart dysfunction associated with pulmonary fibrosis. Thorax. 2014;69(2):123–9.
36. Le Pavec J, Lorillon G, Jais X, Tcherakian C, Feuillet S, Dorfmüller P, et al. Pulmonary Langerhans cell histiocytosis-associated pulmonary hypertension: clinical characteristics and impact of pulmonary arterial hypertension therapies. Chest. 2012;142(5):1150–7.
37. Ahmadi-Simab K, Hellmich B, Gross WL. Bosentan for severe pulmonary arterial hypertension related to systemic sclerosis with interstitial lung disease. Eur J Clin Invest. 2006;36(suppl 3):44–8.
38. Seibold JR, Denton CP, Furst DE, Guillevin L, Rubin LJ, Wells A, et al. Randomized, prospective, placebo-controlled trial of bosentan in interstitial lung disease secondary to systemic sclerosis. Arthritis Rheum. 2010;62(7):2101–8.
39. Furuya Y, Kuwana M. Effect of Bosentan on systemic sclerosis-associated interstitial lung disease ineligible for cyclophosphamide therapy: a prospective open-label study. J Rheumatol. 2011;38(10):2186–92.
40. Baughman RP, Engel PJ, Meyer CA, Barrett AB, Lower EE. Pulmonary hypertension in sarcoidosis. Sarcoidosis Vasc Diffuse Lung Dis. 2006;23(2):108–16.
41. Baughman RP. Pulmonary hypertension associated with sarcoidosis. Arthritis Res Ther. 2007;9(suppl 2):S8.
42. Judson MA, Highland KB, Kwon S, Donohue JF, Aris R, Craft N, et al. Ambrisentan for sarcoidosis associated pulmonary hypertension. Sarcoidosis Vasc Diffuse Lung Dis. 2011;28(2):139–45.

43. Baughman RP, Culver DA, Cordova FC, Padilla M, Gibson KF, Lower EE, et al. Bosentan for sarcoidosis-associated pulmonary hypertension: a double-blind placebo controlled randomized trial. Chest. 2014;145(4):810–7.
44. Krowka MJ, Ahmad S, Andrade J, Nathan SD. A randomized, double-blind, placebo-controlled study to evaluate the safety and efficacy of iloprost inhalation in adults with abnormal pulmonary arterial pressure and exercise limitation associated with idiopathic pulmonary fibrosis. Chest. 2007;132:633S.
45. Brewis MJ, Church AC, Johnson MK, Peacock AJ. Severe pulmonary hypertension in lung disease: phenotypes and response to treatment. Eur Respir J. 2015;46(5):1378–89.
46. Bayer Corporation. Bayer terminates Phase II study with riociguat in patients with pulmonary hypertension associated with idiopathic interstitial pneumonias. May 12, 2016. Retrieved from http://www.prnewswire.com/news-releases/bayer-terminates-phase-ii-study-with-riociguat-in-patients-with-pulmonary-hypertension-associated-with-idiopathic-interstitial-pneumonias-300267616.html.
47. Baughman RP, Judson MA, Lower EE, Highland K, Kwon S, Craft N, et al. Inhaled iloprost for sarcoidosis associated pulmonary hypertension. Sarcoidosis Vasc Diffuse Lung Dis. 2009;26(2):110–20.
48. Nathan SD, King CS. Treatment of pulmonary hypertension in idiopathic pulmonary fibrosis: shortfall in efficacy or trial design? Drug Des Devel Ther. 2014;8:875–85.
49. Nathan SD, Shlobin OA, Ahmad S, Urbanek S, Barnett SD. Pulmonary hypertension and pulmonary function testing in idiopathic pulmonary fibrosis. Chest. 2007;131(3):657–63.
50. Han MK, Bach DS, Hagan PG, Yow E, Flaherty KR, Toews GB, et al. Sildenafil preserves exercise capacity in patients with idiopathic pulmonary fibrosis and right-sided ventricular dysfunction. Chest. 2013;143(6):1699–708.
51. Nathan SD, Shlobin OA, Ahmad S, Koch J, Barnett SD, Ad N, et al. Serial development of pulmonary hypertension in patients with idiopathic pulmonary fibrosis. Respiration. 2008;76(3):288–94.
52. Seeger W, Adir Y, Barbera JA, Champion H, Coghlan JG, Cottin V, et al. Pulmonary hypertension in chronic lung diseases. J Am Coll Cardiol. 2013;62(25 suppl):D109–16.
53. Hamada K, Nagai S, Tanaka S, Handa T, Shigematsu M, Nagao T, et al. Significance of pulmonary arterial pressure and diffusion capacity of the lung as prognosticator in patients with idiopathic pulmonary fibrosis. Chest. 2007;131(3):650–6.
54. Sanchez O, Sitbon O, Jais X, Simonneau G, Humbert M. Immunosuppressive therapy in connective tissue diseases-associated pulmonary arterial hypertension. Chest. 2006;130(1):182–9.
55. Gluskowski J, Hawrylkiewicz I, Zych D, Zielinski J. Effects of corticosteroid treatment on pulmonary haemodynamics in patients with sarcoidosis. Eur Respir J. 1990;3(4):403–7.
56. Sajkov D, Wang T, Saunders NA, Bune AJ, McEvoy RD. Continuous positive airway pressure treatment improves pulmonary hemodynamics in patients with obstructive sleep apnea. Am J Respir Crit Care Med. 2002;165(2):152–8.
57. King C, Nathan SD. Identification and treatment of comorbidities in idiopathic pulmonary fibrosis and other fibrotic lung diseases. Curr Opin Pulm Med. 2013;19(5):466–73.
58. Noth I, Anstrom KJ, Calvert SB, de Andrade J, Flaherty KR, Glazer C, et al. A placebo-controlled randomized trial of warfarin in idiopathic pulmonary fibrosis. Am J Respir Crit Care Med. 2012;186(1):88–95.
59. Ryerson CJ, Cayou C, Topp F, Hilling L, Camp PG, Wilcox PG, et al. Pulmonary rehabilitation improves long-term outcomes in interstitial lung disease: a prospective cohort study. Respir Med. 2014;108(1):203–10.
60. Arcasoy SM, Christie JD, Ferrari VA, Sutton MS, Zisman DA, Blumenthal NP, et al. Echocardiographic assessment of pulmonary hypertension in patients with advanced lung disease. Am J Respir Crit Care Med. 2003;167(5):735–40.
61. Baughman RP, Engel PJ, Nathan S. Pulmonary hypertension in sarcoidosis. Clin Chest Med. 2015;36(4):703–14.

62. Corte TJ, Wells AU, Nicholson AG, Hansell DM, Wort SJ. Pulmonary hypertension in sarcoidosis: a review. Respirology. 2011;16(1):69–77.
63. Barnett CF, Bonura EJ, Nathan SD, Ahmad S, Shlobin OA, Osei K, et al. Treatment of sarcoidosis-associated pulmonary hypertension. A two-center experience. Chest. 2009;135(6):1455–61.
64. Keir GJ, Walsh SL, Gatzoulis MA, Marino PS, Dimopoulos K, Alonso R, et al. Treatment of sarcoidosis-associated pulmonary hypertension: a single centre retrospective experience using targeted therapies. Sarcoidosis Vasc Diffuse Lung Dis. 2014;31(2):82–90.
65. Milman N, Burton CM, Iversen M, Videbaek R, Jensen CV, Carlsen J. Pulmonary hypertension in end-stage pulmonary sarcoidosis: therapeutic effect of sildenafil? J Heart Lung Transplant. 2008;27(3):329–34.
66. Fisher KA, Serlin DM, Wilson KC, Walter RE, Berman JS, Farber HW. Sarcoidosis-associated pulmonary hypertension: outcome with long-term epoprostenol treatment. Chest. 2006;130(5):1481–8.

Chapter 5
Lung Transplantation in Interstitial Lung Disease

Cynthia Kim, Francis Cordova, and Yoshiya Toyoda

Overview

Advanced interstitial lung disease (ILD) that failed medical therapy is a common indication for lung transplantation. The first successful lung transplantation was performed in a patient with idiopathic pulmonary fibrosis. With the implementation of the lung allocation score in 2005, idiopathic pulmonary fibrosis has surpassed chronic obstructive pulmonary disease as the most common indication of lung transplantation. In the context of lung transplantation, interstitial lung diseases can be broadly grouped into idiopathic interstitial pneumonias, interstitial lung disease due to connective tissue disease (CTD), and pulmonary sarcoidosis with or without pulmonary hypertension. Idiopathic pulmonary fibrosis is the most common of the idiopathic interstitial pneumonia, followed by nonspecific interstitial pneumonia. The most common interstitial lung disease due to connective tissue disease that leads to lung transplantation is scleroderma-associated ILD. Others forms of ILD-CTD include rheumatoid arthritis, mixed connective tissue disease, and dermatomyositis/polymyositis.

Interstitial lung diseases confer certain challenges not usually seen in other forms of advanced lung disease that warrant lung transplantation. For instance, IPF can lead to acute exacerbation even with relatively preserved lung function. Acute IPF exacerbation can lead to severe hypoxemia requiring mechanical ventilatory support and in some instances even the need for extracorporeal membrane oxygenator (ECMO). This can lead to deconditioning, hemodynamic instability, and

C. Kim, MD
Department of Medicine, Division of Pulmonary and Critical Care, David Geffen School of Medicine at University of California, Los Angeles, CA, USA

F. Cordova, MD (✉) • Y. Toyoda, MD, PhD
Department of Thoracic Medicine and Surgery, Temple University School of Medicine, 3401 North Broad St, Philadelphia, PA 19140, USA
e-mail: cordovf@tuhs.temple.edu

R.P. Baughman et al. (eds.), *Pulmonary Hypertension and Interstitial Lung Disease*, DOI 10.1007/978-3-319-49918-5_5

extrapulmonary organ dysfunction that will rapidly push the patient out of the transplant window. Patients are often delisted from the active transplant list until they recover. ILD-CTD is often associated with significant extrapulmonary dysfunction that may negatively impact the patient status as a good lung transplant candidate. A good example of this is the presence of severe esophageal dysfunction in patients with scleroderma. Another common comorbidity in this subgroup of patients is the presence of pulmonary hypertension that increases the risk of allograft dysfunction during the immediate postoperative period. In addition, significant coronary artery disease is often uncovered during prelung transplant evaluation even in patients who are asymptomatic. All these pretransplant issues need to be recognized and addressed during pretransplant evaluation in order to minimize postoperative complications and optimize posttransplant outcome. In this chapter, we will discuss when to refer patients with ILD for lung transplant, recognized common comorbidities commonly associated with ILD especially pulmonary hypertension and esophageal dysfunction, discussed the use of ECMO as bridge to transplant, and expected clinical outcome.

Pretransplant Considerations

Timing of Transplant Referral

In general, patients with end-stage lung disease should be considered for referral if there is a high risk of death within 2 years and high probability of surviving after the transplant at least for 5 years [1]. However, it is difficult to make this determination clinically and a significant amount of variation in both presentation and clinical practice exists. The severity and complexity of this disease is reflected in the fact that this group of transplant recipients has a high mortality rate on the transplant list. It should be important to note, especially to the patients with interstitial lung disease, that referral for transplantation is a separate process from listing for transplantation.

The recommendations regarding referral of IPF patients for transplant evaluation state that it should occur as soon as there is radiographic or histopathologic evidence of UIP or fibrosing NSIP. This is in recognition of the poor prognosis associated with this disease, variable clinical progression, and few alternative treatment options. The median survival of patients with UIP is 2–3 years from diagnosis; however, there are a number of patients with preserved lung function who rapidly deteriorate from acute exacerbation. Additionally, it is difficult to determine which patients will follow a normal trajectory versus those that will experience an accelerated decline. Though there are no validated clinical prediction tools for IPF, recognized factors that influence survival include advanced age, low or declining pulmonary function, and concurrent pulmonary hypertension. In addition, a referral should be made with any symptoms of lung compromise such as requirement for oxygen or even the sensation of dyspnea. The full criteria are listed in Table 5.1.

Table 5.1 ILD [1]

Timing of referral for transplant	1. Histopathologic/radiographic evidence of UIP/NSIP regardless of lung function
	2. FVC <80, DLCO <40
	3. Any dyspnea or functional limitation attributable to lung disease
	4. Any oxygen requirement even if only on exertion
Timing of listing	1. Decline in FVC >10% during 6 months of follow up
	2. Decline in DLCO >15% during 6 months of follow up
	3. Desaturation <88%, <250 m on 6 MW of >50 m decline in 6 MW over 6 month period
	4. Pulmonary hypertension on RHC or echo
	5. Hospitalization due to respiratory decline, pneumothorax, or acute exacerbation

Since there are not any good clinical predictor equations for the other interstitial lung diseases, the recommendations for referral are the same as those for IPF provided they have received a reasonable trial of medical therapy. Listing these individuals for transplant varies by transplant center but largely depends upon demonstration of disease progression or instability. The suggested criteria are also listed in Table 5.1.

Comorbidities

Pulmonary Hypertension

Pulmonary hypertension is a common sequela of advanced interstitial lung disease. The etiology of secondary pulmonary hypertension is varied and could be due to progressive parenchymal destruction and loss of vascular bed, the presence of concomitant vasculitis, or hypoxic-induced pulmonary vasoconstriction. In many ILD, the presence of PAH portends poor outcome and often heralds the onset of accelerated decline in functional capacity. Indeed the diagnosis of pulmonary hypertension should trigger referral to lung transplant center. The severity of pulmonary hypertension often dictates whether the patients should receive double or single lung transplant or even combined heart/lung transplant in the presence of overt right heart failure.

Fibrotic sarcoidosis traditionally has similar wait-list mortality similar to IPF but historically has been less likely to receive transplantation [2]. Since wait-list mortality does not correlate linearly with lung function, it is difficult to determine appropriate listing times and there is even less data regarding long-term outcomes with fibrotic sarcoidosis as there is with IPF [3]. Known factors that portend mortality in this population include African American race, the presence of pulmonary hypertension, and oxygen use—all indicative of advanced lung disease [4]. Similarly, another center's experience found that a right atrial pressure >15 mmHg was associated with worsened mortality [5]. Extrapulmonary sarcoid involvement should be well defined prior to transplantation. Some experts have suggested that neurosarcoidosis may present a barrier to transplantation if severe. Additionally, a second organ transplant may be considered for patients with cardiac or hepatic sarcoidosis [6].

Scleroderma patients should also be referred early due to more rapidly progressive disease and high incidence of pulmonary hypertension. In fact, pulmonary fibrosis and pulmonary hypertension are the leading causes of death in systemic scleroderma (SSc) [7]. The systemic nature of scleroderma has led to an idea that these patients perform relatively poorly posttransplant. However, one center has demonstrated similar 2- and 5-year mortality rates as compared to other transplant recipients [8, 9] and show similar rates of acute and chronic rejection as compared to other ILD transplant recipients [10, 11]. However, the authors' caveat is that these results depend on very careful patient selection. Relative contraindications include significant skin breakdown from severe cutaneous disease, a creatinine clearance of less than 50, severe reflux disease and aspiration, and cardiac involvement with arrhythmia. In some centers, an esophageal dysfunction with aperistalsis on manometry is an absolute contraindication to transplant. The unique role of esophageal disorders in pretransplant recipients will be discussed in more detail later. Of the patients that do receive transplantation, the 30-day mortality is ~15%, largely due to graft failure, hemorrhagic stroke, cardiac events, and bacterial infection [12].

Pulmonary hypertension can complicate any interstitial lung disease and has been associated with worsened exercise tolerance independent of lung function, higher mortality, and a risk for acute exacerbations of IPF [13, 14]. Studies show that PH can complicate up to 30–46% of IPF patients on right heart catheterization testing and do not necessarily correlate with measures of lung function [15–17]. Elevated b-type natriuretic peptide and elevated pulmonary vascular resistance both predict early mortality in patients with interstitial lung disease [18, 19]. In addition, some have found a linear correlation between mean right atrial pressure and mortality in IPF [16]. Analysis of the REVEAL database showed that those with CTD-PAH had worse 1-year. survival, higher BNP, and lower 6 MW distances as compared to those with idiopathic disease. In addition, those with systemic sclerosis have the worst prognosis of the group despite having similar hemodynamics [20].

While the widespread use of pulmonary vasodilators has significantly decreased the rate of transplantation for pulmonary arterial hypertension (OPTN 2012 report), these medications have not been able to accomplish the same for ILD-related pulmonary hypertension. Studies with vasodilators in IPF with PH have shown inconsistent improvements in symptoms without any improvement in mortality [21–23]. While presence of pulmonary hypertension is an indication to list someone with interstitial lung disease, many felt that the lung allocation score did not adequately reflect the disease severity of this group. This was also reflected in the fact that PAH patients awaiting transplant have similar wait-list mortality as ILD patients but receive fewer organs. To adjust for this, the lung allocation score was modified in early 2015 to include markers such as mean right atrial pressure, cardiac index, and bilirubin level. A high priority allocation program in France for PH led to significantly decreased wait-list mortality. Future reports will show if the adjusted LAS has had a similar impact in here in the United States. With regards to treatment of CTD-PAH related to systemic lupus erythematosus, mixed connective tissue disease, or Sjogren's syndrome can improve with steroids or immunosuppressive therapy whereas scleroderma-PAH usually does not respond to immunotherapy [24].

Esophageal Dysfunction

There has been a lot of data describing the high frequency of gastroesophageal reflux and probable microaspiration in end-stage lung disease as a likely trigger of lung fibrosis pretransplant and a cause of bronchiolitis obliterans syndrome (BOS) posttransplant. Changes in transdiaphragmatic pressure and possible vagal nerve damage that accompany lung transplant seem to exacerbate this problem as well. One study found that in patients with GERD who had bilateral lung transplant or retransplantation had more delayed gastric emptying and impaired esophageal motility as compared to unilateral transplant recipients [33]. Most centers consider severe untreated GERD and esophageal dysmotility as a contraindication to transplantation. However, small single-center series have demonstrated that surgical correction of GERD with fundoplication can be safely performed both pre- and posttransplant [35] while another center demonstrated slower progression of BOS and fewer episodes of acute rejection in the posttransplant population who had received surgical correction [36]. In a report of 23 patients with scleroderma-ILD, with 12 of 23 patients had esophageal dysfunction, there was no difference in survival and incidence of chronic allograft rejection when compared to other forms of non-connective tissue disease-related interstitial lung disease. Interestingly, the rate of acute rejection was lower in patients with scleroderma. The authors attributed this success to multidisciplinary and proactive care of these patients [11]. It is also our view that successful lung transplantation can be performed in carefully selected scleroderma patients with esophageal dysfunction. Depending on the pulmonary reserve of a particular patient, fundoplication can be performed before or after lung transplantation. Postoperatively, patients with marginal respiratory status often require prolonged NPO and enteral support is initiated through a gastrojejunostomy tube. It is important to note that these patients are cared for by a multidisciplinary team that include speech therapist, nutritionist, gastroenterologist with particular interest in esophageal diseases, transplant physicians, and surgeons.

Contraindications

Lung transplantation is a morbid procedure with many contraindications to candidacy. Examples of absolute contraindications include recent malignancy, chronic infection, and acute medical instability such as sepsis or acute myocardial infarction. However, as our experience with lung transplantation grows, relative contraindications such as age, obesity, and infection with hepatitis C and HIV are being called into question. There is even growing experience with double organ transplantation, which can change the absolute contraindication of untreatable end-organ dysfunction into a relative one.

The recommendations published by ISHLT list 65 years of age as an upper limit for transplantation consideration. However, as life expectancy and experience with transplantation grows, the percentage of transplant recipients over the age of 65 has grown to 24.4% in the 2014 OPTN report. Though these patients are more likely to have comorbidities and have traditionally had worse mortality posttransplant, other studies have shown posttransplant quality of life is similar in all age groups [25]. In fact, pretransplant diagnosis was more important than age in determining quality of life measured, even in the small cohort of patients older than 70. Another study found that decline in functional status trajectory posttransplantation was equal in patients over 65 as for younger patients [26]. The 5-year survival rate for all comers after lung transplantation is roughly 65%, a figure that lags behind that for other organs and makes lung transplantation in essence a palliative procedure in which quality of life is just as important as time of life extended. If this is the case, then there seems to be less reason to exclude older individuals from receiving transplantation. This mirrors our own center's experience with older transplant recipients receiving equal quality-of-life improvement and survival as those younger than 65 years.

Both being underweight and overweight have been associated with an increased risk of death after lung transplantation [27] as well as increased risk of primary graft dysfunction in the early posttransplant period [28]. Obesity is also considered a risk factor for concurrent coronary artery disease and other comorbidities that can complicate transplantation. However, some centers have demonstrated equivalent prognosis for overweight patients (BMI 25–29) as normal weight patients [29]. Additionally, an analysis of 9073 adult lung transplant recipients after adoption of the LAS in 2005 shows that adjusted 1-year mortality for patients of normal weight (BMI 18.5–24.9), overweight (BMI 25–29.9), and class I obesity (BMI 30–34.9) were similar, suggesting that there may be a subpopulation patients with higher BMI that can safely undergo transplantation. That same analysis showed a significant increase in mortality with underweight individuals. Fortunately, weight is largely a modifiable risk factor that may be addressed during the referral process with aggressive nutrition management.

Bridge Therapies to Transplant

Recently, pirfenidone and nintedanib were approved as treatments for idiopathic pulmonary fibrosis by decreasing the rate of decline in lung function as compared to placebo [30, 31]. Pirfenidone is an oral antifibrotic agent whereas nintedanib is a tyrosine kinase inhibitor that blocks multiple targets including vascular endothelial growth factor (VEGF), fibroblast growth factor (FGF), and platelet-derived growth factor (PDGF). While neither medication can reverse fibrosis, the stabilization of disease and reduction in disease progression can potentially prolong the transplant window for these patients with high wait-list mortality. Since these drugs are so new, little is known about the effect of these drugs on lung transplant recipients. There are rat models showing that pirfenidone may even be useful after transplant to limit acute lung allograft injury, presumably through suppression of TNF-a, reduced neutrophil recruitment, and iron accumulation [32]. Small case series have demonstrated that recipients undergoing lung transplantation while on pirfenidone did not have any problems with wound healing or anastomosis breakdown despite the supposed suppression of TGF-b. Other institutions have shown no increased episodes of acute or chronic rejection in patients on pirfenidone pretransplantation [33]. There has also been interest in initiating these medications posttransplantation to manage progressive fibrosis in the remaining lung or as a treatment for restrictive CLAD [34]. As our experience with these medications grows, there will need to be protocols and research addressing the appropriate role for these medications both before and after lung transplantation.

Mechanical bridges to transplantation include invasive ventilation and extracorporeal life support. Transplantation of patients who are mechanically ventilated is controversial due to worsened survival postoperatively. However, these patients simultaneously represent the sickest candidates who have the most urgent need for transplantation. One single-center retrospective analysis showed that survival in patients who required mechanical ventilation without extracorporeal support was 57% at 1 year and escalating therapy and higher simplified acute physiology (SAPS) scores were associated with worse outcome [35]. Recently, there has been increasing experience with extracorporeal support as an alternative to mechanical ventilation which allows the candidate to be awake, non-intubated, and participate in physical therapy while awaiting transplantation [36, 37]. Both veno-venous and veno-arterial ECMO have been employed in this group [38]. In addition, ECMO has also been used successfully for patients with right heart failure from pulmonary hypertension [39]. There has also been experience with a pumpless form of ECS called Novalung that has primarily been employed in cases of refractory hypercapnia in patients awaiting lung transplantation. ECMO also plays a role posttransplant for the treatment of severe PGD [40]. An analysis of UNOS registry from 1987 to 2008 showed that unadjusted survival of transplant recipients who had received mechanical ventilation, ECMO, and no support at 1 year was 62, 50, and 79%, respectively. The authors concluded that while transplantation is worse after mechanical support, it is not prohibitively so and additional risk factors should be considered in deciding to list candidates for transplant. Of note, patients with interstitial lung disease with acute hypoxemic respiratory failure who were treated with mechanical ventilation and ECMO support who were deemed not a candidate for lung transplant have extremely poor prognosis with mortality of 93% [41].

In our lung transplant program, 22 patients received ECMO support as bridge to lung transplantation between February 2012 and October of 2015. The most common recipient diagnosis was acute IPF exacerbation in 18 of 22 listed patients. The average ECMO duration was 15.6 ± 14 days (range 1–60 days). All patients received veno-venous ECMO except for three patients who required VA ECMO for hemodynamic instability and suboptimal oxygenation with VV ECMO. The mean lung allocation score was 89 ± 5. Nine of 22 patients received double lung transplantation and one patient received combined heart lung transplantation. The duration of mechanical ventilation posttransplant was 27 ± 26 days, and length of ICU and hospital stay were 32 ± 16 and 58 ± 33 days, respectively. The 1-year survival was 100%. We believed that ECMO is an acceptable option as a bridge to lung transplantation in select group of patients with severe hypoxemic respiratory failure who failed mechanical ventilation. Its major limitation is finding an appropriate donor organ before the onset of ECMO-related complications. In our experience, factors that may affect difficulty in locating an appropriate donor include small stature, high panel reactive antibodies, and blood type B and AB.

Operative Considerations

Type of Procedure

Single versus Double Lung Transplant

In general practice, there is a preference for bilateral lung transplant when possible, although the clinical benefit of two versus one lung is controversial. An analysis of UNOS registry showed no survival benefit for single versus bilateral lung transplantation when adjusted for baseline differences in COPD patients after the LAS era. Interestingly, those receiving a bilateral transplant seemed to do worse their first year with a higher incidence of primary graft failure whereas those with a single lung transplant had an overall shorter median survival with a higher incidence of death from cancer [42]. Often single lung recipients continue to experience problems from the progressive pathology of the remaining lung. However, issues such as organ shortage, donor and recipient characteristics sometimes necessitate a unilateral lung transplant. A retrospective review of the OPTN database from 2005 to 2007 showed that patients listed for bilateral lung transplant were more likely to die on the transplant list and less likely to receive a transplant [43]. One analysis of UNOS showed that younger patients tended to have better survival with a single lung transplant; however, there was no difference when adjusted for survival at 1-month posttransplant [44]. A retrospective series found that scleroderma patients tended to perform better at 1 year with bilateral lung transplantation; however, this difference was not significant [45].

In the case of concurrent pulmonary hypertension, combined heart–lung transplantation has also been performed. In general, reasons to consider a combined heart–lung transplant over a lung transplant would be irreversible myocardial dysfunction or congenital defects with irreparable valvular or chamber defects in conjunction with lung disease. Most patients with secondary hypertension related to lung disease do well with just lung transplantation with the expectation that the right ventricle will recover provided there is no infarct or fibrotic change [1]. One group found that bilateral lung transplant recipients had similar survival to those with heart–lung transplant with the caveat that sicker patients were preferentially given a heart–lung transplant [46]. Patients with right heart failure who received single lung transplantation tended to have worse outcomes due to reperfusion injury of the transplanted lung and higher incidence of primary graft dysfunction, but it can be accomplished successfully [47]. There is even a case report of a child in Japan who received a living-donor single-lobe lung transplantation for PAH with good graft function 6 years posttransplant [48]. In our center, there has been success with single lung transplant in patients with mild to moderately elevated pulmonary pressures (MAP <35 mmHg) provided the transplanted lung is slightly larger.

In the case of coronary artery disease or valvular defects, concurrent cardiac surgery at the time of lung transplantation is an alternative. Options include a surgical bypass at the time of transplantation or stent with a period of antiplatelet therapy prior to transplantation. In general, PCI is reserved for single lung transplant recipients whose coronary anatomy may not be accessible through a unilateral thoracotomy whereas double lung transplant recipients receive bypass surgery; however, this decision generally requires an individualized multidisciplinary discussion. Single-center retrospective experiences show that both approaches result in comparable outcomes posttransplant in the appropriately selected patient [49–51], although concurrent cardiac surgery may be associated with longer ICU stays and prolonged mechanical ventilation postoperatively [50, 51]. Interestingly, one group noted that long-term freedom from atrial fibrillation more commonly occurs after double than single lung transplant [52].

Posttransplant Considerations

Immunosuppression

The current era of transplantation is made possible by the advances in immunomodulation. Immunosuppressive medications posttransplant consist of induction medications given at the time of surgery and maintenance therapy that is gradually introduced and maintained for the duration of the allograft. Currently, the main induction medications may include a CD-52 antibody named alemtuzumab (Campath) and an anti-IL-2 receptor antibody named basiliximab (Simulect) that are given in conjunction with high-dose corticosteroids. Postoperatively, maintenance immunosuppression is maintained with a three-drug regimen, the backbone of which is a calcineurin inhibitor combined with prednisone, and an antimetabolite [53].

Primary Graft Dysfunction

Primary graft dysfunction (PGD) after lung transplantation is defined as noncardiogenic pulmonary edema occurring within the first 72 h after surgery (Table 5.2). PGD is the leading cause of early posttransplant mortality [54] and is associated

Table 5.2 Grades of primary graft dysfunction

Grade 0	PaO_2/FIO_2 ratio > 300 mmHg, no radiographic evidence of edema
Grade 1	PaO_2/FIO_2 ratio > 300 mmHg, radiographic evidence of edema on CXR
Grade 2	PaO_2/FIO_2 ratio—200–300 mmHg, radiographic evidence of edema on CXR
Grade 3	PaO_2/FIO_2 ratio < 200 mmHg, radiographic evidence of edema on CXR

with increased long-term mortality [28] and long-term rejection [55]. The risk factors vary between studies and many have been inconsistently identified, but common donor risk factors include older donor age and long ischemic time. Commonly implicated recipient risk factors in most studies included elevated mean pulmonary artery pressures and diagnosis of diffuse parenchymal lung disease [28, 54, 56]. The strongest data appears to support recipient pulmonary hypertension as a risk factor; with risk increasing with higher pulmonary pressures [57]. Interestingly, elevated pulmonary artery pressures may also contribute to graft dysfunction of renal transplants recipients [58].

Infection

After PGD, non-CMV infection is a major cause of death in the first month and year posttransplant [59]. Infection can be acquired from the donor, the hospital, or can be reactivation of latent recipient infection. One retrospective series found a donor infection rate of 52%, divided between graft colonization, contamination of preservation fluids, and donor bacteremia in order of prevalence. Despite such frequent contamination, the clinical infection rate was 7.6%, of which the majority was from failure of their prophylaxis regimen [60]. Lung transplant recipients experience one of the highest rates of invasive aspergillosis of the solid organ transplants [61], and routine antifungal prophylaxis is an essential part of posttransplant care. However, significant variation exists in the type and length of regimens [62]. Unlike bacterial infections that appear rapidly, invasive fungal infections tend to occur 3 months after transplant [63]. Lung transplant also carries a higher risk of reactivation tuberculosis as compared with other solid organ recipients, which often carries a higher mortality due to delayed diagnosis and difficulty with regimen selection and adherence [64].

CMV is one of the most common and important causes of posttransplant infection and complications. Pretransplant donor and recipient CMV antibodies are key predictors of subsequent infection and therefore of long-term survival and rejection [65–67]. Survival stratified by CMV status is the poorest when the donor is positive for CMV regardless of the recipient's status, and best when neither the donor nor recipient is positive for CMV. Standard early prophylaxis with antivirals leads to improved outcomes and extra screening of blood transfusions is required for recipients who are CMV negative [68, 69]. Late CMV disease may occur after discontinuation of prophylaxis and does contribute to increased mortality and graft loss in all solid organ transplants [70, 71]. There are two main strategies regarding CMV management posttransplant, one of universal prophylaxis and one of routine surveillance and preemptive therapy. Expert consensus favors universal prophylaxis in high-risk patients, defined as donor positive/recipient negative patients, due to better graft survival and clinical outcomes in small comparison studies [65]. Resistant CMV infections tend to manifest as tissue invasion rather than viremia and cannot necessarily be detected with serum viral loads. Resistance is most commonly conferred by UL97 kinase mutations that confer ganciclovir resistance, whereas the UL54 DNA polymerase mutation may confer resistance to all known antivirals.

Allograft Dysfunction

Acute lung rejection is classified as either cellular or humoral rejection and typically occurs commonly within the first 6 months but can occur any time posttransplant. Since clinical findings of rejection are nonspecific, diagnosis depends upon transbronchial biopsy and histologic evidence of acute rejection. Acute cellular rejection has a well-established histologic grading system; however, antibody-mediated rejection is more difficult to establish histologically and largely depends on evidence of rising titers of donor-specific antibodies, positive C4d stain on biopsy, and evidence of allograft dysfunction. Treatments of acute rejection include high-dose corticosteroids and adjustment of immunosuppressive medications.

Obliterative bronchiolitis (OB), a form of chronic rejection, is a major limitation for prolonged survival after lung transplantation. Histologically, OB is characterized by fibrous obliteration of the small airways and manifest clinically as progressive airflow obstruction known as bronchiolitis obliterans syndrome (BOS). Several risk factors, namely, primary graft dysfunction, CMV mismatch, presence of donor-specific HLA antibodies, recurrent acute cellular rejections, and gastroesophageal reflux have been implicated in the development of OB. Recently, restrictive allograft syndrome, a form of chronic allograft dysfunction that is characterized by simultaneous decline in both FVC and FEV1, and fibrotic changes on the upper lobe with associated bronchiectasis is increasingly recognized, accounting for 25 to 35% of chronic lung allograft dysfunction [72, 73]. Chronic lung allograft dysfunction (CLAD) is a new term to encompass the different chronic rejection phenotype. Obstructive CLAD and restrictive CLAD are used to described BOS and restrictive allograft syndrome, respectively [74]. Why some patients develop obstructive while others develop restrictive CLAD is unclear. Unfortunately, there is no effective therapy for CLAD. Some treatments that may lead to stabilization or partial recovery of lung function include escalation of immune-modulating agents, chronic macrolide treatment, aggressive treatment of gastroesophageal reflux disease including fundoplication, and photopheresis [75].

Lung Function and Exercise Capacity

Patients who received bilateral lung transplant, in the absence of early graft dysfunction or airway complications, will achieve a normal or near normal spirometry. Similarly single lung transplant recipients can also expect approximately 60–70% of predicted normal lung function. In patients with interstitial lung disease, the forced vital capacity at the time of lung transplantation is usually between 30 and 50% of predicted. Consequently, smaller donor lungs are often used and the improvement in posttransplant spirometry depends on the size of the donor lung [76]. On occasion, lobar lung transplant or reduction pneumoplasty can be performed to accommodate larger donor lung. This improvement in lung function after lung transplant usually peaked within 1 year postsurgery. However, despite normal lung function in patients with double lung transplant, the improvement in exercise capacity is similar to patients who received single lung transplant [77]. The suboptimal improvement in exercise capacity compared to normalization of the lung function after bilateral lung transplant has been attributed to myopathy associated with immune suppression medications principally calcineurin inhibitors. Patients are advised to maintain regular exercise program to maintain muscle strength and minimize the effect of drug-induced myopathy.

Survival

Lung transplantation is the only therapy that has been shown to improve survival in patients with IPF. Overall, the median survival following lung transplantation is 5.7 years. The survival at 1 year is 80% and 5 year is 54%. Overall, the median survival for double lung transplant is significantly better compared to single lung transplant (7.1 vs. 4.5 years $p < 0.001$). The primary indication for lung transplant has significant impact on posttransplant survival. The median survival for patients with interstitial lung disease post lung transplant is lower compared to patients with COPD and cystic fibrosis.

Over the last several years, the number of double lung transplant performed worldwide is increasing while the number of single lung transplants performed has plateaued. This is due in part to the better long-term survival conferred by double versus single lung transplant especially in younger recipients. The perceived survival benefit of double versus single lung transplant recipients may in part due to patient selection since younger and healthier patients often received double lung transplant. In recent analysis of the UNOS registry data after the implementation of the lung allocation score, and adjusted for propensity score, double lung transplant was associated with better graft function and survival when compared to single lung transplant in patients with idiopathic pulmonary fibrosis [78]. In contrast, earlier analysis of the same database that included the pre-LAS data that there is no survival advantage with double compared to single lung transplant due to higher hazard ratio for death within the first year posttransplant [42]. Interestingly, there was no difference in survival at 5 years between single and double lung transplant in patients with COPD [78]. The issue with single versus double lung transplant goes beyond survival advantage given the scarcity of the donor organ and the wait-list death between 10 and 20%. In most transplant programs, double is preferred over single lung transplant in younger patients (<60 years old), in patients with moderate to severe pulmonary hypertension, and in the presence of chronic infection related to bronchiectasis.

In patients with CTD-ILD, extrapulmonary involvement is common and can lead to denial of lung transplant as treatment option. This is especially true in patients with systemic sclerosis with esophageal involvement. Recurrent aspirations can lead to early graft dysfunction and obliterative bronchiolitis. In a systematic review of posttransplant outcome in patients with scleroderma, the reported survival range at 1 (59–93%) and 3 years (46–79%) is wide and likely reflect differences in patient selection, the extent and severity of extrapulmonary comorbidities, and posttransplant care among centers. Recurrence of pulmonary fibrosis in the lung allograft has not been reported. The authors concluded that the short- and intermediate-term survival in patients with scleroderma is comparable to patients with idiopathic pulmonary hypertension and other forms of interstitial lung disease [79]. Other investigators reported no difference in survival in patients with interstitial lung disease associated with rheumatoid arthritis and scleroderma compared to patients with IPF [80].

Using the UNOS registry data covering the period of 1991–2009, the survival outcome in CTD-associated ILD was compared to patients with IPF and COPD. The most common ILD-associated CTD included scleroderma (61%), rheumatoid arthritis (13%), polymyositis/dermatomyositis (12%), mixed connective tissue disease (8%), systemic lupus erythematosus (4%), and Sjogren's disease (2%). The 1-year survival for ILD-CTD (73%) was significantly lower compared to IPF (78%) and COPD (83%). The difference in survival was accounted by an increase in mortality at 6 months with a relative risk of 1.7 compared to COPD. The survival advantage narrows at 5 years (CTD-ILD–46%, IPF–47%, and COPD 50%). The increase in mortality within the first year was thought to be due to increased risk of graft dysfunction due to the presence of comorbidities particularly esophageal dysmotility, gastroesophageal reflux disease, neuromuscular weakness, and thromboembolism. Other preoperative factors such as the use of prednisone and other immune suppression therapy may contribute to higher initial perioperative risk. Of note, the rate of acute graft rejection was not increased [81].

Quality of Life

Improvement in the quality of life is one of the major goals of lung transplantation. The significant improvement in lung function after lung transplantation allows resumption of normal life style in majority of lung transplant recipients. Indeed, lung transplantation improves health-related quality of life in patients with end-stage lung disease [82]. In a recent prospective cohort study evaluating the impact of age and diagnosis on health-related quality-of-life benefit following lung transplantation, Singer and others found that older recipients also achieved substantial gain in quality of life after lung transplantation and that age accounts for minimal variability in quality-adjusted survival. Recipient with cystic fibrosis has the highest gain in health-related quality of life, followed by patients with chronic obstructive lung disease and interstitial lung disease [25]. Overall, the improvement in health-related quality of life after lung transplantation is several magnitudes higher compared to other therapies for advanced lung disease including lung volume reduction surgery.

Conclusion

Lung transplantation is an important treatment option for patients with interstitial lung disease, especially with few available alternatives. Though significant advances have been made in the science of transplantation, it remains a complex procedure with many complications and considerations.

References

1. Weill D, Benden C, Corris PA, Dark JH, Davis RD, Keshavjee S, et al. A consensus document for the selection of lung transplant candidates: 2014—an update from the pulmonary transplantation council of the international society for heart and lung transplantation. J Heart Lung Transplant. 2015;34(1):1–15.
2. Shorr AF, Davies DB, Nathan SD. Predicting mortality in patients with sarcoidosis awaiting lung transplantation. Chest J. 2003;124(3):922–8.
3. Patterson KC, Strek ME. Pulmonary fibrosis in sarcoidosis. Clinical features and outcomes. Ann Am Thorac Soc. 2013;10(4):362–70.
4. Shorr AF, Helman DL, Davies DB, Nathan SD. Sarcoidosis, race, and short-term outcomes following lung transplantation. Chest J. 2004;125(3):990–6.
5. Arcasoy SM, Christie JD, Pochettino A, Rosengard BR, Blumenthal NP, Bavaria JE, et al. Characteristics and outcomes of patients with sarcoidosis listed for lung transplantation. Chest J. 2001;120(3):873–80.
6. Shlobin OA, Nathan SD. Management of end-stage sarcoidosis: pulmonary hypertension and lung transplantation. Eur Respir J. 2012;39(6):1520–33. doi:10.1183/09031936.00175511.
7. Lynch JP, Belperio JA, Saggar R, Fishbein MC, Saggar R. Pulmonary hypertension complicating connective tissue disease. Semin Respir Crit Care Med. 2013;34(5):581–99.
8. Shitrit D, Amital A, Peled N, Raviv Y, Medalion B, Saute M, et al. Lung transplantation in patients with scleroderma: case series, review of the literature, and criteria for transplantation. Clin Transplant. 2009;23(2):178–83.
9. Schachna L, Medsger TA, Dauber JH, Wigley FM, Braunstein NA, White B, et al. Lung transplantation in scleroderma compared with idiopathic pulmonary fibrosis and idiopathic pulmonary arterial hypertension. Arthritis Rheum. 2006;54(12):3954–61.
10. Saggar R, Khanna D, Furst DE, Belperio JA, Park GS, Weigt SS, et al. Systemic sclerosis and bilateral lung transplantation: a single centre experience. Eur Respir J. 2010;36(4):893–900. doi:10.1183/09031936.00139809.

11. Sottile PD, Iturbe D, Katsumoto TR, Connolly MK, Collard HR, Leard LA, et al. Outcomes in systemic sclerosis-related lung disease after lung transplantation. Transplantation. 2013;95(7):975–80. doi:10.1097/TP.0b013e3182845f23.
12. De Cruz S, Ross D. Lung transplantation in patients with scleroderma. Curr Opin Rheumatol. 2013;25(6):714–8. doi:10.1097/01.bor.0000434670.39773.a8.
13. Judge EP, Fabre A, Adamali HI, Egan JJ. Acute exacerbations and pulmonary hypertension in advanced idiopathic pulmonary fibrosis. Eur Respir J. 2012;40(1):93–100. doi:10.1183/09031936.00115511.
14. Andersen CU, Mellemkjær S, Hilberg O, Nielsen-Kudsk JE, Simonsen U, Bendstrup E. Pulmonary hypertension in interstitial lung disease: prevalence, prognosis and 6 min walk test. Respir Med. 2012;106(6):875–82.
15. Behr J, Ryu JH. Pulmonary hypertension in interstitial lung disease. Eur Respir J. 2008;31(6):1357–67. doi:10.1183/09031936.00171307.
16. Lettieri CJ, Nathan SD, Barnett SD, Ahmad S, Shorr AF. Prevalence and outcomes of pulmonary arterial hypertension in advanced idiopathic pulmonary fibrosis. Chest J. 2006;129(3):746–52.
17. Shorr AF, Wainright JL, Cors CS, Lettieri CJ, Nathan SD. Pulmonary hypertension in patients with pulmonary fibrosis awaiting lung transplant. Eur Respir J. 2007;30(4):715–21. doi: 09031936.00107206 [pii]
18. Corte TJ, Wort SJ, Gatzoulis MA, Engel R, Giannakoulas G, Macdonald PM, et al. Elevated brain natriuretic peptide predicts mortality in interstitial lung disease. Eur Respir J. 2010;36(4):819–25. doi:10.1183/09031936.00173509.
19. Corte TJ, Wort SJ, Gatzoulis MA, Macdonald P, Hansell DM, Wells AU. Pulmonary vascular resistance predicts early mortality in patients with diffuse fibrotic lung disease and suspected pulmonary hypertension. Thorax. 2009;64(10):883–8. doi:10.1136/thx.2008.112847.
20. Chung L, Liu J, Parsons L, Hassoun PM, McGoon M, Badesch DB, et al. Characterization of connective tissue disease-associated pulmonary arterial hypertension from REVEAL: identifying systemic sclerosis as a unique phenotype. Chest J. 2010;138(6):1383–94.
21. King TE Jr, Behr J, Brown KK, du Bois RM, Lancaster L, de Andrade JA, et al. BUILD-1: a randomized placebo-controlled trial of Bosentan in idiopathic pulmonary fibrosis. Am J Respir Crit Care Med. 2008;177(1):75–81.
22. Raghu G, Behr J, Brown KK, Egan JJ, Kawut SM, Flaherty KR, et al. Treatment of idiopathic pulmonary fibrosis with Ambrisentan: a parallel, randomized trial. Ann Intern Med. 2013;158(9):641–9.
23. Idiopathic Pulmonary Fibrosis Clinical Research Network. A controlled trial of sildenafil in advanced idiopathic pulmonary fibrosis. N Engl J Med. 2010;2010(363):620–8.
24. Hassoun PM. Pulmonary arterial hypertension complicating connective tissue diseases. Semin Respir Crit Care Med. 2009;30(4):429–39.
25. Singer LG, Chowdhury NA, Faughnan ME, Granton J, Keshavjee S, Marras TK, et al. Effects of recipient age and diagnosis on health-related quality-of-life benefit of lung transplantation. Am J Respir Crit Care Med. 2015;192(8):965–73.
26. Genao L, Whitson H, Zaas D, Sanders L, Schmader K. Functional status after lung transplantation in older adults in the Post-Allocation score era. Am J Transplant. 2013;13(1):157–66.
27. Lederer DJ, Wilt JS, D'Ovidio F, Bacchetta MD, Shah L, Ravichandran S, et al. Obesity and underweight are associated with an increased risk of death after lung transplantation. Am J Respir Crit Care Med. 2009;180(9):887–95.
28. Diamond JM, Lee JC, Kawut SM, Shah RJ, Localio AR, Bellamy SL, et al. Clinical risk factors for primary graft dysfunction after lung transplantation. Am J Respir Crit Care Med. 2013;187(5):527–34.
29. Kanasky WF, Anton SD, Rodrigue JR, Perri MG, Szwed T, Baz MA. Impact of body weight on long-term survival after lung transplantation. Chest J. 2002;121(2):401–6.
30. King TE Jr, Bradford WZ, Castro-Bernardini S, Fagan EA, Glaspole I, Glassberg MK, et al. A phase 3 trial of pirfenidone in patients with idiopathic pulmonary fibrosis. N Engl J Med. 2014;370(22):2083–92.

31. Richeldi L, du Bois RM, Raghu G, Azuma A, Brown KK, Costabel U, et al. Efficacy and safety of nintedanib in idiopathic pulmonary fibrosis. N Engl J Med. 2014;370(22):2071–82.
32. Liu H, Drew P, Cheng Y, Visner GA. Pirfenidone inhibits inflammatory responses and ameliorates allograft injury in a rat lung transplant model. J Thorac Cardiovasc Surg. 2005;130(3):852–8.
33. Riddell P, Minnis P, Ging P, Egan J. P242 pirfenidone as a bridge to lung transplantation in patients with progressive IPF. Thorax. 2014;69(Suppl 2):A183.
34. Patterson C, Durheim M, Palmer S, Copeland CF, Snyder L. A national survey of practice and perceptions regarding anti-fibrotic medication in lung transplant recipients. J Heart Lung Transplant. 2016;35(4):S226–7.
35. Gottlieb J, Warnecke G, Hadem J, Dierich M, Wiesner O, Fühner T, et al. Outcome of critically ill lung transplant candidates on invasive respiratory support. Intensive Care Med. 2012;38(6):968–75.
36. Fuehner T, Kuehn C, Hadem J, Wiesner O, Gottlieb J, Tudorache I, et al. Extracorporeal membrane oxygenation in awake patients as bridge to lung transplantation. Am J Respir Crit Care Med. 2012;185:763–8.
37. Rehder KJ, Turner DA, Hartwig MG, Williford WL, Bonadonna D, Walczak RJ Jr, et al. Active rehabilitation during extracorporeal membrane oxygenation as a bridge to lung transplantation. Respir Care. 2013;58(8):1291–8. doi:10.4187/respcare.02155.
38. Olsson KM, Simon A, Strueber M, Hadem J, Wiesner O, Gottlieb J, et al. Extracorporeal membrane oxygenation in nonintubated patients as bridge to lung transplantation. Am J Transplant. 2010;10(9):2173–8.
39. Rosenzweig EB, Brodie D, Abrams DC, Agerstrand CL, Bacchetta M. Extracorporeal membrane oxygenation as a novel bridging strategy for acute right heart failure in group 1 pulmonary arterial hypertension. ASAIO J. 2014;60(1):129–33. doi:10.1097/MAT.0000000000000021.
40. Fischer S, Bohn D, Rycus P, Pierre AF, de Perrot M, Waddell TK, et al. Extracorporeal membrane oxygenation for primary graft dysfunction after lung transplantation: analysis of the extracorporeal life support organization (ELSO) registry. J Heart Lung Transplant. 2007;26(5):472–7.
41. Trudzinski FC, Kaestner F, Schäfers H, Fähndrich S, Seiler F, Böhmer P, et al. Outcome of patients with interstitial lung disease treated with extracorporeal membrane oxygenation for acute respiratory failure. Am J Respir Crit Care Med. 2016;193(5):527–33.
42. Thabut G, Christie JD, Ravaud P, Castier Y, Dauriat G, Jebrak G, et al. Survival after bilateral versus single-lung transplantation for idiopathic pulmonary fibrosis. Ann Intern Med. 2009;151(11):767–74.
43. Nathan SD, Shlobin OA, Ahmad S, Burton NA, Barnett SD, Edwards E. Comparison of wait times and mortality for idiopathic pulmonary fibrosis patients listed for single or bilateral lung transplantation. J Heart Lung Transplant. 2010;29(10):1165–71.
44. Meyer DM, Edwards LB, Torres F, Jessen ME, Novick RJ. Impact of recipient age and procedure type on survival after lung transplantation for pulmonary fibrosis. Ann Thorac Surg. 2005;79(3):950–7.
45. Massad MG, Powell CR, Kpodonu J, Tshibaka C, Hanhan Z, Snow NJ, et al. Outcomes of lung transplantation in patients with scleroderma. World J Surg. 2005;29(11):1510–5.
46. Fadel E, Mercier O, Mussot S, Leroy-Ladurie F, Cerrina J, Chapelier A, et al. Long-term outcome of double-lung and heart-lung transplantation for pulmonary hypertension: a comparative retrospective study of 219 patients. Eur J Cardiothorac Surg. 2010;38(3):277–84. doi:10.1016/j.ejcts.2010.02.039.
47. Kramer MR, Valantine HA, Marshall SE, Starnes VA, Theodore J. Recovery of the right ventricle after single-lung transplantation in pulmonary hypertension. Am J Cardiol. 1994;73(7):494–500.
48. Toyooka S, Sano Y, Yamane M, Oto T, Okazaki M, Kusano KF, et al. Long-term follow-up of living-donor single lobe transplantation for idiopathic pulmonary arterial hypertension in a child. J Thorac Cardiovasc Surg. 2008;135(2):451–2.

49. Sherman W, Rabkin DG, Ross D, Saggar R, Lynch JP, Belperio J, et al. Lung transplantation and coronary artery disease. Ann Thorac Surg. 2011;92(1):303–8.
50. Castleberry A, Martin J, Osho A, Hartwig M, Hashmi Z, Zanotti G, et al. Coronary revascularization in lung transplant recipients with concomitant coronary artery disease. Am J Transplant. 2013;13(11):2978–88.
51. Lee R, Meyers BF, Sundt TM, Trulock EP, Patterson GA. Concomitant coronary artery revascularization to allow successful lung transplantation in selected patients with coronary artery disease. J Thorac Cardiovasc Surg. 2002;124(6):1250–1.
52. Lee R, Meyers BF, Sundt TM, Trulock EP, Patterson GA. Atrial fibrillation following lung transplantation: double but not single lung transplant is associated with long-term freedom from paroxysmal atrial fibrillation. Eur Heart J. 2010;31(22):2774–82. doi:10.1093/eurheartj/ehq224.
53. Thompson ML, Flynn JD, Clifford TM. Pharmacotherapy of lung transplantation: an overview. J Pharm Pract. 2013;26(1):5–13. doi:10.1177/0897190012466048.
54. Lee JC, Christie JD. Primary graft dysfunction. Proc Am Thorac Soc. 2009;6(1):39–46.
55. Daud SA, Yusen RD, Meyers BF, Chakinala MM, Walter MJ, Aloush AA, et al. Impact of immediate primary lung allograft dysfunction on bronchiolitis obliterans syndrome. Am J Respir Crit Care Med. 2007;175(5):507–13.
56. Whitson BA, Nath DS, Johnson AC, et al. Risk factors for primary graft dysfunction after lung transplantation. J Thorac Cardiovasc Surg. 2006;131(1):73–80.
57. Fang A, Studer S, Kawut SM, Ahya VN, Lee J, Wille K, et al. Elevated pulmonary artery pressure is a risk factor for primary graft dysfunction following lung transplantation for idiopathic pulmonary fibrosis. Chest J. 2011;139(4):782–7.
58. Zlotnick DM, Axelrod DA, Chobanian MC, Friedman S, Brown J, Catherwood E, et al. Non-invasive detection of pulmonary hypertension prior to renal transplantation is a predictor of increased risk for early graft dysfunction. Nephrol Dial Transplant. 2010;25(9):3090–6. doi:10.1093/ndt/gfq141.
59. Yusen RD, Edwards LB, Kucheryavaya AY, Benden C, Dipchand AI, Goldfarb SB, et al. The registry of the international society for heart and lung transplantation: thirty-second official adult lung and heart-lung transplantation report—2015; focus theme: early graft failure. J Heart Lung Transplant. 2015;34(10):1264–77.
60. Ruiz I, Gavalda J, Monforte V, Len O, Román A, Bravo C, et al. Donor-to-host transmission of bacterial and fungal infections in lung transplantation. Am J Transplant. 2006;6(1):178–82.
61. Husain S, Paterson D, Studer S, Pilewski J, Crespo M, Zaldonis D, et al. Voriconazole prophylaxis in lung transplant recipients. Am J Transplant. 2006;6(12):3008–16.
62. Neoh C, Snell G, Kotsimbos T, Levvey B, Morrissey CO, Slavin M, et al. Antifungal prophylaxis in lung transplantation—a world-wide survey. Am J Transplant. 2011;11(2):361–6.
63. Pappas PG, Alexander BD, Andes DR, Hadley S, Kauffman CA, Freifeld A, et al. Invasive fungal infections among organ transplant recipients: results of the transplant-associated infection surveillance network (TRANSNET). Clin Infect Dis. 2010;50(8):1101–11. doi:10.1086/651262.
64. Torre-Cisneros J, Doblas A, Aguado JM, San Juan R, Blanes M, Montejo M, et al. Tuberculosis after solid-organ transplant: incidence, risk factors, and clinical characteristics in the RESITRA (Spanish network of infection in transplantation) cohort. Clin Infect Dis. 2009;48(12):1657–65. doi:10.1086/599035.
65. Kotton CN, Kumar D, Caliendo AM, Asberg A, Chou S, Snydman DR, et al. International consensus guidelines on the management of cytomegalovirus in solid organ transplantation. Transplantation. 2010;89(7):779–95. doi:10.1097/TP.0b013e3181cee42f.
66. Snyder LD, Finlen-Copeland CA, Turbyfill WJ, Howell D, Willner DA, Palmer SM. Cytomegalovirus pneumonitis is a risk for bronchiolitis obliterans syndrome in lung transplantation. Am J Respir Crit Care Med. 2010;181(12):1391–6.
67. Christie JD, Edwards LB, Kucheryavaya AY, Benden C, Dipchand AI, Dobbels F, et al. The registry of the international society for heart and lung transplantation: 29th adult lung and heart-lung transplant report-2012. J Heart Lung Transplant. 2012;31(10):1073–86. doi:10.1016/j.healun.2012.08.004.

68. Humar A, Limaye AP, Blumberg EA, Hauser IA, Vincenti F, Jardine AG, et al. Extended valganciclovir prophylaxis in D+/R− kidney transplant recipients is associated with long-term reduction in cytomegalovirus disease: two-year results of the IMPACT study. Transplantation. 2010;90(12):1427–31.
69. Razonable RR, Humar A. Cytomegalovirus in solid organ transplantation. Am J Transplant. 2013;13(s4):93–106.
70. Limaye AP, Bakthavatsalam R, Kim HW, Randolph SE, Halldorson JB, Healey PJ, et al. Impact of cytomegalovirus in organ transplant recipients in the era of antiviral prophylaxis. Transplantation. 2006;81(12):1645–52. doi:10.1097/01.tp.0000226071.12562.1a.
71. Arthurs SK, Eid AJ, Pedersen RA, Kremers WK, Cosio FG, Patel R, et al. Delayed-onset primary cytomegalovirus disease and the risk of allograft failure and mortality after kidney transplantation. Clin Infect Dis. 2008;46(6):840–6. doi:10.1086/528718.
72. Sato M, Waddell TK, Wagnetz U, Roberts HC, Hwang DM, Haroon A, et al. Restrictive allograft syndrome (RAS): a novel form of chronic lung allograft dysfunction. J Heart Lung Transplant. 2011;30(7):735–42.
73. Ofek E, Sato M, Saito T, Wagnetz U, Roberts HC, Chaparro C, et al. Restrictive allograft syndrome post lung transplantation is characterized by pleuroparenchymal fibroelastosis. Mod Pathol. 2013;26(3):350–6.
74. Vos R, Verleden SE, Verleden GM. Chronic lung allograft dysfunction: evolving practice. Curr Opin Organ Transplant. 2015;20(5):483–91.
75. Belperio JA, Weigt SS, Fishbein MC, Lynch JP III. Chronic lung allograft rejection: mechanisms and therapy. Proc Am Thorac Soc. 2009;6(1):108–21.
76. Meyers BF, Lynch JP, Trulock EP, Guthrie T, Cooper JD, Patterson GA. Single versus bilateral lung transplantation for idiopathic pulmonary fibrosis: a ten-year institutional experience. J Thorac Cardiovasc Surg. 2000;120(1):99–107.
77. Bartels MN, Armstrong HF, Gerardo RE, Layton AM, Emmert-Aronson BO, Sonett JR, et al. Evaluation of pulmonary function and exercise performance by cardiopulmonary exercise testing before and after lung transplantation. Chest. 2011;140(6):1604–11.
78. Schaffer JM, Singh SK, Reitz BA, Zamanian RT, Mallidi HR. Single- vs double-lung transplantation in patients with chronic obstructive pulmonary disease and idiopathic pulmonary fibrosis since the implementation of lung allocation based on medical need. JAMA. 2015;313(9):936–48.
79. Khan IY, Singer LG, de Perrot M, Granton JT, Keshavjee S, Chau C, et al. Survival after lung transplantation in systemic sclerosis. A systematic review. Respir Med. 2013;107(12):2081–7.
80. Yazdani A, Singer LG, Strand V, Gelber AC, Williams L, Mittoo S. Survival and quality of life in rheumatoid arthritis–associated interstitial lung disease after lung transplantation. J Heart Lung Transplant. 2014;33(5):514–20.
81. Takagishi T, Ostrowski R, Alex C, Rychlik K, Pelletiere K, Tehrani R. Survival and extrapulmonary course of connective tissue disease after lung transplantation. J Clin Rheumatol. 2012;18(6):283–9.
82. Studer SM, Levy RD, McNeil K, Orens JB. Lung transplant outcomes: a review of survival, graft function, physiology, health-related quality of life and cost-effectiveness. Eur Respir J. 2004;24(4):674–85.
83. Gries CJ, Mulligan MS, Edelman JD, Raghu G, Curtis JR, Goss CH. Lung allocation score for lung transplantation: impact on disease severity and survival. Chest J. 2007;132(6):1954–61.
84. Valapour M, Skeans MA, Smith JM, Edwards LB, Cherikh WS, Callahan ER, et al. Lung. Am J Transplant. 2016;16:141–68.
85. Ley B, Ryerson CJ, Vittinghoff E, Ryu JH, Tomassetti S, Lee JS, et al. A multidimensional index and staging system for idiopathic pulmonary fibrosis. Ann Intern Med. 2012;156(10):684–91.
86. Wells AU, Desai SR, Rubens MB, Goh NS, Cramer D, Nicholson AG, et al. Idiopathic pulmonary fibrosis: a composite physiologic index derived from disease extent observed by computed tomography. Am J Respir Crit Care Med. 2003;167(7):962–9.
87. Marques MB, Tuncer HH. Photopheresis in solid organ transplant rejection. J Clin Apher. 2006;21(1):72–7.

Chapter 6
Pulmonary Hypertension in Idiopathic Interstitial Pneumonias

Simon Bax, Athol Wells, Laura Price, and John Wort

Introduction

The classification of the idiopathic interstitial pneumonias (IIPs) has recently been updated by the ATS and ERS [1] (Table 6.1). Idiopathic pulmonary fibrosis (IPF) is the most common of the IIPs, and data from existing registries suggest that IPF accounts for 17–37% of all interstitial lung disease (ILD) diagnoses [2, 3]. Although estimates of the true incidence and prevalence of IPF are hampered by different methodologies used in epidemiological studies. IPF is a heterogeneous disease with some patients experiencing slow progressive disease, others a much more rapidly progressive disease and others still experiencing periods of stability punctuated by accelerated decline within acute exacerbations. Median survival is just 2–3 years [4]. It is appreciated that the development of pulmonary hypertension (PH) within IPF is common and its development has a dramatic effect both on morbidity and mortality. The desire to improve prognosis and quality of life in patients with IIP-associated PH (IIP–PH) who unfortunately at present have no clinically proven intervention to do so drives clinical research within this difficult area. The study of PH within IIP has predominantly focused upon IPF or mixed patient groups with IIP (which are predominantly made up of IPF patients). Therefore, this chapter focuses predominantly on PH within the IPF population.

S. Bax, BSc, MBBS, MRCP
Royal Brompton Hospital, National Heart and Lung Institute, Imperial College London, London, UK

A. Wells, MBChB, MD, FRACP, FRCP, FRCR
Interstitial Lung Disease Unit, Royal Brompton Hospital, National Heart and Lung Institute, Imperial College London, London, UK

L. Price, BSc, MBChB, MRCP, PhD (✉) • J. Wort, MA, MBBS, PhD, FRCP, FFICM
Pulmonary Hypertension Service, Royal Brompton Hospital, National Heart and Lung Institute, Imperial College London, London, UK

R.P. Baughman et al. (eds.), *Pulmonary Hypertension and Interstitial Lung Disease*, DOI 10.1007/978-3-319-49918-5_6

Table 6.1 Revised ATS/ERS classification of idiopathic interstitial pneumonias [1]

Major idiopathic interstitial pneumonias
Idiopathic pulmonary fibrosis
Idiopathic nonspecific interstitial pneumonia
Respiratory bronchiolitis-interstitial lung disease
Desquamative interstitial pneumonia
Cryptogenic organising pneumonia
Acute interstitial pneumonias
Rare idiopathic interstitial pneumonias
Idiopathic lymphoid interstitial pneumonia
Idiopathic pleuroparenchymal fibroelastosis
Unclassifiable idiopathic interstitial pneumonia

Prevalence

The prevalence of PH in interstitial lung disease ILD is difficult to quantify, both in IPF and in other ILDs. In IPF, it varies greatly according to the severity of pulmonary fibrosis in studied cohorts, with a range of 10–78% in published series. Series with a higher prevalence, ranging from 30 to 45%, consist of reports in patients listed for lung transplantation [5–8], with the presence of PH rising from 38% at initial investigation to 78% at the time of transplantation [8]. By contrast, in the patient cohort enrolled in the ARTEMIS placebo-controlled trial of ambrisentan in mild-to-moderate IPF, right heart catheterisation disclosed that 10% of patients had PH, mostly categorised as Group 3 PH [9]. Thus, PH in IPF includes a subgroup in which PH is a manifestation of advanced ILD, a second subgroup in which PH can be viewed as disproportionate to the severity of ILD, and a significant proportion in which this distinction cannot be made with confidence. It is telling that in IPF, and in ILD in general, the presence of PH has no overall association with the severity of pulmonary function impairment or the severity of pulmonary fibrosis on computed tomography (CT) [5, 10, 11].

The prevalence of PH has not been studied in the other idiopathic interstitial pneumonias (IIPs), but relevant observations have been made in interstitial lung disease associated with connective tissue disease (CTD-ILD), a group of disorders in which all of the IIP histological patterns have been reported. In systemic sclerosis (SSc), the frequency of PH is strongly linked to autoantibody status. Disproportionate PH, akin to isolated PAH, is strongly associated with anti-centromere antibody positivity whereas PH secondary to extensive interstitial fibrosis occurs most often in SSc patients with anti-topoisomerase positivity [12]. This observation is highly relevant to IIPs other than IPF. A significant proportion of patients previously classified as having an IIP can be viewed as having an occult connective tissue disease ("interstitial pneumonitis with autoimmune features"), with the presence of disproportionate PH ("multi-compartment disease") contributing to the definition of this syndrome [13].

The importance of selection bias in influencing PH prevalence in IPF, other IIPs and ILDs in general cannot be overstated. In 246 consecutive Japanese patients with sarcoidosis, the prevalence of pulmonary artery systolic pressure (PASP) >40 mm Hg on Doppler echocardiography was only 5.6% [14] but in a cohort of sarcoidosis patients limited by chronic exertional dyspnoea, the mean pulmonary artery pressure (mPAP) at right heart study exceeded 25 mmHg in 47% of 53 patients [15]. This dichotomy applies also to IPF and other IIPs in the distinction between unselected patients and those with major exercise limitation.

Another important limitation in current prognostic and diagnostic PH series is that in advanced interstitial lung disease, a definitive diagnosis of IPF using current diagnostic guideline criteria cannot be made in a significant proportion of IPF patients. Current series can be subdivided into those containing patients with definite IPF (i.e. with the exclusion of many IPF patients not meeting formal diagnostic criteria) and those containing patients with "fibrotic IIP" (i.e. IPF in most cases, but with minority subgroups of fibrotic NSIP and unclassifiable fibrotic disease). Both approaches have merits and studies of both types are cited in this review.

Prognostic Significance

PH is a malignant prognostic determinant in ILDs, with outcomes studied most frequently in IPF. In an echocardiographic series, median survival was 4.7 years and 4.1 years in IPF patients with echocardiographic PASP of 0–34 mmHg and 35–49 mmHg, respectively, but was only 0.7 years in patients with PASP>50 mmHg [16]. In a cohort containing IPF patients listed for lung transplantation, mortality was 28.8% in those with PH at right heart study compared to 5.5% in those without PH [5]. PH is particularly frequent and has a very poor outcome when IPF coexists with emphysema, probably due to the combined impact of two processes and consequent overall severity of lung disease. In reports of patients with combined pulmonary fibrosis and emphysema, survival of only 30% at 1 year and very poor survival associated with a PASP>75 mmHg have been reported [17, 18].

In patients with IPF undergoing right heart catheterisation, short- not intermediate-term mortality was most strongly linked to increases in pulmonary vascular resistance (PVR) and was also strongly associated with increased mean pulmonary artery pressure and the severity of right ventricular dysfunction on echocardiography (but not to other echocardiographic variables) [19]. These observations were mirrored in a cohort of ILD patients, including a minority with IPF: early mortality was much more strongly linked to a marked increase in PVR than to any other variable at right heart catheterisation or on echocardiography [20]. Recently, increased pulmonary vascular resistance estimated by Doppler echocardiography has been shown to predict mortality in ILD patients [21].

The importance of recognising left heart disease as a contributor to PH has yet to be studied definitively in IPF and other IIPs. However, accumulated clinical experience and reported experience in sarcoidosis PH, taken together, indicate the likely prognostic significance of concurrent cardiac disease. In one sarcoidosis series, outcomes were significantly better in patients with PH due to left heart disease than in the remaining patients with PH, reflecting the efficacy of therapies used to treat left ventricular dysfunction and underlining the importance of distinguishing between these two major PH subgroups [22]. In IPF patients with PH associated with mild-to-moderate disease, an important minority subgroup has WHO Group 2 PH (i.e. PH associated with left heart disease) [23].

Mortality is linked, both in IPF and in other ILDs, to a number of non-invasive markers associated with PH, other than echocardiography. The prognostic significance of elevated brain natriuretic peptide (BNP) levels was first explored in 176 patients with a mixture of chronic pulmonary diseases including a large subset with ILDs of various types [24]. Severe PH (mPAP >35 mm Hg) was diagnosed in over 25% of cases: increasing BNP levels were a risk factor for mortality, independent of pulmonary function impairment or hypoxaemia. In a cohort of 90 patients with a mixture of ILDs, higher BNP concentrations were associated with increased mortality independent of age, gender and pulmonary function impairment [25]. In this study, patients with BNP $\geq$ 20 pmol/L had a 14-fold increase in mortality over patients with BNP < 4 pmol/L. In a review of 131 IPF patients undergoing echocardiography and BNP measurement, increased BNP levels were predictive of mortality with no independent added prognostic value provided by echocardiographic data [26]. It should be stressed, however, that this marker of PH is also a marker of cardiac disease in general, with increased mortality associated with elevated BNP levels in all three series likely to reflect the combined impact of PH and other forms of cardiac disease.

Pulmonary artery size on high resolution computed tomography (HRCT) appears to be a predictor of IPF mortality. In a population of 98 IPF patients, increases in the pulmonary artery diameter/ascending aorta diameter ratio (PA:A ratio) were associated with increased mortality [27]. Patients with a PA:A ratio >1 had a strikingly higher risk of death or transplant, with this threshold found to be an independent adverse prognostic indicator (hazard ratio approximately 4.0).

Pulmonary function variables influenced by the presence of PH also have major prognostic significance in IPF and in other ILDs. The malignant prognostic significance of resting hypoxia has long been recognised. More specific to PH is a reduction in DLco disproportionate to measurements of lung volume. In a fibrotic IIP series, baseline gas transfer coefficient levels (Kco, synonymous with DLco adjusted for VA) were associated with increased early and overall mortality [28]. In two fibrotic IIP series, a six-month decline in Kco was predictive of increased mortality, independent of FVC levels, in two fibrotic IIP series [28, 29] and was associated with an increased likelihood of the development of echocardiographic PH [28].

Severe desaturation during a six minute walk test has been associated with increased mortality in fibrotic IIP, with a desaturation threshold of 88% identified as a malignant prognostic determinant [30, 31]. Differences in mortality above and below this threshold appear to mirror differences in mortality in IPF patients with and without PH.

Diagnosis

The importance of right heart catheterisation (RHC) as a reference standard for the diagnosis of PH applies to PH in patients with ILD. The considerable variability between centres in the threshold for performing RHC is likely to reflect the absence of evidence of treatment benefits from targeted PH treatments in the context of ILD. However, the prognostic significance of proven PH in IPF and other ILDs may be highly influential in determining the timing and priority of lung transplantation. Furthermore, a definite PH diagnosis allows patients to be considered for enrolment in treatment trials or for consideration of targeted therapy on compassionate grounds and in these contexts, the identification of concurrent left heart disease has major management implications. For all these reasons, accurate algorithms are needed in which non-invasive evaluation leads to the appropriate use of diagnostic RHC. The difficulty confronting the ILD clinician is that no single non-invasive test is sufficiently accurate, in isolation, to provide a confident prediction of findings at RHC. Therefore, it is necessary to integrate findings from a number of tests before proceeding to invasive evaluation.

Correlations between echocardiographic findings and RHC data have been examined in a number of series. In IPF, depending upon the PASP threshold examined against RHC data, positive predictive values for PH vary between 35% and 65% (46% if PASP>50 mmHg) with negative predictive values ranging from 65 to 80%. The high false-positive rate indicates that echocardiographic PH is more likely to represent a true positive when the pretest likelihood is high and does not support the routine use of echocardiography at baseline in screening for PH [32]. This conclusion is compatible with echocardiographic-RHC correlations in the largest series published in chronic lung disease, including a large patient subset with a mixture of ILDs [7]. Of 374 patients referred for consideration of lung transplantation, 25% with measurable PASP were considered to have echocardiographic PH (PASP>45 mmHg). At RHC, it transpired that the diagnosis of PH was falsely positive in 48% and that on other, echocardiography overstated PASP by approximately 10 mmHg, although underestimation also occurred in a minority. These findings are broadly similar to those reported in SSc, the other ILD in which echocardiographic-RHC correlations have been examined. Importantly, a consistent finding in a number of reports is that echocardiographic identification of right ventricular dilatation or dysfunction is an invaluable ancillary diagnostic sign, increasing the likelihood that PH is severe.

In an early PH diagnostic study of serum BNP in ILD, BNP levels were increased in 20/39 cases and correlated with increases in mPAP, and reductions in the six-minute walk distance and cardiac output [31]. A BNP threshold of 33 pg/mL had an ROC area under curve of 96% in identifying severe PH (mPAP>35 mm) but this pilot finding in an underpowered cohort requires further evaluation before BNP increases can be used with precision to nuance the perceived likelihood of PH. Currently, accumulated experience indicates that serum BNP estimation may be most helpful when levels are normal and, thus, well below thresholds generally associated with PH in published data. This view is strongly supported in a recent mixed ILD cohort, in which a NT-proBNP <95 ng/L at initial diagnostic evaluation precluded a positive echocardiographic screen for PH [33].

The ancillary CT signs of an increase in the absolute size of the main pulmonary artery [34, 35] and in the ratio of the pulmonary artery diameter to the diameter of the ascending aorta (the PA:A ratio) [36] have both been shown to correlate with increases in the mPAP in general PH cohorts. However, increases in pulmonary artery diameter are not reliably linked to the presence of PH in ILD. In a cross-sectional study of 65 patients with advanced IPF, the diameter of main pulmonary artery did not differ significantly according to the presence or absence of PH [11]. However, in a study of 77 patients with chronic lung disease, including 45 with various forms of ILD, mPAP levels correlated with the PA:A ratio and were most strongly linked to a composite index containing the PA:A ratio and echocardiographic PASP [37]. The discordance between these two series indicates that the reliability of ancillary HRCT signs of PH may depend upon the severity of underlying pulmonary fibrosis.

In IPF, most pulmonary function variables do not differ significantly between patients with and without PH. DLco levels are only a modestly reliable guide to the likelihood of PH as they are influenced by both pulmonary vasculopathy and pulmonary fibrosis. A reduction in DLco that is disproportionate to lung volumes, as captured by a reduction in Kco or an increase in the FVC/DLco ratio has yet to be explored definitively in IPF, although in one IPF cohort, PH was more frequently present when the DLco level was less than 30% and when the FVC level was >70% [6]. However, in SSc, increases in the FVC/DLco ratio have consistently been associated with an increased likelihood of PH, including in patients with overt pulmonary fibrosis [38–40]. This finding that was validated in the prospective DETECT study, in which an algorithm to screen for PH, with a view to selecting patient to undergo RHC, was developed (although it should be stressed that only a minority of patients in this study had clinically significant ILD) [41]. More data are required to evaluate the role of the Kco and FVC/DLco ratio in providing ancillary evidence of PH in ILD, with concurrent smoking-related emphysema likely to be a major confounder [42], an important consideration in IPF.

Six-minute walk data, including the walk distance and severity of oxygen desaturation, are influenced both by pulmonary vasculopathy and by the severity of pulmonary fibrosis. In a cohort with advanced interstitial lung disease of various types, the six minute walk distance was observed to be significantly reduced, and the severity of oxygen desaturation significantly increased, in patients with PH at RHC [43]. Abnormal heart rate recovering following a six minute walk test was predictive of the presence of PH at right heart study in an IPF cohort [44]. However, no discrete diagnostic threshold in any single variable has been validated in a subsequent study. Six-minute walk data are probably most helpful diagnostically when there is an absence of major exercise intolerance or oxygen desaturation, reducing the likelihood of underlying PH.

Overall, the use of non-invasive tools to select ILD patients for RHC is an imprecise exercise. The most widely used approach currently is to base investigation on patients considered to be at higher risk of PH based on the severity of ILD and worsening exercise intolerance. It then appears logical to reconcile findings from a number of tests including echocardiography, HRCT, pulmonary function variables, six-minute walk data and serum BNP estimation.

Pathogenesis of PH in IIP

The current classification of PH associated with ILD (including IIP) is based on perceived common pathophysiology leading to the development of PH; it stresses the presence of lung fibrosis and hypoxia being the major contributory factors [45]. There are several criticisms of this simplified view: First, although ablation of pulmonary vessels ("vascular rarefaction") due to parenchymal destruction is clearly important, there is no direct relationship between the level of fibrosis (and therefore rarefaction), as determined by pulmonary function tests [6, 46] or CT parameters [11], and haemodynamic measurements of pulmonary artery pressure or pulmonary vascular resistance (PVR). Second, most patients with IIP who develop PH are not sufficiently hypoxaemic to explain the level of rise of pulmonary pressure. The pathogenesis of PH in IIP (and other ILDs) is therefore likely to be more complex and includes other causes such as the balance between rarefaction and angiogenesis, true pulmonary vascular remodelling, chronic pulmonary vasoconstriction (other than due to hypoxia), mechanical causes, such as shear stress, as well as important co-morbid conditions such as pulmonary embolism, sleep-disordered breathing and left-sided heart disease.

Rarefaction and Angiogenesis

The observation that vascular remodelling occurred in pulmonary fibrosis was first made in 1963 by Turner-Warwick who demonstrated anastomoses between the systemic and pulmonary micro-vasculature associated with neovascularisation within areas of fibrosis [47], while other studies have reported an overall reduced vascular density [48]. Subsequently, it has been accepted that both phenomena occur in different areas of the same lung [49, 50]. Increased vascularity is seen at the active interface between fibrosis and normal lung parenchyma, and decreased vascularity within areas of fibrosis with abnormally dilated vessels within areas of honeycombing [49]. Indeed, new vessel formation has been shown to be maladaptive with increased irregularity and dilatation [51], and lacking an elastin layer may therefore demonstrate decreased compliance [49], potentially contributing to an increased PVR.

It is not clear what role neovascularisation plays in progression of fibrosis, if any, or whether it remains a by-product of active inflammation. Neovascularisation itself appears to be controlled by a host of angiostatic and angiogenic factors perhaps under the influence of master regulators such as hypoxia initiation factor (HIF) [52] and nuclear factor (NF)-κB [53]. The main factors include vascular endothelial growth factor (VEGF) [54], angiopoetin-1(Ang-1) [55], transforming growth factor (TGF-β1) [56], endostatin [57, 58], pigment epithelium-derived factor (PEDF) [50] and angiopoetin-2 (Ang-2) [55], with their angiogenic or angiostatic roles in IIP summarised in Table 6.2. It is likely that angiogenesis in IIP occurs in response to the observed reduction in capillary density [47], which relates to rarefaction, hypoxic pulmonary vascular remodelling and other causes. This is supported by studies showing that increasing angiostatin levels resulted in reduction of VEGF and led to a worsening of hypoxic PH [59], whereas VEGF overexpression protected against hypoxic PH [60].

Pulmonary Vascular Remodelling

Pulmonary vascular remodelling refers to hyperplasia of the cellular components of the vascular wall, which results in structural wall changes and resulting decreased vascular distensibility and compliance. The layers involved include the intimal layer composed of endothelial cells, the smooth muscle layer or media and the interstitium composed of fibroblasts and extracellular matrix components. As mentioned earlier, hypoxic pulmonary vascular remodelling is likely in all patients with alveolar hypoxia, but further to this, there is heterogeneity in the pattern of remodelling seen in IPF. Farkas et al. reported vessels with isolated medial hyperplasia, vessels with intimal lesions, vessels obstructed with scar tissue and plexiform lesions [61]. Furthermore, it appears that the extent of these changes correlates with the disease activity in surrounding areas [61]. Although the exact pathogenesis of remodelling seen is not known it is likely to be related to a number of factors:

1. Chemokines and cytokines released from damaged/apoptotic endothelial cells, such as endothelin (ET-1), platelet-derived growth factor (PDGF), angiotensin (AT) II and TGF-β1 [61–65];
2. The same factors may be released from the surrounding fibrotic milieu;
3. Increased levels of oxidative stress [66];
4. Reduced production of vasodilators and anti-proliferative molecules such as nitric oxide (NO) and prostacyclin (PGI_2) [61, 62, 64, 67];
5. Increased production of vasoconstrictors and mitogens such as ET-1, thromboxane and AT-II [62, 64];
6. Finally, there is evidence for endothelial cell to mesenchymal cell transition a source for increased numbers of myofibroblasts or vascular smooth muscle cells in remodelled vessels [68–70].

The relative contribution of remodelled vessels to the overall PH phenotype in patients with PH-IIP is crucial as these are potentially amenable to treatment in the same way that pulmonary vasodilators are used to treat pulmonary arterial hypertension (PAH). In fact, this hypothesis has led to a series of clinical trials with variable results to date (see Treatment Section).

Table 6.2 Angiogenic and angiostatic factors in IIP–PH

Angiogenic	Angiostatic
VEGF [54]	Endostatin [57, 58]
Ang-1 [55]	Ang-2 [55]
TGF-β1 [56]	PEDF [58]

The balance between angiogenic and angiostatic factors appears to be important in IIP and appears to vary within areas of the lung. For example, in IPF, VEGF is reduced in broncho-alveolar lavage (BAL) samples from patients from fibrotic regions of the lung and within fibroblastic foci, yet increased in areas of neoangiogenesis (see text later). Pigment epithelium-derived factor (PEDF) is a multifunctional secreted protein that has angiostatic properties and is increased in the fibroblastic foci of IPF patients, with elevated levels been found in BAL samples compared to controls [50]. TGF-β1 has been shown to be co-localised with PEDF in IPF specimens within the overlying epithelium of the fibroblastic focus and within areas of honeycombing, and TGF-β1 increases PEDF expression within fibroblasts [50]. Angiopoetin-1(Ang-1), a critical protein involved in vascular development, stabilises blood vessels by promoting interaction between endothelial cells and surrounding extracellular matrix. Decreased levels of Ang-1 levels have been found in the BAL of IPF patients versus controls [55]. Finally, raised serum levels of endostatin (an angiogenesis inhibitor) are found in patients with IPF [58]. The overall balance therefore seems to favour angiostasis at least within areas of fibrosis. The relationship with this an PH has been suggested by Farkas et al. who demonstrated in rat models of IPF that VEGF levels inversely correlated with pulmonary arterial pressure and endothelial cell apoptosis, and that restoration of VEGF reduced endothelial apoptosis, increased vascularisation and lowered pulmonary artery pressure [61]

VEGF vascular endothelial growth factor, *Ang-1* angiopoetin-1, *TGF-β1* transforming growth factor, *PEDF* pigment epithelium-derived factor, *Ang-2* angiopoetin-2, *BAL* broncho-alveolar lavage

Potential Vasoactive Mediators and Growth Factors

ET-1

ET-1 is responsible for both vasoconstriction and the growth of vascular smooth muscle cells [64]. Levels of ET-1 have found to be increased in the lungs of patients with IPF, with expression strongest in fibrotic areas [71, 72]. Furthermore, in the same patient group, there is a positive correlation of ET-1 concentration in peripheral blood samples of patients with pulmonary pressures [73].

VEGF

As its name suggests VEGF is an angiogenic growth factor responsible for endothelial cell migration during angiogenesis and is important in endothelial cell survival and proliferation; its transcription is mainly induced by hypoxia and TGF-β1 [74, 75]. In keeping with VEGF controlling neoangiogenesis in areas of vascular rarefaction, VEGF levels are increased on immunohistochemistry staining in these areas [49]. VEGF is however reduced in broncho-alveolar lavage fluid from fibrotic regions and especially in fibroblastic foci [49, 50, 76]. Indeed, endothelial cell apoptosis correlates with reduced vascular density and decreased capillary branching [48–50] in these areas.

TGF-β

TGF-β is a profibrotic growth factor, predominantly secreted by macrophages, epithelial cells and fibroblasts [77]. TGF-β1 is likely to contribute to local endothelial cell apoptosis and therefore vascular rarefaction. It also has the potential to cause muscularisation of local pulmonary arteries [50, 78–80].

PDGF

PDGF expression is present on fibroblasts, epithelial cells and platelets [81]. It causes fibroblast proliferation and migration, and also activation of vascular smooth muscle cells and fibroblasts which results in muscularisation and fibrosis of the intimal and adventitial layers [82].

Hypoxia-Related Mechanisms

Although we have argued that hypoxia is not the prime driver of PH in patients with IIP, it cannot be ignored and will certainly factor in patients who have severe parenchymal fibrotic disease, or in those having an acute exacerbation, and may occur intermittently during sleep-disordered breathing or physical exertion. Detailed review of the mechanisms of hypoxia-related vascular remodelling is out of the scope of this chapter and the reader is encouraged to read the recent review by Welsh and Peacock [83].

Sleep-Disordered Breathing

Nocturnal hypoxia is very common in IIP with the majority of prospective studies being performed in IPF; the incidence of obstructive sleep apnoea (OSA) varying from 59 to 90% [84–86]. In fact, nocturnal desaturation is common even in the absence of OSA [87]. Patients with IIP are vulnerable to nocturnal desaturation due to the fact that many patients are on the steep portion of the oxygen–haemoglobin dissociation curve and small changes in arterial oxygen tension result in a large decrease in oxygen saturation; more severe nocturnal hypoxaemia is seen in patients with lower daytime PaO_2 and oxygen saturations [88–90]. Episodes of alveolar hypoventilation induced, in particular, by REM sleep may also play a role in increasing nocturnal hypoxia [91]. Disproportionate nocturnal desaturation has been found in patients with mild ILD and correlated with signs of PH on echocardiogram [92], as well as being an independent predictor of prognosis [84, 92].

Elevated levels of ET-1 have been demonstrated in the blood of patients with ILD and significantly higher levels were found in patients with elevated pulmonary pressures. Levels of ET-1 were measured during sleep and rose in all patients during episodes of desaturation below 90% and correlated with PaO_2 and pulmonary arterial pressure which was measured simultaneously [93]. Repetitive short episodes of hypoxaemia have been demonstrated to increase PVR [94], which may lead to vascular remodelling and propagation of PH. Intermittent nocturnal hypoxia may also reset peripheral chemoreceptors lowering the hypoxic drive and worsening daytime hypoxia, further exacerbating the development of PH.

Left-Sided Heart Disease

The prevalence of left ventricular systolic and diastolic dysfunction increases with advancing age and advancing co-morbidities. Diastolic dysfunction is often overlooked although it has been shown to have a median prevalence of 36% (range 15.8–52.8%) in individuals over the age of 60 [95]. It is an important consideration in patients with IIP given the demographic of patients with the condition. Limited studies have looked specifically in IIP. However, a small, echo-based study ($n = 44$) identified significant LV diastolic dysfunction in 91% of patients with IPF and found no evidence of LV diastolic dysfunction in controls, who were age and sex matched [96]. Furthermore, in a study evaluating the prevalence of pulmonary hypertension in a lung transplant population with IPF (mean FVC 54.6% ± 17.3%) 16.1% demonstrated an elevated pulmonary capillary wedge pressure on RHC [6]. In terms of an underlying aetiology, in patients under evaluation for lung transplantation, 28.8% of 73 patients with IPF had evidence of coronary artery disease, which was associated with worse outcome [97].

Thrombosis

Large epidemiological studies have suggested an association between IPF and vascular thrombotic diseases such as deep vein thrombosis (DVT) and pulmonary embolism (PE) [98–100]. For example, a recent large-scale epidemiological study analysing mortality data demonstrated a 34% higher risk of a venous thromboembolism (VTE) in IPF patients above the background population, and IPF patients with a VTE died earlier than those with IPF alone [74.3 versus 77.4 years in females ($p < 0.0001$); 72.0 versus 74.4 years in males ($p < 0.0001$)] [100]. Supporting these studies, there appears to be a hypercoagulable state in animal models of IPF [101] and patients with IPF [102]. Tissue factor, a trigger of the extrinsic clotting pathway, is raised in BAL of patients with biopsy-proven IPF [102, 103]; plasminogen activator inhibitors are also raised, indicating reduced thrombolysis [103]. In addition, platelets are activated in patients with IPF [104] and d-dimer levels raised [105, 106], suggesting ongoing activation of coagulation and fibrinolysis. A small prospective trial performed baseline and follow-up CT pulmonary angiograms (CTPA) at 3 months in IIP patients without symptoms of PE, where one-third of the patients had evidence of pulmonary emboli on either their baseline or follow-up CTPA [107]. Although no studies as yet document the prevalence of PE in patients presenting with PH-IIP, the observed increase in PE in IIP suggests that this co-morbidity should certainly be excluded in any IIP patient being worked up for PH.

Treatment of IIP–PH

Background

Recent progress has been made in the management of IPF with the use of pirfenidone and nintedanib which reduces the rate of decline in FVC by approximately half in patients with mild-to-moderate disease [108, 109] and a lower risk of subsequent decline in FVC or death in individuals who have progressed on treatment [110]. Unfortunately, at present there is no specific therapy approved for PH associated with IIP, and the evaluation of pulmonary vasodilators in IIP–PH has been punctuated by clinical trials showing a lack of effect on primary outcomes.

The Fifth World Symposium of Pulmonary Hypertension and the European Society of Cardiology/European Respiratory Society PH guidelines [45], and the ATS/ERS guideline for the management of IPF do not advocate the routine use of pulmonary vasodilators [111] in IIP–PH, but suggest further clinical trials before recommendations can be made; however, both advocate optimisation of the underlying disease process and oxygen therapy as the main clinical interventions. In addition, measures to identify and treat co-morbidities that may contribute to a pulmonary hypertensive phenotype should be made.

Basic Principles of Treatment of PH Associated with IIP

Oxygen Therapy

Results from the landmark oxygen trials conducted in patients with COPD [112, 113] have been extrapolated to formulate recommendations for oxygen therapy in many chronic respiratory conditions such as ILD and PH [114]. Without any more specific, up to date studies these recommendations apply therefore to patients with IIP and PH. Patients with IIP–PH should be evaluated for the need for oxygen therapy at rest, on exercise and overnight. As a general rule oxygen saturations should be kept above 90% at all times. In addition, patients should be warned about the risk of travelling to high altitudes (>1500 m) and should be considered for fitness to fly tests for air travel.

Prevent and Treat Exacerbations

Acute exacerbation in IIP represents a period of rapid worsening of symptoms and decline in pulmonary function and is the most common cause of deterioration and death in IPF [115, 116]. Many of the consequences of an acute exacerbation, such as worsening gas exchange, and cytokine release from infection, will potentially lead to increases in pulmonary pressures as well as right ventricular dysfunction. In addition, pulmonary hypertension has been demonstrated to be associated with a higher risk of developing an acute exacerbation and poorer survival [117]. The cause of an acute exacerbation is often not clear and is usually attributed to infection [118], be it viral or bacterial, although an association with air pollution [119] and micro-aspiration [120] has also been demonstrated.

The treatment of an acute exacerbation in IPF is focused upon supportive measures (accepting that no proven intervention exists), such as oxygen therapy, non-invasive ventilation, broad-spectrum antibiotic therapy and careful control of fluid balance. The international evidence-based guidelines on the management of IPF make a weak recommendation for using corticosteroids in an acute exacerbation of IPF [4], stating that they should be used in the majority of patients based upon anecdotal reported benefits and the extremely high mortality associated with an acute exacerbation of IPF. Antifibrotic therapy should be continued if already in use although not commenced during an acute exacerbation [121]. It is desirable although challenging to try and prevent future exacerbations through a combination of annual influenza vaccination in addition to strep pneumonia vaccination and consideration of prophylactic antibiotics when infections are recurrent.

Recognition and Treatment of Coexistent Co-morbidities

Sleep-Discorded Breathing/Nocturnal Desaturation

As mentioned in the Pathogenesis Section, nocturnal desaturation and OSA are common in IIP and likely contribute to the development of PH. Overnight oximetry should be performed in all patients with a clinical suspicion of IIP–PH and sleep studies performed where the history/examination is suggestive of coexistent OSA.

Left Heart Disease

Similarly, ischaemic heart disease and systemic hypertension are common in the patients with IIP–PH. This may lead to left ventricular diastolic dysfunction, which may be a significant driver of PH in these patients. Therefore, all attempts should be made through history, examination and investigations to recognise and treat causes of left heart dysfunction in patients with IIP–PH. ECG and echocardiography are particularly important in terms of investigation as well as careful review of systemic blood pressure. Patients with suspected ischaemic heart disease should be referred to a cardiologist. Systemic blood pressure should be kept under meticulous control and addition of a diuretic may be necessary.

Pulmonary Embolism

Due to the increased prevalence of VTE in IIP as described earlier, it is advisable that IIP patients presenting with pulmonary hypertension, or those with clinical deterioration but stability in fibrosis, be investigated for occult pulmonary emboli. Clinical risk scores to predict PE in large populations include the Wells score, with an area under curve (AUC) of 0.778 (95% CI 0.740–0.818, $p = <0.001$), and the revised Geneva score with an AUC of 0.693 (95% CI 0.653–0.736, $p = <0.001$) [122]. The same scores evaluated in a small study in patients with ILD ($n = 57$, 27 of which had IIP), demonstrate an AUC 0.720 ± 0.083(CI 0.586–0.831), and 0.704 ± 0.081(CI 0.568–0.817) for the Wells score, and revised Geneva score, respectively [107]. The findings suggest clinical risk scores may play a role in predicting pretest probability of coexistent PE, although larger studies in the IIP population are required. The appropriate modality of imaging unfortunately remains undefined in this population, and most patients undergo a CTPA. In a retrospective review of 130 patients with diffuse interstitial lung disease, CTPA was demonstrated to provide adequate opacification of the pulmonary arteries down to the segmental level, whereas in controls without significant parenchymal lung disease was adequate to the sub-segmental level [123]. A recent, small retrospective study evaluated the concordance between CTPA and ventilation perfusion Single Photon Emission Computed Tomography imaging (V/Q-SPECT) in 22 patients with ILD who had clinically deteriorated. In this small study, CTPA detected proximal PE reliably, and the negative VQ scans were also negative on CTPA. V/Q picked up more sub-segmental defects than on CTPA, some of which may have related to areas of fibrosis, although the addition of low dose CT did not, at least in this study, improve the diagnostic accuracy [124]. In practice and previous studies do suggest, however, that the comparison of VQ with areas of fibrosis on CT is useful to determine the aetiology of smaller perfusion defects [125].

In terms of management, at present there is debate as to whether patients (who have a "normal cardiorespiratory reserve") with single sub-segmental defects might benefit from anticoagulation, and a wide variation in clinical practice occurs. A recent general review suggests that withholding anticoagulation may be appropriate in patients who are informed, have negative lower limb Doppler's, are low risk and can have close follow up [126]. Patients with IIP–PH are a high-risk group and anticoagulation is advised. Unfortunately, the choice of anticoagulant is also contentious. Of note, a double-blind, randomised, placebo-controlled trial evaluated a potential survival benefit with warfarin (INR target 2.0 to 3.0) in IPF patients (all-comers). An early safety review revealed not only a lack of benefit, but also that warfarin carried a significantly higher risk of death or decline in FVC by 10% or greater [106]. This increased mortality related to warfarin is postulated to relate to an increased risk of acute exacerbations [127].

We recommend that IIP patients who develop PH due to IIP be evaluated with CTPA (where no contraindications exist) in their workup. In some cases, especially in those with less extensive fibrosis, consider additional V/Q SPECT where clinical suspicion remains high, accepting that there may be false positives especially in sub-segmental vessels. We advocate anticoagulation with novel oral anticoagulants (where appropriate) for all individuals with PE including isolated sub-segmental PE, especially in view of minimising drug interactions. Anticoagulation should be long term unless a clear and reversible provoking factor is present.

Evidence for the Use of Pulmonary Vasodilators

Although the current guidelines do not recommend the routine use of pulmonary vasodilators in patients with IIP–PH, it is worth reviewing the current data. This is summarised in Table 6.3.

Phosphodiesterase Type-5 Inhibitors (PDE-5)

PDE-5 inhibitors (sildenafil and tadalafil) inhibit the degradation of cyclic guanosine monophosphate, which is synthesised by soluble guanylate cyclase in response to nitric oxide (NO), leading to pulmonary vasodilation [22].

There is relevant recent basic science evidence supporting the use of sildenafil in IIP. An ex vivo study of the pulmonary arteries of 18 healthy donors, 9 IPF patients, 8 IPF-PH patients and 4 PH patients was performed to evaluate the vascular effects of sildenafil [128]. Sildenafil relaxed pre-contracted pulmonary arteries in healthy donors and non-PH IPF samples more than in IPF-PH and PH samples. This effect was increased in the presence of an intact endothelium. In addition, sildenafil prevented a TGF-β-induced mesenchymal/myofibroblast phenotype in human pulmonary artery endothelial cells and human pulmonary artery smooth muscle cells, with associated down-regulation of endothelial markers (including eNOS, VEGF) and upregulation of pulmonary PDE5 expression. The same authors also demonstrated in a rat model of bleomycin-induced pulmonary fibrosis and pulmonary hypertension that administration of sildenafil did not worsen ventilation perfusion matching [128].

Table 6.3 Vasodilator studies in IPF and IIP–PH

ILD	Treatment	Duration	Number of patients	Primary endpoint	Echo/RHC	Study result	Type of study	Target	Author/reference
IPF	Bosentan	12 months	154	6MWD	–	No change	R,D,P	IPF	King [147]
IPF	Bosentan	12 months	616	Disease progression	–	No change	R,D,P	IPF	King [140]
IIP	Bosentan	16 weeks	60	↓PVR	RHC	No change	R,D,P	IIP–PH	Corte [142]
IPF	Ambrisentan	35 weeks	492	Disease progression	11% PH	Negative	R,D,P	IPF	Ragu [9]
IPF	Macitentan	12 months	178	FVC	–	No change	R,D,P	IPF	Raghu [141]
IPF	Sildenafil	12 weeks	180	6MWD	–	No change	R,D,P	IPF	Zisman [133]
IPF	Sildenafil	12 weeks	119	6MWD	RVD on echo	Preservation of 6MWD if RVD on echo	R,D,P Sub	IPF with RVSD	Han [134]
Mixed	Sildenafil/tadalafil	3 months	10	–	RHC	↓ PVR, ↑ CI	Open	ILD-PH	Zimmerman [132]
Mixed	Riociguat	12 months	15	Safety	RHC	No Safety concerns	Open	ILD-PH	Hoeper [145]
IIP	Riociguat	26 weeks	147	6MWD	RHC	Negative	R,D,P	IIP–PH	Bayer [146]

6MWD six-minute walk distance, *FVC* change in FVC, *PVR* pulmonary vascular resistance, *RVD* right ventricular dysfunction on echo, *CI* cardiac index, *R* randomised, *D* double blind, *P* placebo controlled, *Open* Open label, *Sub* substudy analysis

Sildenafil has been evaluated in several small, non-randomised, open label populations with proven IIP–PH. First, a small open-label trial (16 patients, 7 with IPF) compared the vasodilatory effects of oral sildenafil and IV prostacyclin after nebulised nitric oxide (10–20 ppm) and demonstrated a 32.5% reduction in PVR (CI: −10.2 to −54.1), with sildenafil. The use of IV prostacyclin was associated with an increased V/Q mismatch and decreased arterial oxygenation, whereas oral sildenafil (and inhaled nitric oxide) maintained V/Q matching and increased arterial oxygenation [129]. Second, another small open-label trial evaluated the effect of sildenafil on 6-minute walk distance (6MWD), and included 14 patients with IPF and PH confirmed by RHC. Eleven patients were able to complete the screening and post-treatment 6MWT. More than half (57%) of the patients improved their 6MWD by > 20%, although there was no control group for comparison. The treatment (over a median follow up of 91 days) was generally well tolerated [130]. Third, a small retrospective review of was also performed in 15 patients with ILD and PH confirmed by either RHC or echocardiography. Following 6 months of sildenafil serum BNP levels were significantly lower and 6MWD improved although there was no change in echocardiographic systolic pulmonary pressure, arterial oxygen saturation or pulmonary function tests [131]. Finally, a small observational pilot study of PDE-5 inhibitors sildenafil or tadalafil in ILD (10 patients, 6 with IPF), importantly in patients with severe degrees of PH but milder degrees of ILD, with evaluation of invasive haemodynamics both at baseline and follow up. Cardiac index was shown to increase significantly and PVR fall with treatment, although no difference was seen in 6MWD, BNP or PFT with treatment [132]. Although a small study, this is an important one to demonstrate haemodynamic improvement in the 'severe PH-milder lung disease' phenotype.

The largest experience of sildenafil in IIP to date has been the double-blind, randomised, placebo-controlled STEP-IPF study. PH was not formally tested for, but the advanced nature of the IPF (DLCO <35%) made its coexistence likely. The primary outcome in this study was a 20% improvement in 6MWT, which was not met. However, several secondary outcome measures were met including an improvement in DLCO, partial pressure of oxygen and oxygen saturations, as well as quality of life measures. An improvement in the former three suggests that sildenafil was having a direct effect on the pulmonary vasculature [133].

All patients underwent a pre-enrolment echocardiogram to exclude significant aortic stenosis as an exclusion factor. Evaluation of the pre-enrolment echo was possible in 119 of 180 patients, and the interaction between right ventricular systolic dysfunction (RVSD) and the effect of sildenafil was evaluated. Patients with RVSD who were on sildenafil experienced a lesser drop (99.3 m $p = 0.01$) in their 6MWD than patients with RVSD who were on placebo [134]. (The minimal clinical important difference for 6MWD in IPF has been demonstrated to be 24–45 m [135]). As well as preserving 6MWD, quality of life scores (St Georges Respiratory Questionnaire) also improved in the sildenafil-treated group [134].

Recently, a retrospective study (using an international registry COMPERA) evaluated patients with IIP and compared them with IPAH patients. There were 151 incident IIP diagnosed patients, who were significantly older than the IPAH patients and had more severely affected lung function (mean DLCO 28.5% predicted for IIP patients versus 50.1% in IPAH). Patients with IIP had lower mean pulmonary artery pressure 37 mmHg versus 45 mmHg, than patients with IPAH, although 79% of the IIP–PH patients met the "severe" PH criteria. Ninety-five per cent of the IIP–PH patients were treated with a single pulmonary vasodilator, 88% of which were a PDE5i. Treatment was associated with a 24.5 m improvement in 6MWD in IIP–PH versus 30 m in IPAH patients, and functional class improved in 22.4% in IIP–PH and 29.5% of IPAH. Patients who improved their 6MWD by at least 20 m or improved in functional class had a better prognosis than patients who did not despite almost identical haemodynamics at baseline. Patients with severe PH were no more likely to show improvements with treatment than patients with lower invasive pulmonary pressures. Interestingly, the authors of this study point out that the primary endpoint from STEP-IPF (increase in 6MWD by 20%) would have been met by 31% within the IIP–PH cohort [136].

Endothelin Receptor Antagonists

Endothelin-1 (ET-1) is a potent vasoconstrictor and promoter of vascular smooth muscle cell proliferation; its role in the pathogenesis of pulmonary arterial hypertension is firmly established [137]. ET-1 is also profibrotic [138], and elevated levels have been demonstrated in patients with IIP [73, 139] and levels have been shown to correlate with pulmonary arterial pressure and in a negative fashion with arterial oxygen content in a small group of patients [73]. ET-1 therefore seems like a very attractive target to prevent progression of the underlying fibrotic process within the lungs and attenuate the development of pulmonary vascular disease.

Endothelin receptor antagonists (ERAs) have been evaluated in a similar fashion to sildenafil in an attempt to prevent time to deterioration in IPF in patients without PH. BUIILD-3 was a large randomised placebo-controlled trial which showed bosentan to be well tolerated in HRCT and biopsy confirmed IPF although no difference was demonstrated with placebo in time to IPF worsening or death (hazard ratio, 0.85 95% CI, 0.66–1.10) [140]. Another study (MUSIC) evaluated 178 patients with biopsy diagnosed IPF (FVC > 50% predicted and DLCO > 30%) in a prospective randomised double-blind placebo-controlled study using macitentan. There was no difference in the primary outcome (change in FVC from baseline up to month 12) or any of the secondary outcomes [141]. Artemis-IPF was a randomised double-blind placebo-controlled trial evaluating the role of ambrisentan in IPF and IPF-PH. The study was stopped following interim analysis as ambrisentan-treated patients were more likely to meet the pre-specified criteria for disease progression. Ten per cent of the group had pulmonary hypertension and sub-analysis of this group demonstrated similar findings although the study was not fully powered for all endpoints in this subgroup [9].

The bosentan in pulmonary hypertension-associated fibrotic idiopathic interstitial pneumonia (B-PHIT) was the first randomised, double-blind placebo-controlled study evaluating PH-specific treatment in IIP–PH. The study failed to show any difference in invasive pulmonary haemodynamics, functional capacity, 6MWD or QOL scores between placebo and bosentan, and subgroup analysis could not demonstrate a group that benefited [142]. However, there was no deterioration in oxygen saturation or oxygen requirement in the study period.

These trials demonstrate a lack of benefit with bosentan and macitentan and the potential for harm with ambrisentan and they are therefore not recommended for use in IIP or IIP–PH.

Prostanoids

Prostacyclin (PGI_2) and its analogues are members of the prostanoid family. PGI_2 inhibits platelet activation and acts as a potent vasodilator. PGI_2 also displays anti-inflammatory and anti-proliferative properties.

Studies involving prostanoids have been small, non-randomised and limited to a short follow-up period with focus on invasive haemodynamics. In one study with 8 ILD patients (only one of which had IPF) with severe underlying pulmonary fibrosis found that inhaled iloprost caused pulmonary vasodilatation with maintenance of gas exchange and systemic arterial pressure whereas intravenous prostacyclin resulted in a significant drop in systemic arterial pressure and a marked increase in ventilation–perfusion mismatching [143].

Guanylate Cyclase Stimulators

Riociguat is a soluble guanylate cyclase stimulator that can synergise with endogenous NO or act independently of NO. It has been shown to improve exercise capacity and haemodynamics in patients with PAH [144]. In a pilot study (open-label, non-blinded, non-randomised) to assess safety and tolerability in patients with mild-to-moderate ILD but moderate-to-severe PH (n = 23, 82% of patients had underlying IIP), riociguat was well tolerated, with 2 of the 23 patients discontinuing the treatment prematurely. In terms of efficacy, PVR decreased, and cardiac output increased, with mean pulmonary pressure remaining unchanged, likely due to a higher cardiac output offsetting the effect of pulmonary vasodilation [145]. As a result of these promising findings a randomised, double-blind placebo-controlled trial on efficacy and safety of riociguat in IIP–PH (RISE-IIP) was commenced in 2014 [146]. Unfortunately, this study has recently been halted prematurely due to increased mortality in the treatment arm. Bayer has recommended that riociguat is not used in this patient group.

In summary, the treatment of IIP–PH is challenging, and evidence of benefit with specific interventions is eagerly awaited to improve patient outcome. PDE-5 inhibitors appear to be the most likely class of drug to improve outcome in IIP–PH, although which patients stand to benefit and at which the stage of the disease (i.e. prior to development of PH or with onset of right ventricular dysfunction) remain unclear.

Conclusion

PH is commonly encountered in IIP and the likelihood of coexistent PH increases as the underlying disease progresses, although its presence is not reliably linked to disease characteristics, which confounds non-invasive detection and underscores the importance of invasive evaluation for confirmation where appropriate. The development of PH is associated with decline in functional status and dramatically worsens prognosis. The underlying aetiology of PH in IIP remains poorly defined and is multifactorial; further study to help develop novel treatment options is highly desirable. The management of PH within IIP at present is predominantly supportive in terms of evaluating for and treating hypoxaemia and other contributory causes of PH. At present there is no evidence to support the use of pulmonary vasodilators, although this remains a very active research area.

References

1. Travis WD et al. An official American Thoracic Society/European Respiratory Society statement: update of the international multidisciplinary classification of the idiopathic interstitial pneumonias. Am J Respir Crit Care Med. 2013;188(6):733–48.
2. Thomeer M, Demedts M, Vandeurzen K. Registration of interstitial lung diseases by 20 centres of respiratory medicine in Flanders. Acta Clin Belg. 2001;56(3):163–72.
3. Tinelli C et al. The Italian register for diffuse infiltrative lung disorders (RIPID): a four-year report. Sarcoidosis Vasc Diffuse Lung Dis. 2005;22(Suppl 1):S4–8.
4. Raghu G et al. An official ATS/ERS/JRS/ALAT statement: idiopathic pulmonary fibrosis: evidence-based guidelines for diagnosis and management. Am J Respir Crit Care Med. 2011;183(6):788–824.
5. Lettieri CJ et al. Prevalence and outcomes of pulmonary arterial hypertension in advanced idiopathic pulmonary fibrosis. Chest. 2006;129(3):746–52.
6. Nathan SD et al. Pulmonary hypertension and pulmonary function testing in idiopathic pulmonary fibrosis. Chest. 2007;131(3):657–63.
7. Arcasoy SM et al. Echocardiographic assessment of pulmonary hypertension in patients with advanced lung disease. Am J Respir Crit Care Med. 2003;167(5):735–40.
8. Nathan SD et al. Serial development of pulmonary hypertension in patients with idiopathic pulmonary fibrosis. Respiration. 2008;76(3):288–94.
9. Raghu G et al. Treatment of idiopathic pulmonary fibrosis with ambrisentan: a parallel, randomized trial. Ann Intern Med. 2013;158(9):641–9.
10. The effect of diffuse fibrosis on reliability of ct signs of ph.pdf.
11. Zisman DA et al. High-resolution chest computed tomography findings do not predict the presence of pulmonary hypertension in advanced idiopathic pulmonary fibrosis. Chest. 2007;132(3):773–9.

12. Nihtyanova SI et al. Prediction of pulmonary complications and long-term survival in systemic sclerosis. Arthritis Rheumatol. 2014;66(6):1625–35.
13. Fischer A et al. An official European Respiratory Society/American Thoracic Society research statement: interstitial pneumonia with autoimmune features. Eur Respir J. 2015;46(4):976–87.
14. Handa T et al. Incidence of pulmonary hypertension and its clinical relevance in patients with sarcoidosis. Chest. 2006;129(5):1246–52.
15. Baughman RP, Engel PJ, Nathan S. Pulmonary hypertension in sarcoidosis. Clin Chest Med. 2015;36(4):703–14.
16. Nadrous HF et al. Pulmonary hypertension in patients with idiopathic pulmonary fibrosis. Chest. 2005;128(4):2393–9.
17. Cottin V et al. Pulmonary hypertension in patients with combined pulmonary fibrosis and emphysema syndrome. Eur Respir J. 2010;35(1):105–11.
18. Mejia M et al. Idiopathic pulmonary fibrosis and emphysema: decreased survival associated with severe pulmonary arterial hypertension. Chest. 2009;136(1):10–5.
19. Rivera-Lebron BN et al. Echocardiographic and hemodynamic predictors of mortality in idiopathic pulmonary fibrosis. Chest. 2013;144(2):564–70.
20. Corte TJ et al. Pulmonary vascular resistance predicts early mortality in patients with diffuse fibrotic lung disease and suspected pulmonary hypertension. Thorax. 2009;64(10):883–8.
21. Yasui K et al. Pulmonary vascular resistance estimated by Doppler echocardiography predicts mortality in patients with interstitial lung disease. J Cardiol. 2016;68(4):300–7.
22. Baughman RP et al. Survival in sarcoidosis-associated pulmonary hypertension: the importance of hemodynamic evaluation. Chest. 2010;138(5):1078–85.
23. Raghu G et al. Pulmonary hypertension in idiopathic pulmonary fibrosis with mild-to-moderate restriction. Eur Respir J. 2015;46(5):1370–7.
24. Leuchte HH et al. Brain natriuretic peptide is a prognostic parameter in chronic lung disease. Am J Respir Crit Care Med. 2006;173(7):744–50.
25. Corte TJ et al. Elevated brain natriuretic peptide predicts mortality in interstitial lung disease. Eur Respir J. 2010;36(4):819–25.
26. Song JW, Song JK, Kim DS. Echocardiography and brain natriuretic peptide as prognostic indicators in idiopathic pulmonary fibrosis. Respir Med. 2009;103(2):180–6.
27. Shin S et al. Pulmonary artery size as a predictor of outcomes in idiopathic pulmonary fibrosis. Eur Respir J. 2016;47(5):1445–51.
28. Corte TJ et al. Pulmonary function vascular index predicts prognosis in idiopathic interstitial pneumonia. Respirology. 2012;17(4):674–80.
29. Peelen L et al. Fibrotic idiopathic interstitial pneumonias: mortality is linked to a decline in gas transfer. Respirology. 2010;15(8):1233–43.
30. Lama VN et al. Prognostic value of desaturation during a 6-minute walk test in idiopathic interstitial pneumonia. Am J Respir Crit Care Med. 2003;168(9):1084–90.
31. Eaton T et al. Six-minute walk, maximal exercise tests: reproducibility in fibrotic interstitial pneumonia. Am J Respir Crit Care Med. 2005;171(10):1150–7.
32. Nathan SD et al. Right ventricular systolic pressure by echocardiography as a predictor of pulmonary hypertension in idiopathic pulmonary fibrosis. Respir Med. 2008;102(9):1305–10.
33. Andersen C et al. NT-proBNP <95 ng/l can exclude pulmonary hypertension on echocardiography at diagnostic workup in patients with interstitial lung disease. Eur Clin Respir J. 2016;3:32027.
34. Kuriyama K et al. CT-determined pulmonary artery diameters in predicting pulmonary hypertension. Investig Radiol. 1984;19(1):16–22.
35. Edwards PD, Bull RK, Coulden R. CT measurement of main pulmonary artery diameter. Br J Radiol. 1998;71(850):1018–20.
36. Ng CS, Wells AU, Padley SP. A CT sign of chronic pulmonary arterial hypertension: the ratio of main pulmonary artery to aortic diameter. J Thorac Imaging. 1999;14(4):270–8.

37. Devaraj A et al. Detection of pulmonary hypertension with multidetector CT and echocardiography alone and in combination. Radiology. 2010;254(2):609–16.
38. Steen V et al. Exercise-induced pulmonary arterial hypertension in patients with systemic sclerosis. Chest. 2008;134(1):146–51.
39. Hsu VM et al. Assessment of pulmonary arterial hypertension in patients with systemic sclerosis: comparison of noninvasive tests with results of right-heart catheterization. J Rheumatol. 2008;35(3):458–65.
40. Launay D et al. Clinical characteristics and survival in systemic sclerosis-related pulmonary hypertension associated with interstitial lung disease. Chest. 2011;140(4):1016–24.
41. Coghlan JG et al. Evidence-based detection of pulmonary arterial hypertension in systemic sclerosis: the DETECT study. Ann Rheum Dis. 2014;73(7):1340–9.
42. Antoniou KM et al. Combined pulmonary fibrosis and emphysema in scleroderma-related lung disease has a major confounding effect on lung physiology and screening for pulmonary hypertension. Arthritis Rheumatol. 2016;68(4):1004–12.
43. Kawut SM et al. Exercise testing determines survival in patients with diffuse parenchymal lung disease evaluated for lung transplantation. Respir Med. 2005;99(11):1431–9.
44. Swigris JJ et al. Heart rate recovery after six-minute walk test predicts pulmonary hypertension in patients with idiopathic pulmonary fibrosis. Respirology. 2011;16(3):439–45.
45. Galiè N et al. 2015 ESC/ERS guidelines for the diagnosis and treatment of pulmonary hypertension. Eur Respir J. 2015;46(4):903–75.
46. Hamada K et al. Significance of pulmonary arterial pressure and diffusion capacity of the lung as prognosticator in patients with idiopathic pulmonary fibrosis. Chest. 2007;131(3):650–6.
47. Turner-Warwick M. Precapillary systemic-pulmonary anastomoses. Thorax. 1963;18:225–37.
48. Renzoni EA et al. Interstitial vascularity in fibrosing alveolitis. Am J Respir Crit Care Med. 2003;167(3):438–43.
49. Ebina M et al. Heterogeneous increase in CD34-positive alveolar capillaries in idiopathic pulmonary fibrosis. Am J Respir Crit Care Med. 2004;169(11):1203–8.
50. Cosgrove GP et al. Pigment epithelium–derived factor in idiopathic pulmonary fibrosis a role in aberrant angiogenesis. Am J Respir Crit Care Med. 2004;170:242–51.
51. Kwon KY, Park KK, Chang ES. Scanning electron microscopic study of capillary change in bleomycin-induced pulmonary fibrosis. J Korean Med Sci. 1991;6(3):234–45.
52. Tzouvelekis A et al. Comparative expression profiling in pulmonary fibrosis suggests a role of hypoxia-inducible factor-1alpha in disease pathogenesis. Am J Respir Crit Care Med. 2007;176(11):1108–19.
53. Strieter RM. Masters of angiogenesis. Nat Med. 2005;11(9):925–7.
54. Ferrara N, Gerber HP, LeCouter J. The biology of VEGF and its receptors. Nat Med. 2003;9(6):669–76.
55. Margaritopoulos GA et al. Investigation of angiogenetic axis Angiopoietin-1 and -2/Tie-2 in fibrotic lung diseases: a bronchoalveolar lavage study. Int J Mol Med. 2010;26(6):919–23.
56. Pertovaara L et al. Vascular endothelial growth factor is induced in response to transforming growth factor-beta in fibroblastic and epithelial cells. J Biol Chem. 1994;269(9):6271–4.
57. Hanumegowda C, Farkas L, Kolb M. Angiogenesis in pulmonary fibrosis: too much or not enough? Chest. 2012;142(1):200–7.
58. Sumi M et al. Increased serum levels of endostatin in patients with idiopathic pulmonary fibrosis. J Clin Lab Anal. 2005;19(4):146–9.
59. Pascaud MA et al. Lung overexpression of angiostatin aggravates pulmonary hypertension in chronically hypoxic mice. Am J Respir Cell Mol Biol. 2003;29(4):449–57.
60. Partovian C et al. Adenovirus-mediated lung vascular endothelial growth factor overexpression protects against hypoxic pulmonary hypertension in rats. Am J Respir Cell Mol Biol. 2000;23(6):762–71.
61. Farkas L et al. VEGF ameliorates pulmonary hypertension through inhibition of endothelial apoptosis in experimental lung fibrosis in rats. J Clin Invest. 2009;119(5):1298–311.

62. Sakao S et al. Apoptosis of pulmonary microvascular endothelial cells stimulates vascular smooth muscle cell growth. Am J Physiol Lung Cell Mol Physiol. 2006;291(3):L362–8.
63. Nathan SD, Noble PW, Tuder RM. Idiopathic pulmonary fibrosis and pulmonary hypertension: connecting the dots. Am J Respir Crit Care Med. 2007;175(9):875–80.
64. Budhiraja R, Tuder RM, Hassoun PM. Endothelial dysfunction in pulmonary hypertension. Circulation. 2004;109(2):159–65.
65. Ask K et al. Targeting genes for treatment in idiopathic pulmonary fibrosis: challenges and opportunities, promises and pitfalls. Proc Am Thorac Soc. 2006;3(4):389–93.
66. Teng RJ et al. Increased superoxide production contributes to the impaired angiogenesis of fetal pulmonary arteries with in utero pulmonary hypertension. Am J Physiol Lung Cell Mol Physiol. 2009;297(1):L184–95.
67. Smith AP, Demoncheaux EA, Higenbottam TW. Nitric oxide gas decreases endothelin-1 mRNA in cultured pulmonary artery endothelial cells. Nitric Oxide. 2002;6(2):153–9.
68. Hashimoto N et al. Endothelial-mesenchymal transition in bleomycin-induced pulmonary fibrosis. Am J Respir Cell Mol Biol. 2010;43(2):161–72.
69. Arciniegas E et al. Perspectives on endothelial-to-mesenchymal transition: potential contribution to vascular remodeling in chronic pulmonary hypertension. Am J Physiol Lung Cell Mol Physiol. 2007;293(1):L1–8.
70. Sakao S et al. VEGF-R blockade causes endothelial cell apoptosis, expansion of surviving CD34+ precursor cells and transdifferentiation to smooth muscle-like and neuronal-like cells. FASEB J. 2007;21(13):3640–52.
71. Giaid A et al. Expression of endothelin-1 in lungs of patients with cryptogenic fibrosing alveolitis. Lancet. 1993;341(8860):1550–4.
72. Saleh D et al. Elevated expression of endothelin-1 and endothelin-converting enzyme-1 in idiopathic pulmonary fibrosis: possible involvement of proinflammatory cytokines. Am J Respir Cell Mol Biol. 1997;16(2):187–93.
73. Trakada G, Spiropoulos K. Arterial endothelin-1 in interstitial lung disease patients with pulmonary hypertension. Monaldi Arch Chest Dis. 2001;56(5):379–83.
74. Voelkel NF, Vandivier RW, Tuder RM. Vascular endothelial growth factor in the lung. Am J Physiol Lung Cell Mol Physiol. 2006;290(2):L209–21.
75. Ramirez-Bergeron DL et al. HIF-dependent hematopoietic factors regulate the development of the embryonic vasculature. Dev Cell. 2006;11(1):81–92.
76. Meyer KC, Cardoni A, Xiang ZZ. Vascular endothelial growth factor in bronchoalveolar lavage from normal subjects and patients with diffuse parenchymal lung disease. J Lab Clin Med. 2000;135(4):332–8.
77. Farkas L et al. Pulmonary hypertension and idiopathic pulmonary fibrosis: a tale of angiogenesis, apoptosis, and growth factors. Am J Respir Cell Mol Biol. 2011;45(1):1–15.
78. Khalil N et al. Enhanced expression and immunohistochemical distribution of transforming growth factor-beta in idiopathic pulmonary fibrosis. Chest. 1991;99(3 Suppl):65s–6s.
79. Bergeron A et al. Cytokine profiles in idiopathic pulmonary fibrosis suggest an important role for TGF-beta and IL-10. Eur Respir J. 2003;22(1):69–76.
80. Zaiman AL et al. Role of the TGF-beta/Alk5 signaling pathway in monocrotaline-induced pulmonary hypertension. Am J Respir Crit Care Med. 2008;177(8):896–905.
81. Fredriksson L, Li H, Eriksson U. The PDGF family: four gene products form five dimeric isoforms. Cytokine Growth Factor Rev. 2004;15(4):197–204.
82. Antoniades HN et al. Platelet-derived growth factor in idiopathic pulmonary fibrosis. J Clin Invest. 1990;86(4):1055–64.
83. Welsh DJ, Peacock AJ. Cellular responses to hypoxia in the pulmonary circulation. High Alt Med Biol. 2013;14(2):111–6.
84. Kolilekas L et al. Sleep oxygen desaturation predicts survival in idiopathic pulmonary fibrosis. J Clin Sleep Med. 2013;9(6):593–601.
85. Pihtili A et al. Obstructive sleep apnea is common in patients with interstitial lung disease. Sleep Breath. 2013;17(4):1281–8.

86. Mermigkis C et al. How common is sleep-disordered breathing in patients with idiopathic pulmonary fibrosis? Sleep Breath. 2010;14(4):387–90.
87. Perez-Padilla R et al. Breathing during sleep in patients with interstitial lung disease. Am Rev Respir Dis. 1985;132(2):224–9.
88. Midgren B et al. Oxygen desaturation during sleep and exercise in patients with interstitial lung disease. Thorax. 1987;42(5):353–6.
89. Clark M et al. A survey of nocturnal hypoxaemia and health related quality of life in patients with cryptogenic fibrosing alveolitis. Thorax. 2001;56(6):482–6.
90. Midgren B. Oxygen desaturation during sleep as a function of the underlying respiratory disease. Am Rev Respir Dis. 1990;141(1):43–6.
91. Fletcher EC et al. Pulmonary vascular hemodynamics in chronic lung disease patients with and without oxyhemoglobin desaturation during sleep. Chest. 1989;95(4):757–64.
92. Corte TJ et al. Elevated nocturnal desaturation index predicts mortality in interstitial lung disease. Sarcoidosis Vasc Diffuse Lung Dis. 2012;29(1):41–50.
93. Trakada G et al. Endothelin-1 levels in interstitial lung disease patients during sleep. Sleep Breath. 2003;7(3):111–8.
94. Talbot NP et al. Two temporal components within the human pulmonary vascular response to approximately 2 h of isocapnic hypoxia. J Appl Physiol (1985). 2005;98(3):1125–39.
95. van Riet EE et al. Epidemiology of heart failure: the prevalence of heart failure and ventricular dysfunction in older adults over time. A systematic review. Eur J Heart Fail. 2016;18(3):242–52.
96. Papadopoulos CE et al. Left ventricular diastolic dysfunction in idiopathic pulmonary fibrosis: a tissue Doppler echocardiographic [corrected] study. Eur Respir J. 2008;31(4):701–6.
97. Nathan SD et al. Prevalence and impact of coronary artery disease in idiopathic pulmonary fibrosis. Respir Med. 2010;104(7):1035–41.
98. Hubbard RB et al. The association between idiopathic pulmonary fibrosis and vascular disease: a population-based study. Am J Respir Crit Care Med. 2008;178(12):1257–61.
99. Sode BF et al. Venous thromboembolism and risk of idiopathic interstitial pneumonia: a nationwide study. Am J Respir Crit Care Med. 2010;181(10):1085–92.
100. Sprunger DB et al. Pulmonary fibrosis is associated with an elevated risk of thromboembolic disease. Eur Respir J. 2012;39(1):125–32.
101. Wygrecka M et al. Cellular origin of pro-coagulant and (anti)-fibrinolytic factors in bleomycin-injured lungs. Eur Respir J. 2007;29(6):1105–14.
102. Fujii M et al. Relevance of tissue factor and tissue factor pathway inhibitor for hypercoagulable state in the lungs of patients with idiopathic pulmonary fibrosis. Thromb Res. 2000;99(2):111–7.
103. Kotani I et al. Increased procoagulant and antifibrinolytic activities in the lungs with idiopathic pulmonary fibrosis. Thromb Res. 1995;77(6):493–504.
104. Fahim A et al. Increased platelet binding to circulating monocytes in idiopathic pulmonary fibrosis. Lung. 2014;192(2):277–84.
105. Kinder BW, Collard HR, King Jr TE. Anticoagulant therapy and idiopathic pulmonary fibrosis. Chest. 2006;130(1):302–3.
106. Noth I et al. A placebo-controlled randomized trial of warfarin in idiopathic pulmonary fibrosis. Am J Respir Crit Care Med. 2012;186(1):88–95.
107. Luo Q et al. Prevalence of venous thromboembolic events and diagnostic performance of the wells score and revised geneva scores for pulmonary embolism in patients with interstitial lung disease: a prospective study. Heart Lung Circ. 2014;23(8):778–85.
108. Noble PW et al. Pirfenidone in patients with idiopathic pulmonary fibrosis (CAPACITY): two randomised trials. Lancet. 2011;377(9779):1760–9.
109. Richeldi L et al. Efficacy of a tyrosine kinase inhibitor in idiopathic pulmonary fibrosi. N Engl J Med. 365(12):1079–87.
110. Nathan SD et al. Effect of continued treatment with pirfenidone following clinically meaningful declines in forced vital capacity: analysis of data from three phase 3 trials in patients with idiopathic pulmonary fibrosis. Thorax. 2016;71(5):429–35.

111. Raghu G et al. An official ATS/ERS/JRS/ALAT clinical practice guideline: treatment of idiopathic pulmonary fibrosis. An update of the 2011 clinical practice guideline. Am J Respir Crit Care Med. 2015;192(2):e3–19.
112. Long term domiciliary oxygen therapy in chronic hypoxic cor pulmonale complicating chronic bronchitis and emphysema. Report of the Medical Research Council Working Party. Lancet. 1981;1(8222):681–6.
113. Continuous or nocturnal oxygen therapy in hypoxemic chronic obstructive lung disease: a clinical trial. Nocturnal Oxygen Therapy Trial Group. Ann Intern Med. 1980;93(3):391–8.
114. Hardinge M et al. British Thoracic Society guidelines for home oxygen use in adults. Thorax. 2015;70(Suppl 1):i1–43.
115. Kim DS et al. Acute exacerbation of idiopathic pulmonary fibrosis: frequency and clinical features. Eur Respir J. 2006;27(1):143–50.
116. Song JW et al. Acute exacerbation of idiopathic pulmonary fibrosis: incidence, risk factors and outcome. Eur Respir J. 2011;37(2):356–63.
117. Judge EP et al. Acute exacerbations and pulmonary hypertension in advanced idiopathic pulmonary fibrosis. Eur Respir J. 2012;40(1):93–100.
118. Huie TJ et al. A detailed evaluation of acute respiratory decline in patients with fibrotic lung disease: aetiology and outcomes. Respirology. 2010;15(6):909–17.
119. Johannson KA et al. Acute exacerbation of idiopathic pulmonary fibrosis associated with air pollution exposure. Eur Respir J. 2014;43(4):1124–31.
120. Lee JS et al. Bronchoalveolar lavage pepsin in acute exacerbation of idiopathic pulmonary fibrosis. Eur Respir J. 2012;39(2):352–8.
121. Maher TM et al. Development of a consensus statement for the definition, diagnosis, and treatment of acute exacerbations of idiopathic pulmonary fibrosis using the delphi technique. Adv Ther. 2015;32(10):929–43.
122. Shen JH et al. Comparison of the Wells score with the revised Geneva score for assessing suspected pulmonary embolism: a systematic review and meta-analysis. J Thromb Thrombolysis. 2016;41(3):482–92.
123. Wijesekera NT et al. Image quality of computed tomographic pulmonary angiography for suspected pulmonary embolus in patients with diffuse interstitial lung disease. J Thorac Imaging. 2012;27(3):156–63.
124. Leuschner G et al. Suspected pulmonary embolism in patients with pulmonary fibrosis: discordance between ventilation/perfusion SPECT and CT pulmonary angiography. Respirology. 2016;21(6):1081–7.
125. Strickland NH et al. Cause of regional ventilation-perfusion mismatching in patients with idiopathic pulmonary fibrosis: a combined CT and scintigraphic study. AJR Am J Roentgenol. 1993;161(4):719–25.
126. Peiman S et al. Subsegmental pulmonary embolism: a narrative review. Thromb Res. 2016;138:55–60.
127. Alagha K et al. Warfarin should be banned in ipf.pdf. Am J Respir Crit Care Med. 2015;191:958–60.
128. Milara J et al. Vascular effects of sildenafil in patients with pulmonary fibrosis and pulmonary hypertension: an ex vivo/in vitro study. Eur Respir J. 2016;47(6):1737–49.
129. Ghofrani HA et al. Sildenafil for treatment of lung fibrosis and pulmonary hypertension: a randomised controlled trial. Lancet. 2002;360(9337):895–900.
130. Collard HR, Anstrom KJ, Schwarz MI, Zisman DA. Sildenafil improves walk distance in idiopathic pulmonary fibrosis. Chest. 2007;131(3):897–9.
131. Corte TJ et al. The use of sildenafil to treat pulmonary hypertension associated with interstitial lung disease. Respirology. 2010;15(8):1226–32.
132. Zimmermann GS et al. Haemodynamic changes in pulmonary hypertension in patients with interstitial lung disease treated with PDE-5 inhibitors. Respirology. 2014;19(5):700–6.
133. Zisman DA et al. A controlled trial of sildenafil in advanced idiopathic pulmonary fibrosis. N Engl J Med. 2010;363(7):620–8.

134. Han MK et al. Sildenafil preserves exercise capacity in patients with idiopathic pulmonary fibrosis and right-sided ventricular dysfunction. Chest. 2013;143(6):1699–708.
135. du Bois RM et al. Six-minute-walk test in idiopathic pulmonary fibrosis: test validation and minimal clinically important difference. Am J Respir Crit Care Med. 2011;183(9):1231–7.
136. Hoeper MM et al. Pulmonary hypertension in patients with chronic fibrosing idiopathic interstitial pneumonias. PLoS One. 2015;10(12):e0141911.
137. Giaid A et al. Expression of endothelin-1 in the lungs of patients with pulmonary hypertension. N Engl J Med. 1993;328(24):1732–9.
138. Ross B, D'Orleans-Juste P, Giaid A. Potential role of endothelin-1 in pulmonary fibrosis: from the bench to the clinic. Am J Respir Cell Mol Biol. 2010;42(1):16–20.
139. Uguccioni M et al. Endothelin-1 in idiopathic pulmonary fibrosis. J Clin Pathol. 1995;48(4):330–4.
140. King Jr TE et al. BUILD-3: a randomized, controlled trial of bosentan in idiopathic pulmonary fibrosis. Am J Respir Crit Care Med. 2011;184(1):92–9.
141. Raghu G et al. Macitentan for the treatment of idiopathic pulmonary fibrosis: the randomised controlled MUSIC trial. Eur Respir J. 2013;42(6):1622–32.
142. Corte TJ et al. Bosentan in pulmonary hypertension associated with fibrotic idiopathic interstitial pneumonia. Am J Respir Crit Care Med. 2014;190(2):208–17.
143. Olschewski H et al. Inhaled prostacyclin and iloprost in severe pulmonary hypertension secondary to lung fibrosis. Am J Respir Crit Care Med. 1999;160(2):600–7.
144. Ghofrani HA et al. Riociguat for the treatment of pulmonary arterial hypertension. N Engl J Med. 2013;369(4):330–40.
145. Hoeper MM et al. Riociguat for interstitial lung disease and pulmonary hypertension: a pilot trial. Eur Respir J. 2013;41(4):853–60.
146. Bayer. Efficacy and safety of riociguat in patients with symptomatic pulmonary hypertension (PH) associated with idiopathic interstitial pneumonia's (IIP) (RISE-IIP). https://clinicaltrials.gov/ct2/show/, NCT02138825.
147. King Jr TE et al. BUILD-1: a randomized placebo-controlled trial of bosentan in idiopathic pulmonary fibrosis. Am J Respir Crit Care Med. 2008;177(1):75–81.

Chapter 7
Sarcoidosis-Associated Pulmonary Hypertension: Diagnosis and Treatment

Robert P. Baughman and Elyse E. Lower

Introduction

Sarcoidosis-associated pulmonary hypertension (SAPH) is included in Group 5 of the World Health Organization (WHO) categories of pulmonary hypertension [1]. Group 5 was established to include a variety of conditions with multifactorial pathogenesis of pulmonary hypertension that cannot meet the criteria of the other four categories. Group 5 is often problematic as SAPH and several other conditions in this group often have features of some of the other four WHO diagnostic groups and more than one may coexist in the same patient. SAPH is an important consideration in a known sarcoidosis patient who has persistent dyspnea.

Causes of SAPH

Several potential factors are noted in Table 7.1 that can lead to pulmonary hypertension in a sarcoidosis patient. Left ventricular dysfunction can elevate the pulmonary artery occluding pressure (PAOP) to greater than 15 mmHg (PH/LVD). This can be the result of reduced left ventricular ejection fraction (LVEF) from sarcoidosis cardiomyopathy [2, 3]. In addition, sarcoidosis patients may experience heart failure with preserved ejection fraction (HF-PEF). The reduced LVEF can be verified by

R.P. Baughman, MD (✉) • E.E. Lower, MD
Department of Medicine, University of Cincinnati Medical Center, Cincinnati, OH, USA
e-mail: bob.baughman@uc.edu

R.P. Baughman et al. (eds.), *Pulmonary Hypertension and Interstitial Lung Disease*, DOI 10.1007/978-3-319-49918-5_7

Table 7.1 Causes of pulmonary hypertension in sarcoidosis

• Cardiac
– Cardiomyopathy with reduced LVEF
– Heart failure with preserved ejection fraction
• Vascular
– Granulomatous angiitis (arterial and venous)
– Pulmonary veno-occlusive disease
– Compression of pulmonary vasculature
– Intimal fibrosis and medial hypertrophy
• Parenchymal lung disease
– Pulmonary fibrosis with obliteration of lung tissue
• Hypoxia-induced pulmonary hypertension
• Systemic disease
– Sarcoidosis-associated cirrhosis and portopulmonary hypertension

cardiac imaging such as MRI which may also identify infiltration of the myocardium with preserved LVEF [4]. Diastolic dysfunction may occur due to granulomatous infiltration of heart or comorbidities of sarcoidosis such as diabetes or systemic hypertension [5]. In one study of 130 persistently dyspneic sarcoidosis patients [6], right heart catheterization revealed PH/LVD in 20 patients (Fig. 7.1). Of these, only seven (35%) had documented reduced left ventricular systolic function. The survival was significantly better for those with PH/LVD than those patients with precapillary PH [6].

Vascular disease from sarcoidosis can also create pulmonary hypertension. Intimal fibrosis, medial hypertrophy, and changes in vascular tone have been reported with SAPH [7, 8]. Additionally granulomatous angiitis has also been reported. One study of open lung biopsies in 128 sarcoidosis patients identified some form of angiitis in 88 (69%) patients [9]. Venous disease was seen in over 90% of the angiitis cases with a third experiencing both arterial and venous involvement. In contrast, arterial involvement alone was seen in less than 10% of angiitis cases. A similar finding was reported in explants from sarcoidosis patients undergoing lung transplant [10]. Pulmonary veno-occlusive disease (PVOD) can be found [10] and its presence has clinical implications, since patients with PVOD may develop pulmonary edema when treated with some pulmonary vasodilators such as prostanoids [11]. While PVOD has been reported in up to a third of patients with SAPH [10], pulmonary edema associated with prostanoid therapy is much less frequently encountered [12, 13].

Direct compression of the pulmonary vasculature can also lead to pulmonary hypertension. Although simple hilar adenopathy may be causing direct compression, pulmonary hypertension is more likely associated with mediastinal fibrosis [14, 15]. While direct compression was felt to be a rare complication [14–16] one prospective series found 8 of 72 (11%) sarcoidosis patients had severe proximal

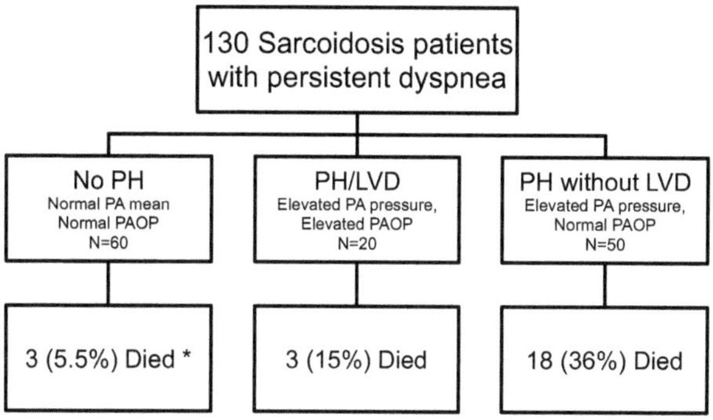

Fig. 7.1 Outcome of right heart catheterization of 130 sarcoidosis patients with persistent dyspnea. Patients were divided into three groups: *No PH*: normal PA mean and PAOP pressure, *PH/LVD*: elevated PA mean and PAOP, and *PH without LVD*: elevated PA mean and normal PAOP. (*Asterisk*) The observed mortality for all three groups was significantly higher for those with elevated PA mean and normal PAOP [6]

pulmonary artery stenosis [17]. In that series, patients were evaluated with echocardiography and computer tomographic pulmonary angiography, and all SAPH cases were confirmed by right heart catheterization. Not all cases of fibrosing mediastinitis are due to sarcoidosis. In one series of fibrosing mediastinitis-associated pulmonary hypertension, only half of cases were due to sarcoidosis [15]. Other conditions to consider include infections such as histoplasmosis and tuberculosis as well as mediastinal radiation [15, 18].

Pulmonary fibrosis occurs in 10–20% of sarcoidosis patients [19, 20]. The fibrosis may lead not only to destruction of lung parenchyma but also pulmonary vasculature involvement (Fig. 7.2). In addition to fibrosis, airway distortion, traction bronchiectasis, and emphysematous changes may be seen [21]. The destruction of lung tissue can also lead to hypoxia, which can further contribute to pulmonary hypertension. While patients with SAPH often have pulmonary fibrosis, a significant proportion of patients with SAPH have less advanced chest X-ray changes [22, 23]. Not all patients with SAPH have fibrotic chest x-ray. Figure 7.3 compares the Scadding chest X-ray stage [19] of patients with and without SAPH in two large series of sarcoidosis patients evaluated for pulmonary hypertension [22, 23].

Sarcoidosis is a multiorgan disease which affects the liver in at least 25% of sarcoidosis patients [24, 25]. While most cases are mild [24], severe liver involvement with cirrhosis can occur [26]. Cirrhosis due to sarcoidosis rarely develops hepatopulmonary syndrome and pulmonary hypertension [27, 28].

Because the clinical scenarios can vary greatly, expert evaluation is required to determine the exact cause of the pulmonary hypertension in sarcoidosis patients. This evaluation includes pulmonary function testing, chest imaging, laboratory evaluation, and right heart catheterization.

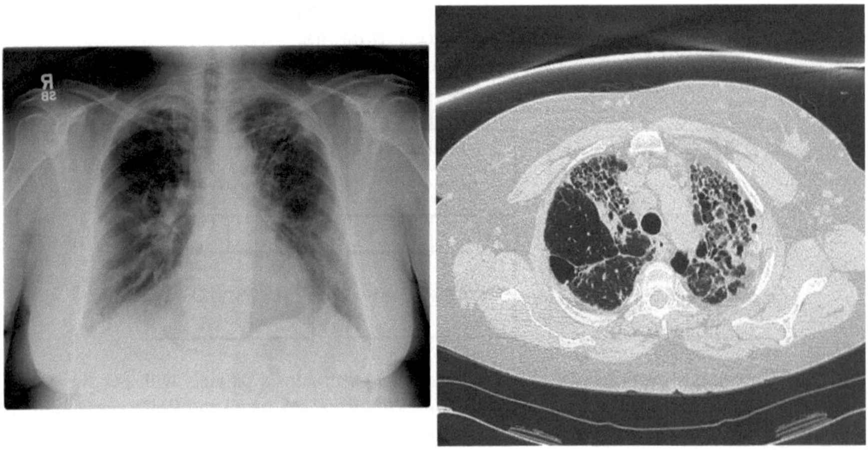

Fig. 7.2 Chest X-ray and computer tomography of sarcoidosis patient with pulmonary fibrosis and sarcoidosis-associated pulmonary hypertension

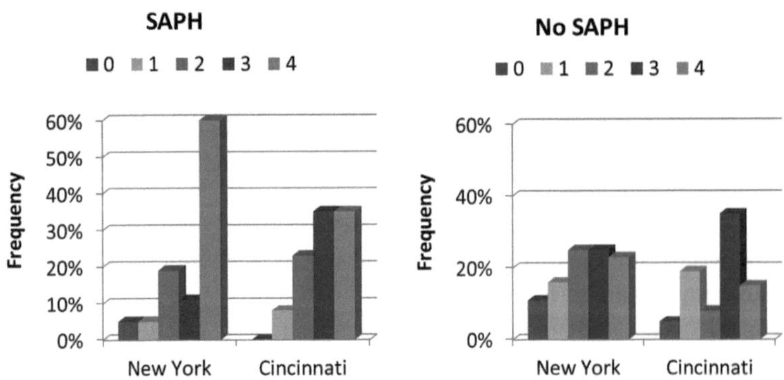

Fig. 7.3 The Scadding chest X-ray stage [19] of patients with and without SAPH for two large series of sarcoidosis patients evaluated for pulmonary hypertension (New York [23] and Cincinnati [22]

Frequency of SAPH

The frequency of pulmonary hypertension in sarcoidosis depends on the studied population. Table 7.2 reveals the prevalence of SAPH in the general sarcoidosis population [29–32], moderate to severely dyspneic sarcoidosis patients [6, 12, 23, 33], or sarcoidosis patients listed for lung transplant [34, 35]. Most studies include patients with both precapillary and left ventricular dysfunction. As shown in Fig. 7.1, about 20% of patients with SAPH have elevated pressures due to left ventricular disease [6]. Screening for pulmonary hypertension was performed by various methods in these studies and in only a few studies did all patients underwent right heart catheterization [6, 34, 35]. In other studies, screening was performed by

Table 7.2 Prevalence of pulmonary hypertension in sarcoidosis[a]

Clinic	Percentage with SAPH (%)	Diagnosis confirmed by
All patients in clinic		
Kyoto [32]	6	Echocardiography
London [43]	11	Right heart catheterization
Detroit [30]	16	Right heart catheterization
Riyadh [29]	20.8	Echocardiography
Persistently dyspneic patients		
Milan [33]	55	Right heart catheterization
New York [23]	52	Echocardiography
Chicago [12]	56.5	Right heart catheterization
Cincinnati [6]	60[a]	Right heart catheterization
Lung transplant list		
Washington [35]	72	Right heart catheterization
Copenhagen [34]	79	Right heart catheterization

[a]Includes both precapillary and pulmonary hypertension due to left ventricular dysfunction

echocardiography with a right heart catheterization performed only to confirm pulmonary hypertension [23, 29–31]. Other studies reported only echocardiography results. Regardless of the screening technique used, the overall prevalence of SAPH was similar for each of these groups.

As revealed in Table 7.3, several of Table 7.2 studies examined potential risk factors for SAPH. Many of the features were studied in some but not all reports. The "typical" patient with SAPH will have pulmonary fibrosis, a reduced diffusing capacity of the lung for carbon monoxide (DLCO), and desaturation with exercise. In one large registry of SAPH, a significant negative correlation was identified between DLCO percent predicted (Fig. 7.4a) and PA mean but no significant relationship was seen between FVC percent predicted and PA mean (Fig. 7.4b). This probably reflects that the reduction in DLCO is usually more prominent than the reduction in lung volume [31]. This "out of proportion" reduction in DLCO has also been noted in scleroderma-associated pulmonary hypertension [36]. It is not clear whether this ratio may also be useful in identifying sarcoidosis patients with SAPH.

Diagnosis of SAPH

The first step in detecting SAPH is simple: think about it. Pulmonary hypertension often presents with nonspecific symptoms including dyspnea. Because sarcoidosis is a multifaceted disease, reduced exercise capacity may be due to multiple causes, such as parenchymal or airway lung disease, direct cardiac dysfunction, skeletal muscle disease, neurologic disease, or even fatigue or depression [37]. Our approach in diagnosing SAPH is detailed in Table 7.4.

Table 7.3 Features associated with sarcoidosis-associated pulmonary hypertension

• Pulmonary fibrosis on chest X-ray [23, 31–33]
• Reduced forced vital capacity [6, 23, 30, 32]
• Reduced DLCO [6, 23, 30–32]
• Reduced six minute walk distance [30, 41, 66]
• Hypoxemia especially after six minute walk test [30, 66]
• Older age [31]

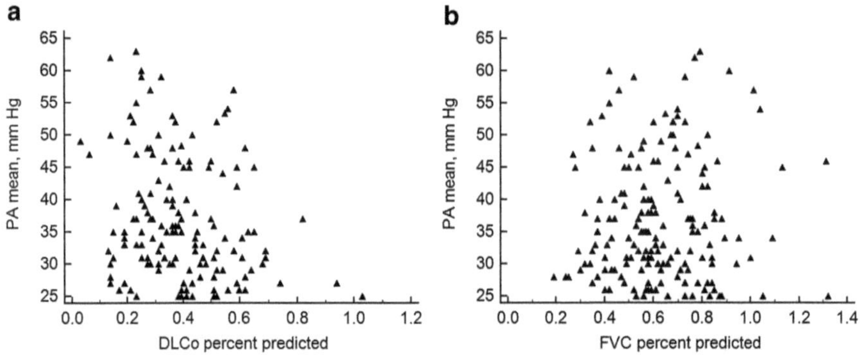

Fig. 7.4 (**a**) There was a significant negative correlation between the DLCO percent predicted versus PA mean (Rho = −0.235, $p < 0.005$). (**b**) There was no correlation between FVC percent predicted and PA mean ($p > 0.05$). Data from registry for sarcoidosis-associated pulmonary hypertension (ReSAPH), presented at American Thoracic Society 2016

The initial evaluation remains questioning about dyspnea, which can be quantified by standardized questionnaires [38]. One commonly used system is the American Thoracic Society/Medical Resource Council questionnaire, which allows one to identify mild, moderate, or severe dyspnea. This questionnaire has adequately stratified patients with sarcoidosis or idiopathic pulmonary fibrosis [39, 40]. Another standard questionnaire is the Borg score, which is often used in conjunction with the six minute walk (6MW) test. The 6MW walk is also useful for evaluating dyspnea. The 6MW distance is shorter in patients with SAPH [41]. Hypoxia, especially with exertion, is a common feature [30] and should lead to further evaluation for SAPH. The hypoxia from pulmonary hypertension is often due to shunting, which may be worsened with vasodilator therapy [8]. Clinically significant worsening of shunting is relatively rare after vasodilator therapy [42]. Hypoxia may also be due to underlying parenchymal lung disease from the sarcoidosis.

As shown in Fig. 7.4a, there is a negative correlation between DLCO and PA mean pressure [22, 43]. In addition, SAPH is more frequently encountered in patients with a disproportionate reduction in DLCO [36]. A reduced DLCO is a strong predictor of pulmonary hypertension, especially in a patient without pulmonary fibrosis [31].

Table 7.4 Evaluation for possible sarcoidosis-associated pulmonary hypertension

• *Initial evaluation*: Presence of one or more feature
– Complaint of moderate or greater dyspnea with exertion
– Hypoxia at rest or with exercise
– Reduced DLCO out of proportion to reduction of lung volumes
– Significant pulmonary fibrosis on chest roentgenogram
Computer tomography scan showing significant pulmonary fibrosis
• *Screening*: Presence of one or more feature from Initial Evaluation leads to
– Echocardiography showing estimated systolic pulmonary artery pressure of greater than 35 mmHg
– Evidence of right ventricular dysfunction
Echocardiography
Magnetic resonance imaging
– Six minute walk
Desaturation by more than 5%
– Computer tomography scan showing either
Main pulmonary artery to aorta ratio of greater than one
Main pulmonary artery >29 mm
• *Confirmation and classification of pulmonary hypertension*: If any screening tests positive
– Right heart catheterization

As shown in Fig. 7.3, patients with SAPH are far more likely to have pulmonary fibrosis on chest X-ray than the general sarcoidosis population [23, 33]. However, there is considerable overlap and the lack of pulmonary fibrosis does not rule out pulmonary hypertension [22, 31]. Pulmonary fibrosis can also be detected by computer tomography (CT) scanning. The CT scan can be very sensitive to minimal scarring as a residual for sarcoidosis. Walsh et al. proposed that the presence of 20% or more fibrosis on CT scan be considered significant pulmonary fibrosis [20].

The presence of one or more of the features listed in Table 7.4 during initial evaluation is present, one should proceed with screening for pulmonary hypertension. The two tests most commonly used to screen for pulmonary hypertension are echocardiography and 6MW test. While less commonly employed as an exclusive screening tool, the results of CT scan may also be a useful screening test.

The echocardiogram is the most commonly used noninvasive tool for assessing for pulmonary hypertension regardless of cause. However, the echocardiogram has been shown to have significant limitations in patients with interstitial lung disease including sarcoidosis, with PA systolic pressure often over- or underestimated [44, 45]. However, for patients with an estimated PA systolic pressure of >50 mmHg, most will have significant pulmonary hypertension by catheterization [6, 45]. In addition, one study of SAPH found that an elevated PA systolic pressure by echocardiogram of 50 mmHg or more was associated with increased mortality [6]. It is important to remember that the echocardiogram is not able to distinguish between precapillary and postcapillary pulmonary hypertension.

Right ventricular function can also be assessed noninvasively and the presence of right ventricular dysfunction is suggestive of SAPH [33]. The tricuspid annular plane systolic excursion (TAPSE), a well-described measure of right ventricular performance which can be measured by echocardiography and has been shown to be abnormal in some cases of SAPH [43]. Magnetic resonance imaging (MRI) has also been reported as effective in assessing right ventricular dysfunction [46]. A recent study evaluated RV function in 50 consecutive sarcoidosis patients undergoing cardiac MRI for clinical reasons [47]. Using sensitive measures of RV dysfunction, the investigators found abnormal results in more than half of the patients studied. RV dysfunction was most common in patients with parenchymal lung disease, left ventricular dysfunction, and pulmonary hypertension, but four patients had no cause identified [47].

The 6MW test is another commonly used test to assess dyspnea and screen for pulmonary hypertension and is shorter in SAPH than other sarcoidosis patients [41]. However, there is considerable overlap. This is in part because of the multiple factors in sarcoidosis that can affect exercise performance including parenchymal lung disease, muscle involvement, and fatigue from the sarcoidosis [37]. Another test for screening for pulmonary hypertension is desaturation during the 6MW test [30]. However, not all SAPH patients desaturate [41] so this test cannot be used to exclude pulmonary hypertension.

As computer tomography (CT) has been applied more widely to advanced pulmonary disease, information regarding possible pulmonary hypertension can be assessed [48]. The size of the pulmonary artery can be readily evaluated by the CT scan. A main pulmonary artery of greater than 29 mm or a PA main to aorta ratio of greater than one has been proposed as highly suggestive of pulmonary hypertension [49] including those with interstitial lung disease [50]. In sarcoidosis, the presence of an increased ratio can suggest pulmonary hypertension [51] but the ratio does not seem to correlate with the level of pulmonary hypertension [22].

If one or more of the screening tests are supportive of pulmonary hypertension, one should confirm the diagnosis with right heart catheterization. There are several reasons to perform a right heart catheterization. It has been shown that the prognosis is significantly different between those with precapillary pulmonary hypertension and pulmonary hypertension due to diastolic dysfunction [6]. Right heart catheterization also allows one to accurately characterize cardiac output and determine pulmonary vascular resistance. These are important aspects of prognosis and treatment of SAPH.

Treatment

The treatment of SAPH can follow the general approach summarized in Fig. 7.5. The first step is to treat hypoxia either at rest or with exercise with supplemental oxygen. Patients with sarcoidosis also have an increased risk for sleep apnea and nocturnal desaturation [52, 53]. Nocturnal desaturation is associated with increased mortality in interstitial lung disease [54]. Treatment may improve symptoms and

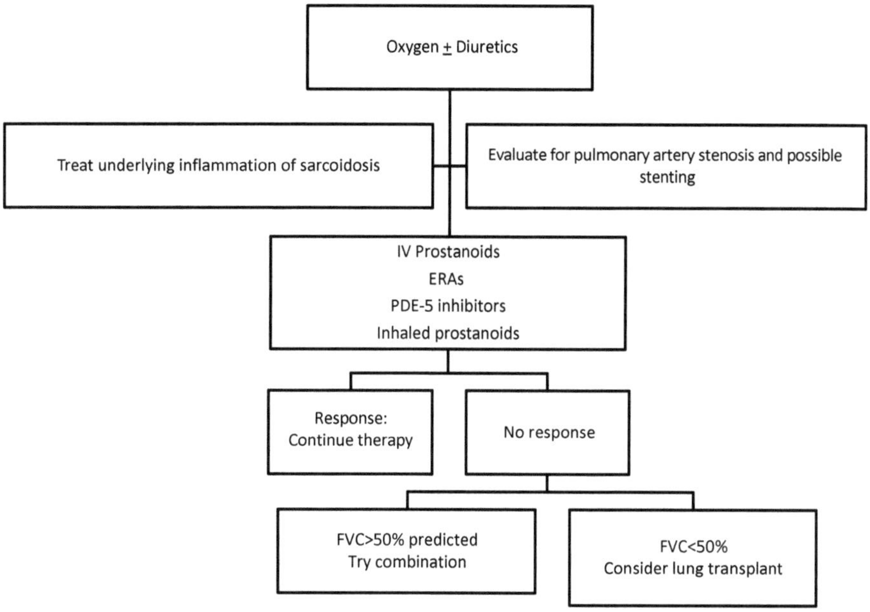

Fig. 7.5 Proposed algorithm for treating precapillary sarcoidosis-associated pulmonary hypertension. *IV* intravenous, *ERAs* endothelin receptor antagonists, *PDE-5* phosphodiesterase 5, *FVC* forced vital capacity

outcome. Diuretic therapy may also improve symptoms of right heart dysfunction in patients with pulmonary hypertension.

One should also evaluate for pulmonary artery stenosis. Mediastinal adenopathy and fibrosis can lead to pulmonary hypertension and can often be detected by CT scan. In some cases, there may be some response to anti-inflammatory therapy such as glucocorticoids [14, 16]. However, anti-inflammatory therapy does not improve the vascular narrowing in all cases [14, 15]. Some of these patients may respond to pulmonary artery stenting and/or steroids [55]. In one study of 32 patients with SAPH identified by echocardiography, eight (25%) had large vessel narrowing [17]. The authors treated these patients with dilation/stenting and corticosteroids. All patients were doing well at least 3 months after interventional treatment.

The recommendations for pharmacologic treatment of SAPH are based on case series and examining the results of treatment trials in other pulmonary hypertension conditions [56]. Many of the older agents for idiopathic pulmonary hypertension have been studied in SAPH, but there is limited information regarding newer agents.

Prostacyclins: Intravenous epoprostenol was the first drug to be shown to effectively treat precapillary pulmonary hypertension [57]. This regimen is usually reserved for patients with moderate-to-severe pulmonary hypertension because of toxicity and cost [49]. For SAPH, there have been reports of intravenous epoprostenol for both short-term [8] and long-term treatment [12, 13]. Fisher et al. [13] began six SAPH patients with epoprostenol and five were still on treatment more than 1 year later. Two patients had severe complications during initiation of therapy: one had a cardiac arrest and the other required mechanical ventilation. The second patient experienced pulmonary edema, possibly due to a component of veno-occlusive disease as part of the SAPH. Nonetheless, that patient was eventually able to tolerate long-term therapy with epoprostenol. This overall positive response was confirmed by a recent, retrospective study by Bonham et al. [12] They treated 13 patients with prostaglandins, 7 with epoprostenol, and 6 with trepostinil, with 9 of 13 still alive after 1 year of therapy. Repeat catheterizations were performed on 10 of 13 patients. There was a significant improvement in cardiac output and pulmonary vascular resistance but not in mean pulmonary artery pressure. The authors did not comment on changes in 6MW distance.

Inhaled iloprost has also been studied in SAPH. Use of iloprost in SAPH has been limited because of the high rate of complications (mostly cough). In one prospective study of 22 patients treated with inhaled iloprost [58], only 15 completed the full 16 weeks of therapy. In that study, repeat right heart catheterization demonstrated improved hemodynamics in only six of these patients and only three patients improved their 6MW distance by more than 30 m. However, most patients reported an improvement in quality of life in this open-label trial.

Endothelin receptor antagonists (ERA): Bosentan has been the most widely studied ERA in treatment for SAPH. This includes retrospective case series employing the drug as a single agent [22, 59, 60] or in combination with other agents [22, 43, 60]. A double-blind, placebo-controlled trial of bosentan as single agent for SAPH has been reported [42]. There was a significant improvement in both mean pulmonary artery pressure and pulmonary vascular resistance for the bosentan-treated patients with no change for the placebo group. Unfortunately, there was no significant improvement in the 6MW distance during the 16 weeks of the study. Also, there were no significant changes in quality of life measures after treatment with bosentan compared to the placebo-treated group.

Ambrisentan is another ERA reported as a treatment for SAPH [43]. In a prospective, open-label trial of ambrisentan for SAPH, Judson et al. reported an improvement in reported quality of life but no change in 6MW distance after 24 weeks of therapy [61]. In a study of patients with idiopathic pulmonary fibrosis, ambrisentan was associated with worse outcome compared to placebo [62].

PDE-5 inhibitors: The use of sildenafil and tadalafil has been reported in some case series in SAPH [43, 60]. In one retrospective series, sarcoidosis patients listed for lung transplant who were found to have SAPH were treated with sildenafil had improvement in mean pulmonary artery pressure [34]. This study did not find a significant change in the 6MW distance. On the other hand, two groups have reported on the use of sildenafil alone or in combination with other agents [43, 60]. While not reporting on the outcome of treatment with sildenafil exclusively, the authors found that their "real world" use of this drug was associated with an overall improvement in various parameters including pulmonary hemodynamics [60], 6MW distance [43, 60], and TAPSE [43].

Overall outcome of pharmacologic treatment of SAPH: To date, there is no clear-cut PAH-specific therapy that has proven efficacy or approval for treatment of

Table 7.5 Outcomes improved by pharmacologic treatment of SAPH

Class/Drug	Evidence	Results
Prostacyclines		
Epoprostenol	CS [12, 13]	Clinical improvement [7, 13]
	CR [7, 8]	Improved hemodynamics [12]
Inhaled iloprost	PCS [58]	Improved hemodynamics [58]
		Improved quality of life measures [58]
Endothelin receptor antagonists		
Bosentan	DBPC [42]	Clinical improvement [22, 43, 60]
	CS [22, 43, 60]	Improved hemodynamics [42]
Ambrisentan	PCS [61]	Improved quality of life measures [61]
Phosphodiesterase inhibitor		
Sildenafil	CS [34]	Improved hemodynamics [67]
Combination drug therapy		
Various drugs	CS [12, 22, 43, 60]	Clinical improvement [12, 22, 43, 60]
		Improved hemodynamics [60]
		Improved 6MW distance [12, 43, 60]

CS case series, *CR* case reports, *PCS* prospective case series, *DBPC* double blind, placebo controlled

SAPH. Nonetheless, a meta-analysis found that pharmacologic treatment of SAPH was associated with improvement in pulmonary hemodynamics and quality of life [63]. Table 7.5 lists various potential treatments for sarcoidosis with some of the outcomes. Improvement in clinical status was reported in almost all reports. Some studies performed repeat right heart catheterization and found improved hemodynamics in some but not all patients. In two series, measures of right ventricular dysfunction such as TAPSE and N-terminal pro-B type natriuretic peptide were reported as improved [12, 43]

In some series, quality of life instruments were used to assess response to therapy. Quality of life instruments may be useful in assessing the impact of therapy. There is no agreement on a single quality of life instrument specific for pulmonary arterial hypertension [64]. In the reported studies of treatment for SAPH, improvement in quality of life using the general instruments short form 36 (SF-36) and Saint George Respiratory Questionnaire (SGRQ) has been reported in two open-label prospective trials [58, 61]. However, there was no significant improvement in quality of life compared to placebo in the only double-blind trial reported to date in SAPH using these instruments [42]. Future trials using more specific questionnaires may provide more information.

Changes in pulmonary hemodynamics have not always led to improvement in 6MW distance. The three studies that reported an improvement in 6MW distance were all retrospective studies in which the clinicians changed therapy based on initial response [12, 43, 60]. The treatment used in these studies is consistent with recommendations for treatment of group 1 pulmonary arterial hypertension [49].

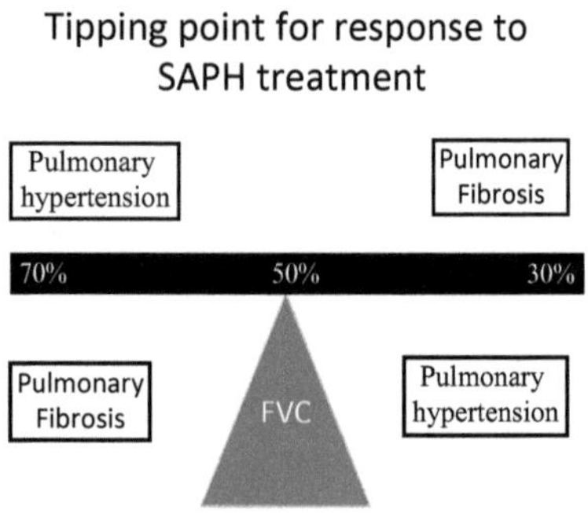

Fig. 7.6 Tipping point for when treatment for pulmonary hypertension will be no longer effective due to extent of pulmonary fibrosis

In those studies reporting an improvement in 6MW distance [12, 43, 60], not all patients had improved 6MW distance. A reduced forced vital capacity (FVC) is an independent risk factor for reduced 6MW distance [41]. For patients with a very low FVC, the treatment of pulmonary hypertension will have little impact on their clinical outcome and 6MW distance. On the other hand, those with minimal fibrosis will likely respond to pulmonary hypertension therapy as assessed by 6MW distance. Figure 7.6 proposes that there is a "tipping point" in the degree of pulmonary fibrosis in patients with SAPH. In the study by Barnett et al., patients with a FVC % predicted above the median (51%) were much more likely to improve their 6MW distance with treatment of pulmonary hypertension [60]. In an open-label extension of the bosentan trial SAPH, Culver et al. reported that a subgroup of patients had a >50 m improvement in 6MW distance after 32–48 weeks of treatment with bosentan [65]. All the patients who responded had an initial FVC of 60%.

In conclusion, recognition of SAPH requires that one think of the diagnosis. A right heart catheterization should be considered in all cases of potential SAPH. Treatment of SAPH should consider issues such as pulmonary artery narrowing and severely reduced lung tissue. Further trials regarding the impact of therapy for SAPH are needed.

References

1. Simonneau G, Robbins IM, Beghetti M, Channick RN, Delcroix M, Denton CP, et al. Updated clinical classification of pulmonary hypertension. J Am Coll Cardiol. 2009;54(1 Suppl):S43–54.
2. Mehta D, Lubitz SA, Frankel Z, Wisnivesky JP, Einstein AJ, Goldman M, et al. Cardiac involvement in patients with sarcoidosis: diagnostic and prognostic value of outpatient testing. Chest. 2008;133(6):1426–35.
3. Pabst S, Hammerstingl C, Grau N, Kreuz J, Grohe C, Juergens UR, et al. Pulmonary arterial hypertension in patients with sarcoidosis: the Pulsar single center experience. Adv Exp Med Biol. 2013;755:299–305.
4. Crouser ED, Ono C, Tran T, He X, Raman SV. Improved detection of cardiac sarcoidosis using magnetic resonance with myocardial T2 mapping. Am J Respir Crit Care Med. 2014;189(1):109–12.

5. Martusewicz-Boros MM, Boros PW, Wiatr E, Roszkowski-Sliz K. What comorbidities accompany sarcoidosis? A large cohort (n=1779) patients analysis. Sarcoidosis Vasc Diffuse Lung Dis. 2015;32(2):115–20.
6. Baughman RP, Engel PJ, Taylor L, Lower EE. Survival in sarcoidosis associated pulmonary hypertension: the importance of hemodynamic evaluation. Chest. 2010;138:1078–85.
7. Barst RJ, Ratner SJ. Sarcoidosis and reactive pulmonary hypertension. Arch Intern Med. 1985;145(11):2112–4.
8. Preston IR, Klinger JR, Landzberg MJ, Houtchens J, Nelson D, Hill NS. Vasoresponsiveness of sarcoidosis-associated pulmonary hypertension. Chest. 2001;120(3):866–72.
9. Rosen Y, Moon S, Huang CT, Gourin A, Lyons HA. Granulomatous pulmonary angiitis in sarcoidosis. Arch Pathol Lab Med. 1977;101(4):170–4.
10. Nunes H, Humbert M, Capron F, Brauner M, Sitbon O, Battesti JP, et al. Pulmonary hypertension associated with sarcoidosis: mechanisms, haemodynamics and prognosis. Thorax. 2006;61(1):68–74.
11. Montani D, Achouh L, Dorfmuller P, Le PJ, Sztrymf B, Tcherakian C, et al. Pulmonary veno-occlusive disease: clinical, functional, radiologic, and hemodynamic characteristics and outcome of 24 cases confirmed by histology. Medicine (Baltimore). 2008;87(4):220–33.
12. Bonham CA, Oldham JM, Gomberg-Maitland M, Vij R. Prostacyclin and oral vasodilator therapy in sarcoidosis-associated pulmonary hypertension: a retrospective case series. Chest. 2015;148(4):1055–62.
13. Fisher KA, Serlin DM, Wilson KC, Walter RE, Berman JS, Farber HW. Sarcoidosis-associated pulmonary hypertension: outcome with long-term epoprostenol treatment. Chest. 2006;130(5):1481–8.
14. Toonkel RL, Borczuk AC, Pearson GD, Horn EM, Thomashow BM. Sarcoidosis-associated fibrosing mediastinitis with resultant pulmonary hypertension: a case report and review of the literature. Respiration. 2010;79(4):341–5.
15. Seferian A, Steriade A, Jais X, Planche O, Savale L, Parent F, et al. Pulmonary hypertension complicating fibrosing mediastinitis. Medicine (Baltimore). 2015;94(44):e1800.
16. Hasegawa K, Ohno S, Takada M, Ogino H, Shiotsu S, Takumi C, et al. Sarcoidosis complicated with major pulmonary artery obstruction and stenosis. Intern Med. 2012;51(19):2775–80.
17. Liu L, Xu J, Zhang Y, Fang L, Chai Y, Niu M, et al. Interventional therapy in sarcoidosis-associated pulmonary arterial stenosis and pulmonary hypertension. Clin Respir J. 2016; doi:10.1111/crj.12435.
18. Davis AM, Pierson RN, Loyd JE. Mediastinal fibrosis. Semin Respir Infect. 2001;16(2):119–30.
19. Scadding JG. Prognosis of intrathoracic sarcoidosis in England. Br Med J. 1961;2(5261):1165–72.
20. Walsh SL, Wells AU, Sverzellati N, Keir GJ, Calandriello L, Antoniou KM, et al. An integrated clinicoradiological staging system for pulmonary sarcoidosis: a case-cohort study. Lancet Respir Med. 2014;2(2):123–30.
21. Nunes H, Uzunhan Y, Gille T, Lamberto C, Valeyre D, Brillet PY. Imaging of sarcoidosis of the airways and lung parenchyma and correlation with lung function. Eur Respir J. 2012;40(3):750–65.
22. Baughman RP, Engel PJ, Meyer CA, Barrett AB, Lower EE. Pulmonary hypertension in sarcoidosis. Sarcoidosis Vasc Diffuse Lung Dis. 2006;23:108–16.
23. Sulica R, Teirstein AS, Kakarla S, Nemani N, Behnegar A, Padilla ML. Distinctive clinical, radiographic, and functional characteristics of patients with sarcoidosis-related pulmonary hypertension. Chest. 2005;128(3):1483–9.
24. Cremers J, Drent M, Driessen A, Nieman F, Wijnen P, Baughman R, et al. Liver-test abnormalities in sarcoidosis. Eur J Gastroenterol Hepatol. 2012;24:17–24.
25. Kahi CJ, Saxena R, Temkit M, Canlas K, Roberts S, Knox K, et al. Hepatobiliary disease in sarcoidosis. Sarcoidosis Vasc Diffuse Lung Dis. 2006;23(2):117–23.
26. Fetzer DT, Rees MA, Dasyam AK, Tublin ME. Hepatic sarcoidosis in patients presenting with liver dysfunction: imaging appearance, pathological correlation and disease evolution. Eur Radiol. 2016;26(9):3129–37.

27. Gupta S, Faughnan ME, Prud'homme GJ, Hwang DM, Munoz DG, Kopplin P. Sarcoidosis complicated by cirrhosis and hepatopulmonary syndrome. Can Respir J. 2008;15(3):124–6.
28. Salazar A, Mana J, Sala J, Landoni BR, Manresa F. Combined portal and pulmonary hypertension in sarcoidosis. Respiration. 1994;61(2):117–9.
29. Alhamad EH, Idrees MM, Alanezi MO, Alboukai AA, Shaik SA. Sarcoidosis-associated pulmonary hypertension: Clinical features and outcomes in Arab patients. Ann Thorac Med. 2010;5(2):86–91.
30. Bourbonnais JM, Samavati L. Clinical predictors of pulmonary hypertension in sarcoidosis. Eur Respir J. 2008;32(2):296–302.
31. Rapti A, Kouranos V, Gialafos E, Aggeli K, Moyssakis J, Kallianos A, et al. Elevated pulmonary arterial systolic pressure in patients with sarcoidosis: prevalence and risk factors. Lung. 2013;191(1):61–7.
32. Handa T, Nagai S, Miki S, Fushimi Y, Ohta K, Mishima M, et al. Incidence of pulmonary hypertension and its clinical relevance in patients with sarcoidosis. Chest. 2006;129(5):1246–52.
33. Rizzato G, Pezzano A, Sala G, Merlini R, Ladelli L, Tansini G, et al. Right heart impairment in sarcoidosis: haemodynamic and echocardiographic study. Eur J Respir Dis. 1983;64(2):121–8.
34. Milman N, Burton CM, Iversen M, Videbaek R, Jensen CV, Carlsen J. Pulmonary hypertension in end-stage pulmonary sarcoidosis: therapeutic effect of sildenafil? J Heart Lung Transplant. 2008;27(3):329–34.
35. Shorr AF, Helman DL, Davies DB, Nathan SD. Pulmonary hypertension in advanced sarcoidosis: epidemiology and clinical characteristics. Eur Respir J. 2005;25(5):783–8.
36. Steen V, Medsger TA Jr. Predictors of isolated pulmonary hypertension in patients with systemic sclerosis and limited cutaneous involvement. Arthritis Rheum. 2003;48(2):516–22.
37. Baughman RP, Lower EE. Six-minute walk test in managing and monitoring sarcoidosis patients. Curr Opin Pulm Med. 2007;13(5):439–44.
38. Mahler DA, Wells CK. Evaluation of clinical methods for rating dyspnea. Chest. 1988;93(3):580–6.
39. Baughman RP, Drent M, Kavuru M, Judson MA, Costabel U, Du BR, et al. Infliximab therapy in patients with chronic sarcoidosis and pulmonary involvement. Am J Respir Crit Care Med. 2006;174(7):795–802.
40. Papiris SA, Daniil ZD, Malagari K, Kapotsis GE, Sotiropoulou C, Milic-Emili J, et al. The Medical Research Council dyspnea scale in the estimation of disease severity in idiopathic pulmonary fibrosis. Respir Med. 2005;99(6):755–61.
41. Baughman RP, Sparkman BK, Lower EE. Six-minute walk test and health status assessment in sarcoidosis. Chest. 2007;132(1):207–13.
42. Baughman RP, Culver DA, Cordova FC, Padilla M, Gibson KF, Lower EE, et al. Bosentan for sarcoidosis associated pulmonary hypertension: A double-blind placebo controlled randomized trial. Chest. 2014;145:810–7.
43. Keir GJ, Walsh SL, Gatzoulis MA, Marino PS, Dimopoulos K, Alonso R, et al. Treatment of sarcoidosis-associated pulmonary hypertension: A single centre retrospective experience using targeted therapies. Sarcoidosis Vasc Diffuse Lung Dis. 2014;31(2):82–90.
44. Arcasoy SM, Christie JD, Ferrari VA, Sutton MS, Zisman DA, Blumenthal NP, et al. Echocardiographic assessment of pulmonary hypertension in patients with advanced lung disease. Am J Respir Crit Care Med. 2003;167(5):735–40.
45. Nathan SD, Shlobin OA, Barnett SD, Saggar R, Belperio JA, Ross DJ, et al. Right ventricular systolic pressure by echocardiography as a predictor of pulmonary hypertension in idiopathic pulmonary fibrosis. Respir Med. 2008;102(9):1305–10.
46. Frank H, Globits S, Glogar D, Neuhold A, Kneussl M, Mlczoch J. Detection and quantification of pulmonary artery hypertension with MR imaging: results in 23 patients. AJR Am J Roentgenol. 1993;161(1):27–31.
47. Patel MB, Mor-Avi V, Murtagh G, Bonham CA, Laffin LJ, Hogarth DK, et al. Right heart involvement in patients with sarcoidosis. Echocardiography. 2016;10
48. Hennebicque AS, Nunes H, Brillet PY, Moulahi H, Valeyre D, Brauner MW. CT findings in severe thoracic sarcoidosis. Eur Radiol. 2005;15(1):23–30.

49. Galie N, Humbert M, Vachiery JL, Gibbs S, Lang I, Torbicki A, et al. 2015 ESC/ERS Guidelines for the diagnosis and treatment of pulmonary hypertension: The Joint Task Force for the Diagnosis and Treatment of Pulmonary Hypertension of the European Society of Cardiology (ESC) and the European Respiratory Society (ERS): Endorsed by: Association for European Paediatric and Congenital Cardiology (AEPC), International Society for Heart and Lung Transplantation (ISHLT). Eur Respir J. 2015;46(4):903–75.
50. Ng CS, Wells AU, Padley SP. A CT sign of chronic pulmonary arterial hypertension: the ratio of main pulmonary artery to aortic diameter. J Thorac Imaging. 1999;14(4):270–8.
51. Huitema MP, Spee M, Vorselaars VM, Boerman S, Snijder RJ, van Es HW, et al. Pulmonary artery diameter to predict pulmonary hypertension in pulmonary sarcoidosis. Eur Respir J. 2015;47:673–6.
52. Patterson KC, Huang F, Oldham JM, Bhardwaj N, Hogarth DK, Mokhlesi B. Excessive daytime sleepiness and obstructive sleep apnea in patients with sarcoidosis. Chest. 2013;143(6):1562–8.
53. Turner GA, Lower EE, Corser BC, Gunther KL, Baughman RP. Sleep apnea in sarcoidosis. Sarcoidosis. 1997;14:61–4.
54. Corte TJ, Wort SJ, Talbot S, Macdonald PM, Hansel DM, Polkey M, et al. Elevated nocturnal desaturation index predicts mortality in interstitial lung disease. Sarcoidosis Vasc Diffuse Lung Dis. 2012;29(1):41–50.
55. Hamilton-Craig CR, Slaughter R, McNeil K, Kermeen F, Walters DL. Improvement after angioplasty and stenting of pulmonary arteries due to sarcoid mediastinal fibrosis. Heart Lung Circ. 2009;18(3):222–5.
56. Baughman RP, Engel PJ, Nathan S. Pulmonary hypertension in sarcoidosis. Clin Chest Med. 2015;36(4):703–14.
57. Barst RJ, Rubin LJ, Long WA, McGoon MD, Rich S, Badesch DB, et al. A comparison of continuous intravenous epoprostenol (prostacyclin) with conventional therapy for primary pulmonary hypertension. The Primary Pulmonary Hypertension Study Group. N Engl J Med. 1996;334(5):296–302.
58. Baughman RP, Judson MA, Lower EE, Highland K, Kwor S, Craft N, et al. Inhaled iloprost for sarcoidosis associated pulmonary hypertension. Sarcoidosis Vasc Diffuse Lung Dis. 2009;26:110–20.
59. Foley RJ, Metersky ML. Successful treatment of sarcoidosis-associated pulmonary hypertension with bosentan. Respiration. 2008;75(2):211–4.
60. Barnett CF, Bonura EJ, Nathan SD, Ahmad S, Shlobin OA, Osei K, et al. Treatment of sarcoidosis-associated pulmonary hypertension: a two-center experience. Chest. 2009;135:1455–61.
61. Judson MA, Highland KB, Kwon S, Donohue JF, Aris R, Craft N, et al. Ambrisentan for sarcoidosis associated pulmonary hypertension. Sarcoidosis Vasc Diffuse Lung Dis. 2011;28(2):139–45.
62. Raghu G, Behr J, Brown KK, Egan JJ, Kawut SM, Flaherty KR, et al. Treatment of idiopathic pulmonary fibrosis with ambrisentan: a parallel, randomized trial. Ann Intern Med. 2013;158(9):641–9.
63. Dobarro D, Schreiber BE, Handler C, Beynon H, Denton CP, Coghlan JG. Clinical characteristics, haemodynamics and treatment of pulmonary hypertension in sarcoidosis in a single centre, and meta-analysis of the published data. Am J Cardiol. 2013;111(2):278–85.
64. Chen H, Taichman DB, Doyle RL. Health-related quality of life and patient-reported outcomes in pulmonary arterial hypertension. Proc Am Thorac Soc. 2008;5(5):623–30.
65. Culver DA, Baughman RP, Cordova FC, Padilla M, Gibson K, Lower EE, et al. Effect of prolonged treatment of bosentan on sarcoidosis associated pulmonary hypertension. Am J Respir Crit Care Med. Presented at American Thoracic Society May 2013. 2013 (Ref Type: Abstract).
66. Alhamad EH, Shaik SA, Idrees MM, Alanezi MO, Isnani AC. Outcome measures of the 6 minute walk test: relationships with physiologic and computed tomography findings in patients with sarcoidosis. BMC Pulm Med. 2010;10:42. doi:10.1186/1471-2466-10-42.:42-10.
67. Milman N, Graudal N, Loft A, Mortensen J, Larsen J, Baslund B. Effect of the TNFalpha inhibitor adalimumab in patients with recalcitrant sarcoidosis: a prospective observational study using FDG-PET. Clin Respir J. 2011;30:10–699X.

Chapter 8
Hypersensitivity Pneumonitis

Moisés Selman, Ivette Buendía-Roldán, Carmen Navarro, and Miguel Gaxiola

Introduction

Hypersensitivity pneumonitis (HP), also known as extrinsic allergic alveolitis, is a complex syndrome of varying intensity, clinical presentation, and natural history [1, 2]. Numerous provocative agents have been described around the world, including, mammalian and avian proteins, fungi, thermophilic bacteria, and certain small molecular weight chemical compounds (Table 8.1). Importantly, new HP antigens are being constantly described. For example, in the last 15 years evidence accumulate supporting that *Mycobacterium avium complex* (MAC), often from hot tub exposure, may provoke the disease [3, 4]. Therefore, in the presence of acute respiratory illness or a patient with a clinical behavior of an interstitial lung disease, clinicians should always consider HP in the spectrum of the differential diagnosis and should carefully search for any potential source of HP-related antigens.

The incidence and prevalence of HP remains largely unknown. Much of the epidemiological information has been derived from studies of farmers and bird fanciers and primary from acute cases. Both, prevalence and incidence of HP vary considerably around the world, depending upon disease definitions and diagnosis, intensity of exposure to offensive antigens, geographical and local conditions, cultural practices, and genetic risk factors. Farmer's lung disease is one of the most common forms of HP, affecting variable percentages of the farming population. For example, the mean annual incidence of farmer's lung among the entire farming population (standardized for age and sex to the total population in Finland in 1975) was 44 per 100,000 persons in farming [5]. However, more recent studies indicate that the incidence of farmer's lung is now in decline [6].

M. Selman, MD (✉) • I. Buendía-Roldán, MSc • C. Navarro, MD • M. Gaxiola, MD
Instituto Nacional de Enfermedades Respiratorias, Dr. Ismael Cosío Villegas,
Tlalpan 4502, CP 14080 México DF, Mexico
e-mail: mselmanl@yahoo.com.mx; moiselman@salud.gob.mx; ivettebu@yahoo.com.mx; mcnavigo@yahoo.com; miguelog@yahoo.com

R.P. Baughman et al. (eds.), *Pulmonary Hypertension and Interstitial Lung Disease*, DOI 10.1007/978-3-319-49918-5_8

Table 8.1 Identified agents that cause hypersensitivity pneumonitis

Disease	Antigen	Source
Fungal and bacterial		
Farmer's lung	*Saccharopolyspora rectivirgula, Thermoactinomyces vulgaris, Absidia corymbifera*	Moldy hay, grain, silage
Mushroom worker's lung	*Thermoactinomyces sacchari*	Moldy mushroom compost
Malt worker's lung	*Aspergillus fumigatus, Aspergillus clavus*	Moldy barley
Woodworker's lung	*Alternaria* sp., wood dust	Oak, cedar, and mahogany dust, pine and spruce pulp
Maple bark strippers' lung	*Cryptostroma corticale*	Moldy maple bark
Cheese washers' lung	*Penicillium casei*	Moldy cheese
Sewage worker's lung	*Cephalosporium*	Sewer
Sequiosis	*Pullularia*	Moldy sawdust
Stipatosis	*Aspergillus fumigatus*	Esparto fibers
Suberosis	*Penicillium frequentans, Aspergillus fumigatus*	Cork dust
Harwood lung	*Paecilomyces*	Hardwood processing plant
Bagassosis	*Thermoactinomyces sacchari*	Moldy sugarcane
Sauna taker's lung	*Aureobasidium* sp., *Pullularia*	Contaminated sauna water
Ventilation/humidifier lung	*Thermoactinomyces vulgaris, Thermoactinomyces sacchari, Thermoactinomyces candidus*	Contaminated forced-air systems; water reservoirs
Metal working fluid-associated HP	*Mycobacterium immunogenum*	Metal working fluids
Sax lung	*Candida albicans*	Saxophone
Hot tub lung	*Mycobacterium avium complex*	Hot tubs; swimming pools, whirlpools
Summer-type pneumonitis	*Trichosporon cutaneum*	Contaminated old houses
HP in peat moss processing plant workers	*Monocillium* sp. *Penicillium citreonigrum*	Peat moss processing plants
Animal proteins		
Pigeon breeder's disease	Avian droppings, feathers, serum	Parakeets, budgerigars, pigeons, chickens, turkeys
Furrier's lung	Animal-fur dust	Animal pelts
Animal handler's lung; Laboratory worker's lung	Rats, gerbils	Urine, serum, pelts proteins
Pituitary snuff taker's lung	Pork	Pituitary snuff
Chemical compounds		
Pauli's reagent alveolitis	Sodium diazobenzene sulfate	Laboratory reagent
Chemical worker's lung	Isocyanates; trimellitic anhydride	Polyurethane foams, spray paints, special glues
Epoxy resin lung	Phthalic anhydride	heated epoxy resin
Pyrethrum pneumonitis	Pyrethrum	Insecticide

A study estimating the incidence of HP in the UK showed that between 1991 and 2003 the incident rate for this disorder was stable at approximately 0.9 cases per 100,000 person-years [7]. Data from a European survey suggest that HP constitutes 4–13% of all interstitial lung diseases [8]. In general, the prevalence of HP is difficult to estimate accurately because it represents a group of syndromes with different causative agents, and because epidemiologic studies lack uniform diagnostic criteria. Overall, the prevalence and incidence of HP are low, in part because a number of individuals with mild HP are not detected and patients with subacute and chronic disease are misdiagnosed as suffering other type of interstitial lung disease.

It is well known that HP occurs more frequently in nonsmokers than in cigarette smokers under similar risk exposure [9–11]. However, when the disease occurs in smokers it seems to be characterized by an insidious and chronic presentation with a worst clinical outcome [12].

Pathogenic Mechanisms

The pathogenesis of HP is complex and probably involves the coexistence of genetic and/or environmental risk factors with the exposure to the offending HP antigen. The nature of the genetic predisposition is unknown, but susceptibility associated to the major histocompatibility complex (MHC) class II alleles has been reported [13]. More recently, it was shown that HP patients had a significant increase in the frequency of the immunoproteasome catalytic subunit (PSMB8) KQ genotype as well as of the allele Gly-637 and the genotypes Asp-637/Gly-637 and Pro-661/Pro-661 of the subunit of the transporter associated with antigen processing TAP1 compared to matched controls [14, 15]. PSMB8 participates in the degradation of ubiquitinated proteins generating peptides presented by MHC class I molecules while TAP transports peptides for loading on to class I MHC molecules that present them to cytotoxic T lymphocytes.

Some other host processes may also contribute as a risk factor. In this context, it has been recently reported that female HP patients show increased frequency of microchimerism, that is, the presence of circulating cells transferred from one genetically distinct individual to another [16]. In this study, fetal microchimeric cells was also revealed in bronchoalveolar lavage and lung tissues of HP patients demonstrating that these cells traffic to and home the lungs. However, the putative role of these microchimeric fetal cells in the HP lungs is presently unknown, although they seem to increase the severity of the disease.

Viral infections involving common respiratory viruses, primarily Influenza A, and the exposure to a second inhalatory injury (i.e., pesticides) may also have a promoting effect enhancing the development of HP [17, 18].

The mechanisms of hypersensitivity lung damage involve both humoral and cellular processes depending on the clinical presentation. Inflammation in the acute episodes seems to be provoked by immune-complexes deposit, which may explain the 4–8 h late onset of symptoms after massive antigen inhalation. Supporting this concept are the findings of activated complement components, activated blood neutrophils, and bronchoalveolar lavage neutrophilia in patients with acute HP and in those studied few hours/days after antigen inhalation challenge [19–21].

By contrast, subacute and chronic HP appears to be mediated by an exaggerated T-cell-mediated response and actually, a striking increase of T-lymphocytes characterizes this disorder. The mechanisms implicated in the T-cell alveolitis are not completely understood but appear to include increased T-cell recruitment and migration, increased proliferation in the local microenvironment, and decreased programmed cell death [1, 22–26]. A recent global gene expression study identified a variety of genes typically associated with inflammation, T cell activation, and immune responses in the lungs of patients with subacute/chronic disease [27]. Genes related to T-lymphocyte activation included Src-like-adaptor 2, CD2, components of the T cell receptor complex (CD3-D, and -E), and the alpha chain of CD8. Likewise, MHC class II transactivator, the master regulator of MHC class II expression, and several genes encoding MHC class I and II molecules were also overexpressed. Several chemokines such as CXCL9 and CXCL10 which are involved in the recruitment of activated T cells and NK cells were upregulated. CXCR4 and CCR5 and their ligands CCL5 and CCL4 were overexpressed as well suggesting that the recruiting/homing program for lung lymphocytes involves multiple chemokines.

Clinical Behavior

The clinical features of the disease are usually similar, regardless of the type of the inhaled dust. In general, three overlapping clinical forms are recognized: acute, subacute, and chronic [1]. The nature of the antigen, as well as the intensity and frequency of antigen exposure influences the clinical presentation.

Acute HP

This form of HP usually follows a heavy exposure to an offending agent. Acute presentation is characterized by an abrupt onset of symptoms few hours after intermittent and intense antigen exposure. Patients present fever, chills, dyspnea, chest tightness, and dry or mildly productive cough. Removal from exposure to the provoking antigen results in improvement of symptoms within hours to days and complete resolution of clinical and radiographic findings within several weeks. However, the disease often recurs after the next inhalation of the causative antigen. Occasionally, respiratory failure mimicking adult respiratory distress syndrome may occur requiring intensive unit care management [28]. Acute HP behaves similar to an acute respiratory infection provoked by virus or mycoplasma [1]. In farmers, the differential diagnosis must include the organic dust toxic syndrome (ODTS) provoked by exposure to bacterial endotoxins and fungal toxins of moldy hay [29].

In contrast to patients with acute HP, ODTS patients have no precipitins to antigens of molds and usually present with normal clinical findings upon respiratory examination and chest radiographs. ODTS is usually self-limiting, with symptoms rarely exceeding 36 h.

Subacute HP

Subacute HP is characterized by progressive dyspnea and cough occurring during weeks or few months after continued exposure. Patients often display fever, fatigue, anorexia, and weight loss. Some improvement of symptoms is noticed if patients avoid further exposure, but takes longer than with the acute form of the disease (weeks to months), and usually pharmacological treatment is necessary.

Chronic HP

Chronic HP may exhibit different clinical behaviors [30–34]. One subgroup of patients evolves to interstitial lung fibrosis after recurrent acute episodes (chronic recurrent HP); other subgroup of patients presents slowly progressive chronic fibrotic disease with no history of acute/subacute episodes (chronic insidious HP), and finally a third subgroup may progress to a chronic obstructive lung disease. The reasons for these different outcomes (fibrosis versus emphysema) are unknown but it may be related with the characteristics of the inhaled antigen, the type of exposure, cigarette smoking status, and the genetic background. Pulmonary fibrosis is the general outcome of chronic HP induced by avian antigens while emphysematous lung lesions are observed in farmers exposed to thermophilic bacteria and fungi.

Subacute HP as well as chronic recurrent and insidious HP may mimic virtually any interstitial lung disease and the diagnosis may be extremely difficult. Differential diagnosis of subacute HP includes some lung infections such as miliary tuberculosis or histoplasmosis, as well as noninfectious granulomatous lung disorders like sarcoidosis. Also, several idiopathic interstitial pneumonias such as lymphoid interstitial pneumonia, cryptogenic organizing pneumonia, and idiopathic nonspecific interstitial pneumonia should be considered. Chronic HP (primarily the insidious form) may be misdiagnosed as idiopathic pulmonary fibrosis (IPF) or other advanced fibrotic lung disorder if a careful history and specific studies are not carried out [30, 31]. In this context, a recent study has shown that almost half of the patients previously diagnosed as IPF were subsequently diagnosed with chronic hypersensitivity pneumonitis, and most of these cases were attributed to exposure of occult avian antigens from commonly used feather bedding [32]. The authors conclude that chronic HP can be diagnosed in patients with clinical and HRCT findings of usual interstitial pneumonia meeting any one of the following three criteria: (1) Positive bronchial challenge testing (this criterion is reinforced by often coinciding with positivity of specific IgG). (2) Specific IgG positivity and surgical lung biopsy sample compatible with HP or greater than 20% lymphocytes in BAL fluids. (3) Surgical lung biopsy sample or explanted lung showing histopathological features or characteristics of subacute HP [32].

Tachypnea and bibasilar dry crackles are common findings in any clinical presentation of HP. Patients with chronic insidious or recurrent HP may develop digital clubbing, pulmonary arterial hypertension, and even Cor pulmonale [1, 35].

Chest Imaging

The chest radiograph is useful to know that the patient has some kind of interstitial lung disease. However, it is generally nonspecific. Also, the sensitivity of chest radiographs for detecting HP seems to have steadily declined over the last decades [36], and patients with acute and occasionally mild subacute HP may exhibit normal chest x-ray. When abnormal, chest radiographs show nodular opacities with ground-glass attenuation in acute/subacute presentations while the chronic stages are characterized by a predominantly reticular pattern which may evolve to honeycombing changes.

Findings on High-Resolution Computed Tomography (HRCT)

Acute HP is characterized by a diffuse and hazy increase of parenchymal density (ground-glass attenuation) and occasionally by patchy or widespread air space consolidation [33]. Patients with subacute HP show areas of ground-glass opacities, small poorly defined centrilobular nodules, and mosaic attenuation (Fig. 8.1a, b; [37–39]). A CT scan obtained at the end of expiration is useful to detect patchy air trapping images. The micronodular pattern consists of poorly defined micronodules, usually of less than 5 mm in diameter, with a centrilobular distribution that affect both the central and peripheral portions of the lung. Chronic fibrotic HP is characterized by the presence of reticular opacities superimposed on findings of subacute HP. Reticulation may evolve to honeycombing, mainly in chronic patients that show slowly progressive (insidious) disease [Fig. 8.2, [30, 40]]. In these cases, the disease may mimic idiopathic pulmonary fibrosis. Patients with chronic farmer's lung show more frequently emphysematous changes than interstitial fibrosis [33, 34]. HRCT features that best differentiate chronic HP from NSIP included evidence of secondary lobular areas of decreased attenuation and vascularity, extensive upper lobe involvement, and the presence of centrilobular nodules. In contrast, findings that best differentiated NSIP includes relative subpleural sparing, absence of centrilobular ground-glass nodules, absence of honeycombing, and lack of air trapping. Finally, findings that best distinguish IPF from chronic HP include honeycombing without subpleural sparing or centrilobular nodules [41].

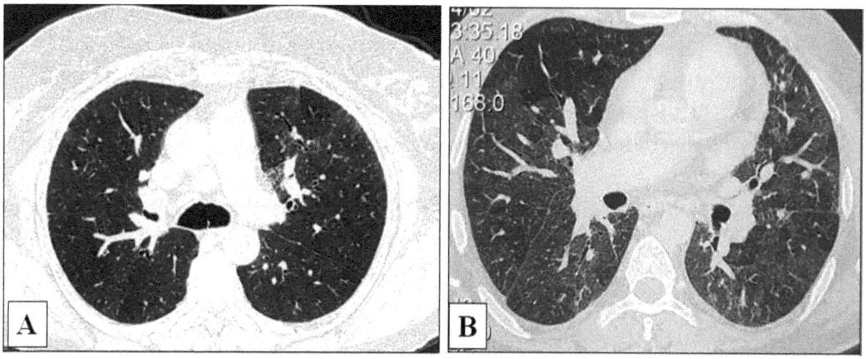

Fig. 8.1 (**a**) High-resolution computed tomography image showing bilateral poorly defined centrilobular nodules and ground-glass opacities in a HP patient with subacute presentation. (**b**) HRCT illustrates ground-glass opacities and areas of decreased attenuation (mosaic pattern) that are typical findings in subacute disease

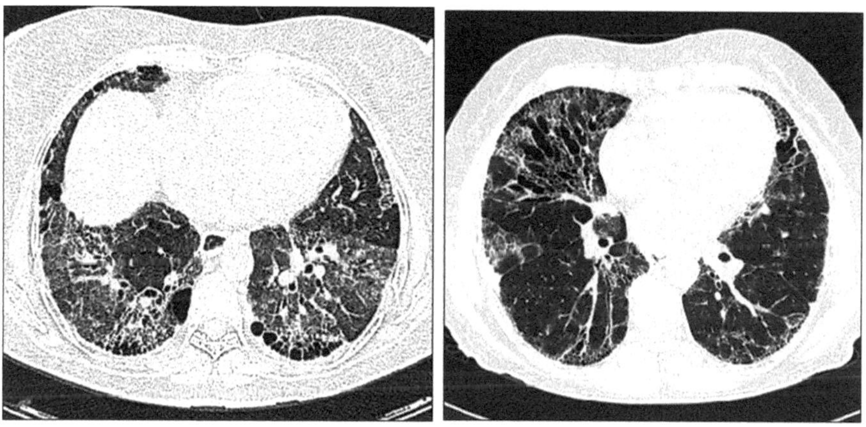

Fig. 8.2 HRCT scan of a patient with chronic HP. It can be observed bilateral reticular opacities, traction bronchiectasis, and subpleural microcysts. Idiopathic pulmonary fibrosis is the usual differential diagnosis

Physiologic Abnormalities

The main purpose of the pulmonary function tests is to determine the severity of the lung impairment. HP is characterized by a restrictive ventilatory defect with a reduction of forced vital capacity and total lung capacity [42]. The static expiratory pressure–volume curve is downward and rightward shifted of the normal curve, showing a decrease in lung compliance over the entire range of the reduced inspiratory capacity [43]. However, these changes are neither specific nor diagnostic for HP because similar abnormalities are revealed in most interstitial lung diseases.

Patients display impaired gas exchange characterized by hypoxemia which usually worsens with exercise and increased alveolar-arterial oxygen gradient [P(A-a) O2]. Patients with mild disease or in the early stages may present normoxemia at rest, but exercise always reveals hypoxemia. Diffusing capacity of carbon monoxide (DL_{CO}) is typically reduced being a good predictor of arterial oxygen desaturation during exercise.

Some degree of obstruction of the peripheral airways, as suggested by a decrease in the maximum to mid-flow rates and in the ratio of dynamic to static lung compliance, may be present due to bronchiolitis [44]. However, small airways obstruction is usually not detected by functional tests [45]. Nevertheless, in chronic farmer's lung, functional defects reflecting airways obstruction and emphysematous lesions can be noticed [34].

The correlation between pulmonary functional abnormality and the severity or prognosis of HP is poor. Patients with a severe decrease in lung volume and DL_{CO} may recover fully, whereas others with relatively mild functional abnormalities at the onset of disease may develop progressive pulmonary fibrosis or airway obstruction and emphysematous changes [1].

Hemodynamic Measurements

Several studies dealing with the effect of lung inflammation/fibrosis on pulmonary arterial vessels, hemodynamic, and cardiac function in HP have been recently reported. Previously (mostly from case reports), a marked pulmonary arterial hypertension (PAH) has been found in acute/subacute patients, where pulmonary embolism was suspected [46–50]. In an old study dealing with ten HP patients and performed with right heart catheterization, it was found that all patients had PAH and increased pulmonary arterial resistance [51]. Abnormal pulmonary artery diastolic pressure/pulmonary wedge pressure difference was noticed in most of the patients. Hemodynamic abnormalities correlated with arterial oxygen saturation and furthermore, a significant improvement was observed after oxygen breathing. Interestingly, all patients showed vascular abnormalities on samples of lung tissues. Most of them displayed medial hypertrophy in arteries and arterioles while in some of them cellular intimal proliferation in the smallest muscular arteries and intimal fibrosis were also seen. The study was performed in Mexico City at 2240 m altitude, and the authors concluded that alveolar hypoxia produced by HP, presumably enhanced by living at a high altitude, provoke pulmonary hypertension.

Other studies dealing with the histopathologic changes in HP have also reported vascular abnormalities including intimal hyperplasia and some muscle hypertrophy in chronic cases [52].

In our center we reviewed the clinical records of 87 patients with chronic HP in which an echocardiography was performed as part of their clinical evaluation. One-third of the patients exhibited increased pulmonary artery systolic pressure (Fig. 8.3). Higher defect in gas exchange was the only parameter that correlated with the

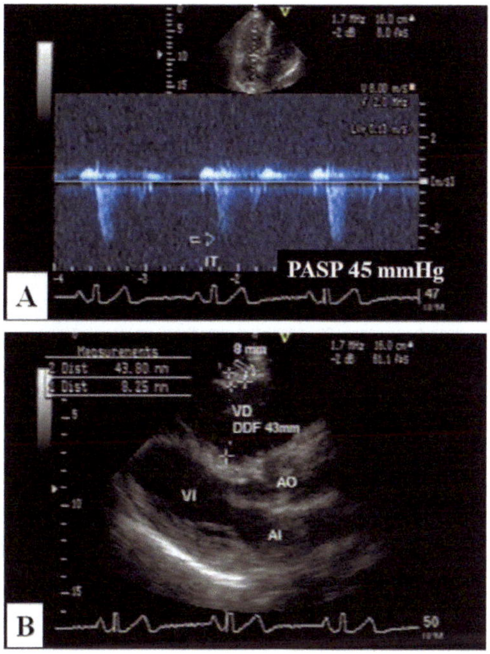

Fig. 8.3 Echocardiography in HP patients showing tricuspid insufficiency and increased pulmonary artery systolic pressure (**a**) and dilatation and hypertrophy of right ventricle (**b**)

Table 8.2 Oxygen saturation in patients with and without pulmonary arterial hypertension

	Without PAH (n = 57)	With PAH (n = 30)	P
PaO_2 (mmHg)	50 ± 10	45 ± 9	0.03
Rest SpO_2%	85 ± 7	80 ± 9	0.01
PASP	25 ± 4.7	51 ± 18.3	0.0001

PaO_2 arterial pressure of oxygen, *SpO_2* pulse oximetry, *PASP* pulmonary artery systolic pressure

presence of PAH (Table 8.2). Alveolar hypoxia may lead to vasoconstriction of small pulmonary arteries (hypoxic pulmonary hypertension) and right heart failure. Hypoxic pulmonary vasoconstriction contributes to ventilation–perfusion matching in the lung by diverting blood flow to oxygen-rich areas. With prolonged hypoxia, small pulmonary arteries suffer a process described as pulmonary vascular remodeling characterized primarily by thickening of the smooth vascular layer with neointima formation, medial thickening, inflammatory cell recruitment, and endothelial dysfunction. Both hypoxic vasoconstriction and architectural remodeling contribute to the development of progressive pulmonary hypertension.

It is important to take into account, however, that our study was performed with echocardiography that compared with right heart catheterism may give inaccurate measurement of systolic pulmonary artery pressure, mainly in patients with advanced lung disease leading to considerable overdiagnosis of pulmonary hypertension [53].

In a similar study, 73 patients with chronic HP and available Doppler echocardiography data were evaluated. Pulmonary hypertension (sPAP ≥ 50 mmHg) was detected in 14 patients (19%) and was associated with a greater risk of death. Patients with pulmonary hypertension were older and had a significantly decreased PaO_2. There was a weak correlation between pulmonary function parameters and the underlying sPAP, for FVC, FEV_1, and PaO_2 and inversely with $PaCO_2$ [54].

A more recent study assessed the hemodynamic changes in chronic HP by right heart catheterization. A prevalence of 44% of precapillary pulmonary hypertension was observed and the correlation with the pulmonary function tests suggested that the severity of pulmonary hypertension is proportional to the severity of lung alterations because it was more frequent among patients with lower lung function and hypoxemia [54]. Moreover, the dynamic exercise evaluation using cardiopulmonary exercise testing showed that patients with precapillary PAH had lower values than did the patients without PAH for FVC, DLCO, and PaO_2 [55].

Diagnostic Appraisal and Additional Tools for Difficult Cases

In general, the criteria for HP diagnosis should include a high index of suspicion by the clinician when dealing with an interstitial lung disease. In any case of an acute respiratory illness, or a subacute/chronic ILD, clinicians should always consider HP in the spectrum of the differential diagnosis and should carefully search for any potential source of HP-related antigens. Although the disease seems to be less frequent in children, it should be considered in any child with recurrent or unexplained respiratory symptoms [56, 57].

A key consideration in acute HP is the important improvement of a flu-like syndrome after removing the patient from the suspected environment and worsening after reexposure. Similar improvement although less dramatic can be also observed in the subacute form.

In a multicenter study that included a cohort of 400 patients (116 with HP and 284 with other interstitial lung disease), six significant clinical predictors of HP were identified [58]: (1) exposure to a known offending antigen, (2) positive precipitating antibodies to the offending antigen, (3) recurrent episodes of symptoms, (4) inspiratory crackles on physical examination, (5) symptoms occurring 4–8 h after exposure, and (6) and weight loss.

As mentioned, HRCT plays a central role for diagnosis. The acute form is characterized by ground-glass attenuation and confluent opacities. The subacute form is distinguished by centrilobular nodules, areas of ground-glass attenuation, a mosaic perfusion pattern, and air trapping on expiratory imaging. The chronic phase is characterized by irregular reticular opacities superimposed to some subacute changes and with associated architectural distortion.

Following are other important tests to evaluate patients with suspected HP:

Specific antibodies: Precipitating IgG antibodies against the offending antigens can be identified in the patient's serum. However, a percent of exposed but asymptomatic individuals (mostly with a high degree of exposure) may also have positive serum precipitins [59–62]. Perhaps more important from the clinical point of view is that in a number of patients with chronic insidious HP circulating specific antibodies are not detected [30]. Therefore, the absence of serum precipitins does not rule out HP while the presence of them does not rule in. Ideally, it will be better to obtain a sample of the suspected causative agent from the original source and test it against the patient's blood.

Bronchoalveolar lavage (BAL): BAL may give important supportive evidence for diagnosis of HP because it is a highly sensitive tool to detect the alveolitis [1, 27, 63, 64]. The disease (in any of its clinical presentations) is characterized by a remarkable increment of lymphocytes, usually greater than 30% and often exceeding 50% of the inflammatory cells recovered (Fig. 8.4). However, as mentioned for the presence of specific antibodies, the presence of an alveolar lymphocytosis by itself does not establish the diagnosis because asymptomatic, exposed individuals can also have increased numbers of lymphocytes in their BAL [65]. Also, similar levels can be found in infectious and noninfectious granulomatous diseases such as sarcoidosis, berylliosis, or miliary tuberculosis.

It is the general belief that the main lymphocyte subset that increases is the $CD8^+$ with the subsequent decrease of BAL $CD4^+/CD8^+$ ratio to less than 1.0 [66]. However, a number of studies have found that CD4+ T-cells are increased with the consequent increased CD4+/CD8+ ratio [67, 68]. Several circumstances seem to explain this variability including the clinical form (acute, subacute, or chronic), cigarette smoking habit, type/dose of inhaled antigen, and the time elapsed since antigen exposure. A predominant increase of CD8+ seems to occur in nonsmokers

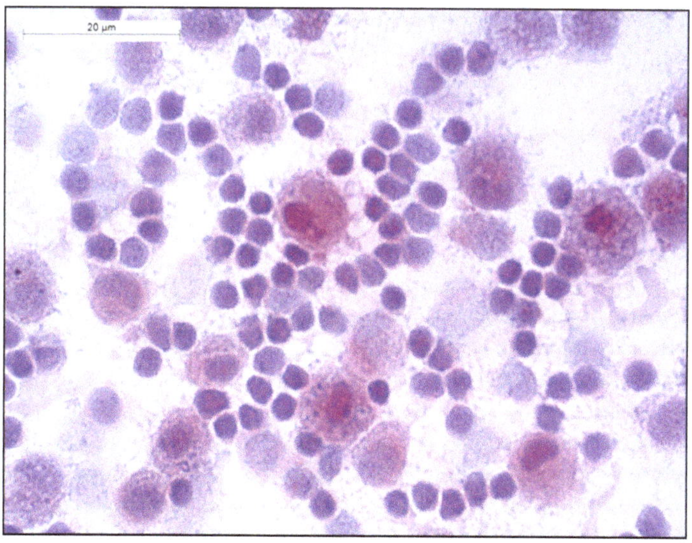

Fig. 8.4 Bronchoalveolar lavage from a patient with subacute HP. Most of the obtained cells are lymphocytes (hematoxylin & eosin, original magnification 20×)

with acute/subacute HP, while an increase of CD4+ is frequently found in smokers or those with chronic/fibrotic forms of the disease.

BAL neutrophils are usually elevated in acute cases and after recent antigen exposure [69]. Therefore, an increase in BAL lymphocytes and neutrophils in a patient with an acute respiratory syndrome is strongly indicative of HP. Also, a modest but significant increase of neutrophils is detected in advanced disease [70].

As well, several studies have reported slight but considerable increase of plasma cells mainly after recent exposure [71]. This finding together with the increase in T-lymphocytes may help to distinguish HP from others ILD [72]. Also, a small but significant increase of mast cells has been reported in HP [73, 74].

Antigen-induced lymphocyte proliferation: In vitro proliferation of peripheral and bronchoalveolar lymphocytes to avian antigens has been assayed for diagnostic and research purposes [30, 75]. Importantly, this test resulted to be positive in more than 90% of the recurrent and insidious cases of chronic pigeon breeder's disease where the presence of circulating antibodies may be negative [30]. Experiments also demonstrated that a positive stimulation index was usually 2.0 or higher. In a more recent study, it was found that antigen-induced lymphocyte proliferation in peripheral blood or bronchoalveolar lavage cells was positive in all the studied patients with chronic HP presumably caused by feather duvets [76].

Lung biopsy: Histopathological confirmation of the diagnosis is required in a number of subacute and chronic cases. It is critical that the pathologist is informed when HP is being considered; the findings are often subtle and must be interpreted with knowledge of the clinical presentation. This is particularly important because we now know that a relatively large number of patients with subacute or chronic HP may exhibit a different histological pattern, including nonspecific interstitial pneumonia [NSIP, [77]], cryptogenic organizing pneumonia (COP), or even usual interstitial pneumonia (UIP)-like changes.

Classical histopathologic findings include small, poorly formed noncaseating bronchiolocentric granulomas (Fig. 8.5a, b; [78]). These poorly defined aggregates of epithelioid macrophages are often associated with multinucleated giant cells. There is also a patchy mononuclear cell infiltration (predominantly lymphocytes and plasma cells) of the alveolar walls, typically in a bronchiolocentric distribution. Bronchiolar abnormalities are usually present although they may differ according to the type of HP. Thus, in farmer's lung it has been described proliferative bronchiolitis obliterans [79], while in pigeon breeder's disease peribronchiolar inflammation/fibrosis with smooth muscle hypertrophy and extrinsic narrowing of the small airways are usually found [45]. Occasionally, classic BOOP-like lesions are described [80, 81].

Chronic stage is characterized by variable degrees of interstitial fibrosis (Fig. 8.6a, b). In these cases, the presence of giant cells, poorly formed granulomas, or inflammatory features of subacute HP may corroborate the diagnosis of HP [30, 31, 82]. It has been proposed that three different patterns of fibrosis may occur: (a) predominantly peripheral fibrosis in a patchy pattern with architectural distortion and fibroblast foci resembling usual interstitial pneumonia, (b) temporal and geographic homogeneous interstitial fibrosis resembling fibrotic NSIP, and (c) irregular

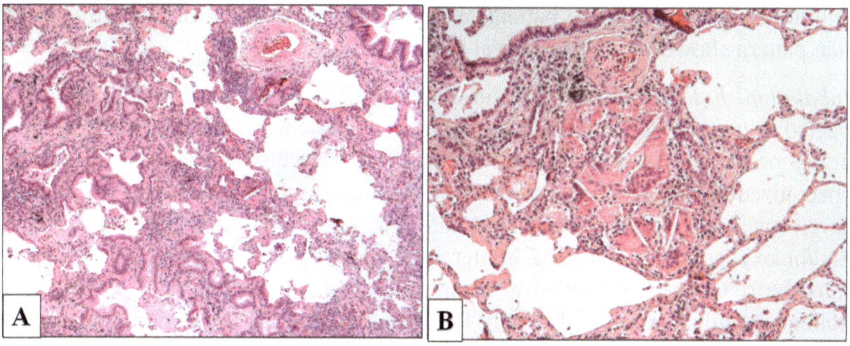

Fig. 8.5 (**a**) Photomicrograph of histopathologic specimen of a patient with subacute hypersensitivity pneumonitis showing diffuse, chronic lymphocytic inflammatory infiltrate (H&E 10×). (**b**) Another patient with subacute disease showing a granulomatous lesion with several multinucleated giant cells (H & E, 40×)

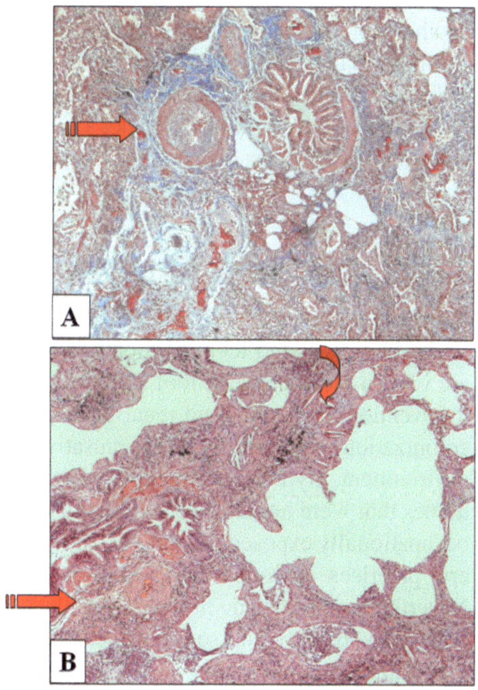

Fig. 8.6 (**a**, **b**) Photomicrographs of histopathologic samples from two patients with chronic HP showing collagen deposit [(**a**) Masson's trichrome, 10×] and honeycomb changes [(**b**) H & E, 10×]. It can be noticed the vascular remodeling (arrows). There is moderate inflammatory infiltrate and a small granuloma [(**b**) curved arrow]

peribronchiolar fibrosis [83]. Other features of chronic HP are alveolar epithelial cell hyperplasia and thickened arterioles [84]. Recently, our group reported that chronic HP may display seven morphological patterns including the "typical" one (characteristics already discussed), nonspecific interstitial pneumonia (NSIP-pattern), usual interstitial pneumonia (UIP-like pattern), mixed pattern, organizing pneumonia (OP-like pattern), airway-centered interstitial fibrosis (ACIF-pattern), and nonclassified. UIP-like patients exhibited the worst survival rate while NSIP-like pattern showed the best survival [85].

Inhalation challenge test: Reexposure of the patients to the environment of the suspected agent may be recommended. Inhalation challenge in the hospital is not generally performed because lack of standardized antigens and limited access to a specialized setting to conduct the study. A positive challenge is characterized by fever, malaise, headache, peripheral and BAL neutrophilia, and decrease of FVC and/or oxygen saturation 8–12 h after exposure [75, 86, 87]. Inhalation challenge must be rigorously controlled to avoid an exaggerated reaction. In addition, the patient should be monitored closely for at least 24 h. Occasionally, the patient may present a two-stage reaction with an immediate, transient wheezing and a decrease in the FEV1 which is followed in 4–6 h by decrease in FVC, fever, and leukocytosis.

In our experience, false-positive results are obtained in approximately 15% of patients with other ILD but not in avian antigen exposed subjects, suggesting that provocation test can identify patients with HP in the majority of the cases [86]. In another more recent study, specific provocation test was performed in 59 patients with HP induced by avian antigens, and in 20 healthy pigeon keepers and 20 patients with diffuse interstitial lung disease other than HP as controls. The test was positive in 54 of the 59 patients with bird breeder's lung and negative in all controls; the authors concluded that the test had a sensitivity of 92% and a specificity of 100% [88].

Treatment and Prognosis

Early diagnosis, and identification and avoidance of the inciting antigen exposure are vital in the management of HP. In acute form avoidance alone may be sufficient intervention. In a study, no recurrence of summer-type HP was noticed when the colonization by *T. cutaneum*, the causative agent, was eliminated from the domestic environment. By contrast, recurrence was observed in all patients who resided in homes that were not cleaned or in homes where cleaning was not adequate [89]. In occupationally exposed individuals, the risk of HP can be reduced by adapting modern practices and conditions that reduce the content of causative antigens. Nevertheless, in chronic fibrotic HP patients subsequent antigen avoidance may not reverse the disease and some of them show progressive worsening and eventually die from the disease.

Prednisone is indicated in subacute/chronic presentations, although long-term efficacy of these agents has yet to be determined. An optional approach consists of 0.5 mg per kg per day of prednisone for a month, followed by a gradual reduction until a maintenance dose of 10–15 mg per day is reached. Prednisone is discontinued when the patient is considered to be healed (or after a substantial improvement of symptoms and functional abnormalities) or when there is no clinical and/or functional response. Inhaled corticosteroids have been suggested for acute/subacute cases but long-term experience is insufficient.

Reports in pediatric HP are scanty. In one study, monthly courses of high dose of intravenous methylprednisolone were used [90]. Additionally, oral prednisolone was employed in most cases, and according to severity, other immunosuppressive drugs such as azathioprine or cyclosporine were added. Most children improved, and no mortality was observed. In chronic advanced HP in adults, we also have explored the combination of prednisone plus azathioprine with some encouraging results. However, there is no solid published experience so far.

Since pulmonary hypertension may negatively influence the outcome, treatment with antihypertensive drugs such as sildenafil or iloprost may be considered on individual basis.

Progressive lung scarring that characterizes chronic advanced HP has no effective therapy, and lung transplantation should be recommended [1]. In a recent study, the survival posttransplant was evaluated in chronic HP and compared with IPF [91]. Survival at 1, 3, and 5 years after lung transplant was significantly better in HP (96%, 89%, and 89% versus 86%, 67%, and 49% in IPF). HP subjects manifested a reduced adjusted risk of death compared to IPF subjects. Interestingly, the diagnosis of hypersensitivity pneumonitis was made at explant in 16% of the patients emphasizing the diagnostic complexity of this disease when clinicians face a patient with chronic advanced interstitial lung disorder.

The prognosis of this disease for patients displaying the acute and subacute presentations is favorable (in the absence of further exposure) and most patients heal or display a significant improvement with some residual respiratory functional abnormalities remaining.

By contrast, patients with chronic HP, primarily pigeon breeder's disease, may evolve to interstitial fibrosis showing a high rate of mortality with median survivals of 5 and 7 years, respectively [31, 92].

Patients with farmer's lung, mainly those that experience recurrent acute attacks, develop more often a syndrome similar to chronic obstructive pulmonary diseases with airflow obstruction and emphysema, but survival data are unavailable [34, 93].

References

1. Selman M, Pardo A, King Jr TE. Hypersensitivity pneumonitis: insights in diagnosis and pathobiology. Am J Respir Crit Care Med. 2012;186:314–24.
2. Fink JN, Ortega HG, Reynolds HY, Cormier YF, Fan LL, Franks TJ, et al. Needs and opportunities for research in hypersensitivity pneumonitis. Am J Respir Crit Care Med. 2005;171:792–8.
3. Marras TK, Wallace Jr RJ, Koth LL, Stulbarg MS, Cowl CT, Daley CL. Hypersensitivity pneumonitis reaction to Mycobacterium avium in household water. Chest. 2005;127:664–71.
4. Martinez S, McAdams HP, Batchu CS. The many faces of pulmonary nontuberculous mycobacterial infection. AJR Am J Roentgenol. 2007;189:177–86.
5. Terho EO, Heinonen OP, Lammi S, Laukkanen V. Incidence of clinically confirmed farmer's lung in Finland and its relation to meteorological factors. Eur J Respir Dis Suppl. 1987;152:47–56.

6. Arya A, Roychoudhury K, Bredin CP. Farmer's lung is now in decline. Ir Med J. 2006;99:203–5.
7. Solaymani-Dodaran M, West J, Smith C, Hubbard R. Extrinsic allergic alveolitis: incidence and mortality in the general population. QJM. 2007;100:233–7.
8. Thomeer MJ, Costabe U, Rizzato G, Poletti V, Demedts M. Comparison of registries of interstitial lung diseases in three European countries. Eur Respir J Suppl. 2001;32:114s–8s.
9. Arima K, Ando M, Ito K, Sakata T, Yamaguchi T, Araki S, et al. Effect of cigarette smoking on prevalence of summer-type hypersensitivity pneumonitis caused by Trichosporon cutaneum. Arch Environ Health. 1992;47:274–8.
10. Cormier Y, Israël-Assayag E, Bédard G, Duchaine C. Hypersensitivity pneumonitis in peat moss processing plant workers. Am J Respir Crit Care Med. 1998;158:412–7.
11. Dalphin JC, Debieuvre D, Pernet D, Maheu MF, Polio JC, Toson B, et al. Prevalence and risk factors for chronic bronchitis and farmer's lung in French dairy farmers. Br J Ind Med. 1993;50:941–4.
12. Ohtsuka Y, Munakata M, Tanimura K, Ukita H, Kusaka H, Masaki Y, et al. Smoking promotes insidious and chronic farmer's lung disease, and deteriorates the clinical outcome. Intern Med. 1995;34:966–71.
13. Camarena A, Juárez A, Mejía M, Estrada A, Carrillo G, Falfán R, et al. Major histocompatibility complex and tumor necrosis factor-alpha polymorphisms in pigeon breeder's disease. Am J Respir Crit Care Med. 2001;163:1528–33.
14. Camarena A, Aquino-Galvez A, Falfán-Valencia R, Sánchez G, Montaño M, Ramos C, et al. PSMB8 (LMP7) but not PSMB9 (LMP2) gene polymorphisms are associated to pigeon breeder's hypersensitivity pneumonitis. Respir Med. 2010;104:889–94.
15. Aquino-Galvez A, Camarena A, Montaño M, Juarez A, Zamora AC, González-Avila G, et al. Transporter associated with antigen processing (TAP) 1 gene polymorphisms in patients with hypersensitivity pneumonitis. Exp Mol Pathol. 2008;84:173–7.
16. Bustos ML, Frías S, Ramos S, Estrada A, Arreola JL, Mendoza F, et al. Local and circulating microchimerism is associated with hypersensitivity pneumonitis. Am J Respir Crit Care Med. 2007;176:90–5.
17. Cormier Y, Samson N, Israel-Assayag E. Viral infection enhances the response to Saccharopolyspora rectivirgula in mice prechallenged with this farmer's lung antigen. Lung. 1996;174:399–407.
18. Hoppin JA, Umbach DM, Kullman GJ, Henneberger PK, London SJ, Alavanja MC, et al. Pesticides and other agricultural factors associated with self-reported farmer's lung among farm residents in the Agricultural Health Study. Occup Environ Med. 2007;64:334–41.
19. Fournier E, Tonnel AB, Gosset P, Wallaert B, Ameisen JC, Voisin C. Early neutrophil alveolitis after antigen inhalation in hypersensitivity pneumonitis. Chest. 1985;88:563–6.
20. Yoshizawa Y, Nomura A, Ohdama S, Tanaka M, Morinari H, Hasegawa S. The significance of complement activation in the pathogenesis of hypersensitivity pneumonitis; sequential changes of complement components and chemotactic activities in bronchoalveolar lavage fluids. Int Arch Allergy Appl Immunol. 1988;87:417–23.
21. Vogelmeier C, Krombach F, Munzing S, Konig G, Mazur G, Beinert T, et al. Activation of blood neutrophils in acute episodes of farmer's lung. Am Rev Respir Dis. 1993;148:396–400.
22. Laflamme C, Israel-Assayag E, Cormier Y. Apoptosis of bronchoalveolar lavage lymphocytes in hypersensitivity pneumonitis. Eur Respir J. 2003;21:225–31.
23. Ohtsuka M, Yoshizawa Y, Naitou T, Yano H, Sato T, Hasegawa S. The motility of lung lymphocytes in hypersensitivity pneumonitis and sarcoidosis. Am J Respir Crit Care Med. 1994;149(2 Pt1):455–9.
24. Dakhama A, Israel-Assayag E, Cormier Y. Role of interleukin-2 in the development and persistence of lymphocytic alveolitis in farmer's lung. Eur Respir J. 1998;11:1281–6.
25. Trentin L, Migone N, Zambello R, di Celle PF, Aina F, Feruglio C, et al. Mechanisms accounting for lymphocytic alveolitis in hypersensitivity pneumonitis. J Immunol. 1990;145: 2147–54.

26. Dakhama A, Israel-Assayag E, Cormier Y. Altered immunosuppressive activity of alveolar macrophages in farmer's lung disease. Eur Respir J. 1996;9:1456–62.
27. Selman M, Pardo A, Barrera L, Estrada A, Watson SR, Wilson K, et al. Gene expression profiles distinguish idiopathic pulmonary fibrosis from hypersensitivity pneumonitis. Am J Respir Crit Care Med. 2006;173:188–98.
28. Da Broi U, Orefice U, Cahalin C, Bonfreschi V, Cason L. ARDS after double extrinsic exposure hypersensitivity pneumonitis. Intensive Care Med. 1999;25:755–7.
29. Seifert SA, Von Essen S, Jacobitz K, Crouch R, Lintner CP. Organic dust toxic syndrome: a review. J Toxicol Clin Toxicol. 2003;41:185–93.
30. Ohtani Y, Saiki S, Sumi Y, Inase N, Miyake S, Costabel U, et al. Clinical features of recurrent and insidious chronic bird fancier's lung. Ann Allergy Asthma Immunol. 2003;90:604–10.
31. Pérez-Padilla R, Salas J, Chapela R, Sánchez M, Carrillo G, Pérez R, et al. Mortality in Mexican patients with chronic pigeon breeders lung compared to those with usual interstitial pneumonia. Am Rev Respir Dis. 1993;148:49–53.
32. Morell F, Villar A, Montero MÁ, Muñoz X, Colby TV, Pipvath S, et al. Chronic hypersensitivity pneumonitis in patients diagnosed with idiopathic pulmonary fibrosis: a prospective case-cohort study. Lancet Respir Med. 2013;1:685–94.
33. Cormier Y, Brown M, Worthy S, Racine G, Muller NL. High-resolution computed tomographic characteristics in acute farmer's lung and in its follow-up. Eur Respir J. 2000;16:56–60.
34. Erkinjuntti-Pekkanen R, Rytkonen H, Kokkarinen JI, Tukiainen HO, Partanen K, Terho EO. Long-term risk of emphysema in patients with farmer's lung and matched control farmers. Am J Respir Crit Care Med. 1998;158:662–5.
35. Sansores R, Salas J, Chapela R, Barquin N, Selman M. Clubbing in hypersensitivity pneumonitis. Its prevalence and possible prognostic role. Arch Intern Med. 1990;150:1849–51.
36. Hodgson MJ, Parkinson DK, Karpf M. Chest x-rays in hypersensitivity pneumonitis: a meta-analysis of secular trend. Am J Ind Med. 1989;16:5–53.
37. Glazer CS, Rose CS, Lynch DA. Clinical and radiologic manifestations of hypersensitivity pneumonitis. J Thorac Imaging. 2002;17:261–72.
38. Small JH, Flower CD, Traill ZC, Gleeson FV. Air trapping in extrinsic allergic alveolitis on computed tomography. Clin Radiol. 1996;51:684–8.
39. Silva CI, Churg A, Muller NL. Hypersensitivity pneumonitis: spectrum of high-resolution CT and pathologic findings. AJR Am J Roentgenol. 2007;188:334–44.
40. Akira M. High-resolution CT in the evaluation of occupational and environmental disease. Radiol Clin North Am. 2002;40:43–59.
41. Silva CI, Müller NL, Lynch DA, Curran-Everett D, Brown KK, Lee KS, et al. Chronic hypersensitivity pneumonitis: differentiation from idiopathic pulmonary fibrosis and nonspecific interstitial pneumonia by using thin-section CT. Radiology. 2008;246:288–97.
42. Du Wayne Schmidt C, Jensen RL, Christensen LT, Crapo RO, Davis JJ. Longitudinal pulmonary function changes in pigeon breeders. Chest. 1988;93:359–63.
43. Sansores R, Pérez-Padilla R, Pare P, Selman M. Exponential analysis of the lung pressure-volume curve in patients with chronic pigeon breeder's lung. Chest. 1992;101:1352–6.
44. Pérez J, Selman M, Rubio H, Ocaña H, Chapela R. Relationship between lung inflammation or fibrosis and frequency dependence of compliance in interstitial pulmonary diseases. Respiration. 1987;52:254–62.
45. Pérez-Padilla R, Gaxiola M, Salas J, Mejía M, Ramos C, Selman M. Bronchiolitis in chronic pigeon breeder's disease. Morphologic evidence of a spectrum of small airway lesions in hypersensitivity pneumonitis induced by avian antigens. Chest. 1996;110:371–7.
46. McKeown PF, Walsh SJ, Menown IB. Images in cardiology: an unusual case of right ventricular dilatation. Heart. 2005;91:1147.
47. Krasniuk EP, Petrova IS, Pilinskii VV. Exogenous allergic alveolitis in workers engaged in the manufacture of pepsin. Lik Sprava. 2001;4:168–71.
48. Gainet M, Chaudemanche H, Westeel V, Lounici A, Dubiez A, Depierre A, et al. A misleading form of hypersensitivity pneumonitis. Rev Mal Respir. 2000;17:987–9.

49. Ostergaard JR. Reversible pulmonary arterial hypertension in a 6-year-old girl with extrinsic allergic alveolitis. Acta Paediatr Scand. 1989;78:145–8.
50. Ceviz N, Kaynar H, Olgun H, Onbas O, Misirligil Z. Pigeon breeder's lung in childhood: is family screening necessary? Pediatr Pulmonol. 2006;41:279–82.
51. Lupi-Herrera E, Sandoval J, Bialostozky D, Seoane M, Martinez ML, Bonetti PF, et al. Extrinsic allergic alveolitis caused by pigeon breeding at a high altitude (2,240 meters). Hemodynamic behavior of pulmonary circulation. Am Rev Respir Dis. 1981;124:602–7.
52. Seal RM, Hapke EJ, Thomas GO, Meek JC, Hayes M. The pathology of the acute and chronic stages of farmer's lung. Thorax. 1968;23:469–89.
53. Arcasoy SM, Christie JD, Ferrari VA, Sutton MS, Zisman DA, Blumenthal NP, et al. Echocardiographic assessment of pulmonary hypertension in patients with advanced lung disease. Am J Respir Crit Care Med. 2003;167:735–40.
54. Koschel DS, Cardoso C, Wiedemann B, Höffken G, Halank M. Pulmonary hypertension in chronic hypersensitivity pneumonitis. Lung. 2012;190:295–302.
55. Oliviera R, Pereira C, Ramos R, Ferreira E, Messina C, Kuranishi L, et al. A haemodynamic study of pulmonary hypertension in chronic hypersensitivity pneumonitis. Eur Respir J. 2014;44:415–24.
56. Nacar N, Kiper N, Yalcin E, Dogru D, Dilber E, Ozcelik U, et al. Hypersensitivity pneumonitis in children: pigeon breeder's disease. Ann Trop Paediatr. 2004;24:349–55.
57. Stauffer Ettlin M, Pache JC, Renevey F, Hanquinet-Ginter S, Guinand S, Barazzone Argiroffo C. Bird breeder's disease: a rare diagnosis in young children. Eur J Pediatr. 2006; 165:55–61.
58. Lacasse Y, Selman M, Costabel U, Dalphin JC, Ando M, Morell F, et al. Clinical diagnosis of hypersensitivity pneumonitis. Am J Respir Crit Care Med. 2003;168:952–8.
59. Hébert J, Beaudoin J, Laviolette M, Beaudoin R, Bélanger J, Cormier Y. Absence of correlation between the degree of alveolitis and antibody levels to Micropolysporum faeni. Clin Exp Immunol. 1985;60:572–8.
60. Pinon JM, Geers R, Lepan H, Pailler S. Immunodetection by enzyme-linked immuno-filtration assay (ELIFA) of IgG, IgM, IgA and IgE antibodies in bird breeder's disease. Eur J Respir Dis. 1987;71:164–9.
61. Fink JN. Epidemiologic aspects of hypersensitivity pneumonitis. Monogr Allergy. 1987;21:59–69.
62. Dalphin JC, Toson B, Monnet E, Pernet D, Dubiez A, Laplante JJ, et al. Farmer's lung precipitins in Doubs (a department of France): prevalence and diagnostic value. Allergy. 1994;49:744–50.
63. Welker L, Jörres RA, Costabel U, Magnussen H. Predictive value of BAL cell differentials in the diagnosis of interstitial lung diseases. Eur Respir J. 2004;24:1000–6.
64. Cormier Y, Bélanger J, LeBlanc P, Laviolette M. Bronchoalveolar lavage in farmers' lung disease: diagnostic and physiological significance. Br J Ind Med. 1986;43:401–5.
65. Cormier Y, Belanger J, Laviolette M. Persistent bronchoalveolar lymphocytosis in asymptomatic farmers. Am Rev Respir Dis. 1986;133:843–7.
66. Semenzato G. Immunology of interstitial lung diseases: cellular events taking place in the lung of sarcoidosis, hypersensitivity pneumonitis and HIV infection. Eur Respir J. 1991;4:94–102.
67. Murayama J, Yoshizawa Y, Ohtsuka M, Hasegawa S. Lung fibrosis in hypersensitivity pneumonitis. Association with CD4+ but not CD8+ cell dominant alveolitis and insidious onset. Chest. 1993;104:38–43.
68. Ando M, Konishi K, Yoneda R, Tamura M. Difference in the phenotypes of bronchoalveolar lavage lymphocytes in patients with summer-type hypersensitivity pneumonitis, farmer's lung, ventilation pneumonitis, and bird fancier's lung: report of a nationwide epidemiologic study in Japan. J Allergy Clin Immunol. 1991;87:1002–9.
69. Drent M, van Velzen-Blad H, Diamant M, Wagenaar SS, Hoogsteden HC, van den Bosch JM. Bronchoalveolar lavage in extrinsic allergic alveolitis: effect of time elapsed since antigen exposure. Eur Respir J. 1993;6:1276–81.

70. Pardo A, Barrios R, Gaxiola M, Segura-Valdez L, Carrillo G, Estrada A, et al. Increase of lung neutrophils in hypersensitivity pneumonitis is associated with lung fibrosis. Am J Respir Crit Care Med. 2000;161:1698–704.
71. Drent M, Velzen-Blad H, Diamant M, Wagenaar SS, Donckerwolck-Bogaert M, van den Bosch JM. Differential diagnostic value of plasma cells in bronchoalveolar lavage fluid. Chest. 1993;103:1720–4.
72. Drent M, Wagenaar SS, Velzen-Blad H, Mulder PG, Hoogsteden HC, van den Bosch JM. Relationship between plasma cell levels and profile of bronchoalveolar lavage fluid in patients with subacute extrinsic allergic alveolitis. Thorax. 1993;48:835–9.
73. Laviolette M, Cormier Y, Loiseau A, Soler P, Leblanc P, Hance AJ. Bronchoalveolar mast cells in normal farmers and subjects with farmer's lung. Diagnostic, prognostic, and physiologic significance. Am Rev Respir Dis. 1991;144:855–60.
74. Miadonna A, Pesci A, Tedeschi A, Bertorelli G, Arquati M, Olivieri D. Mast cell and histamine involvement in farmer's lung disease. Chest. 1994;105:1184–9.
75. Ohtani Y, Kojima K, Sumi Y, Sawada M, Inase N, Miyake S, et al. Inhalation provocation tests in chronic bird fancier's lung. Chest. 2000;118:1382–9.
76. Inase N, Ohtani Y, Sumi Y, Umino T, Usui Y, Miyake S, et al. A clinical study of hypersensitivity pneumonitis presumably caused by feather duvets. Ann Allergy Asthma Immunol. 2006;96:98–104.
77. Vourlekis JS, Schwarz MI, Cool CD, Tuder RM, King TE, Brown KK. Nonspecific interstitial pneumonitis as the sole histologic expression of hypersensitivity pneumonitis. Am J Med. 2002;112:490–3.
78. Coleman A, Colby TV. Histologic diagnosis of extrinsic allergic alveolitis. Am J Surg Pathol. 1988;12:514–8.
79. Reyes CN, Wenzel FJ, Lawton BR, Emanuel DA. The pulmonary pathology of farmer's lung disease. Chest. 1982;81:142–6.
80. Ohtani Y, Saiki S, Kitaichi M, Usui Y, Inase N, Costabel U, et al. Chronic bird fancier's lung: histopathological and clinical correlation. An application of the 2002 ATS/ERS consensus classification of the idiopathic interstitial pneumonias. Thorax. 2005;60:665–71.
81. Herraez I, Gutierrez M, Alonso N, Allende J. Hypersensitivity pneumonitis producing a BOOP-like reaction: HRCT/pathologic correlation. J Thorac Imaging. 2002;17:81–3.
82. Hayakawa H, Shirai M, Sato A, Yoshizawa Y, Todate A, Imokawa S, et al. Clinicopathological features of chronic hypersensitivity pneumonitis. Respirology. 2002;7:359–64.
83. Churg A, Muller NL, Flint J, Wright JL. Chronic hypersensitivity pneumonitis. Am J Surg Pathol. 2006;30.201–8.
84. Khalil N, Churg A, Muller N, O'Connor R. Environmental, inhaled and ingested causes of pulmonary fibrosis. Toxicol Pathol. 2007;35:86–96.
85. Gaxiola M, Buendía-Roldán I, Mejia M, Carrillo G, Estrada A, Navarro MC, et al. Morphologic diversity of chronic pigeon breeder's disease: clinical features and survival. Respir Med. 2011;105:608–14.
86. Ramirez-Venegas A, Sansores RH, Pérez-Padilla R, Carrillo G, Selman M. Utility of a provocation test for diagnosis of chronic pigeon breeder's disease. Am J Respir Crit Care Med. 1998;158:862–9.
87. Reynolds SP, Jones KP, Edwards JH, Davies BH. Inhalation challenge in pigeon breeder's disease: BAL fluid changes after 6 hours. Eur Respir J. 1993;6:467–76.
88. Morell F, Roger A, Reyes L, Cruz MJ, Murio C, Muñoz X. Bird fancier's lung: a series of 86 patients. Medicine (Baltimore). 2008;87:110–30.
89. Yoshida K, Ando M, Sakata T, Araki S. Prevention of summer-type hypersensitivity pneumonitis: effect of elimination of Trichosporon cutaneum from the patient's homes. Arch Environ Health. 1989;44:317–22.
90. Buchvald F, Petersen BL, Damgaard K, Deterding R, Langston C, Fan LL, et al. Frequency, treatment, and functional outcome in children with hypersensitivity pneumonitis. Pediatr Pulmonol. 2011;46:1098–107.

91. Kern RM, Singer JP, Koth L, Mooney J, Golden J, Hays S, et al. Lung transplantation for hypersensitivity pneumonitis. Chest. 2014;189:A5172. [Epub ahead of print]
92. Vourlekis JS, Schwarz MI, Cherniack RM, Curran-Everett D, Cool CD, Tuder RM, et al. The effect of pulmonary fibrosis on survival in patients with hypersensitivity pneumonitis. Am J Med. 2004;116:662–8.
93. Cormier Y, Bélanger J. Long-term physiologic outcome after acute farmer's lung. Chest. 1985;87:796–800.

Chapter 9
Interstitial Lung Disease-Associated Pulmonary Hypertension in the Connective Tissue Disorders

Debabrata Bandyopadhyay, Tanmay S. Panchabhai, and Kristin B. Highland

Abbreviations and Acronyms

6MWD	Six-minute walk distance
6MWT	Six-minute walk test
AA	Ascending aorta
Ao	Aorta
ANA	Antinuclear antibodies
APAH	Associated pulmonary arterial hypertension
cGMP	Cyclic guanyl monophosphate
CTD	Connective tissue disease
CTGF	Connective tissue disease-associated growth factor
CTPA	Coaxial tomography with pulmonary angiogram
DAD	Diffuse alveolar damage
DIP	Desquamative interstitial pneumonia
DLco	Diffusion capacity
ET	Endothelin
FVC	Forced vital capacity
HRCT	High resolution coaxial tomography
ILD	Interstitial lung disease
IGF	Insulin-like growth factor
LIP	Lymphocytic interstitial pneumonia

D. Bandyopadhyay, MD, MRCP
Department of Thoracic Medicine, Geisinger Medical Center, Danville, PA, USA

T.S. Panchabhai, MD
Norton Thoracic Institute, St Joseph's Medical Center, Phoenix, AZ, USA

K.B. Highland, MD, MSCR (✉)
Department of Pulmonary and Critical Care Medicine, Respiratory Institute, Cleveland Clinic Foundation, 9500 Euclid Avenue, Desk A90, Cleveland, OH 44195, USA
e-mail: highlak@ccf.org

R.P. Baughman et al. (eds.), *Pulmonary Hypertension and Interstitial Lung Disease*, DOI 10.1007/978-3-319-49918-5_9

MCTD	Mixed connective tissue disease
MPAD	Main pulmonary artery diameter
mPAP	Mean pulmonary artery pressure
MRI	Magnetic resonance imaging
NO	Nitric oxide
NSIP	Nonspecific interstitial pneumonia
NT Pro-BNP	N-terminal B-type natriuretic peptide
OP	Organizing pneumonia
PA	Pulmonary artery
PAH	Pulmonary arterial hypertension
PDGF	Platelet-derived growth factor
PH	Pulmonary hypertension
PM/DM	Polymyositis/dermatomyositis
PVR	Pulmonary vascular resistance
RA	Rheumatoid arthritis
RNP	Ribonucleoprotein
sGC	Soluble guanyl cyclase
SLE	Systemic lupus erythematosus
SSc	Systemic sclerosis
TGF β	Transforming growth factor beta
TR	Tricuspid regurgitation
UIP	Usual interstitial pneumonia
VMI	Ventricular mass index

Introduction

Pulmonary hypertension (PH) is an incurable condition that is associated with high morbidity and morbidity. In most cases, PH eventually leads to right ventricular hypertrophy followed by dilation, right ventricular failure, and death. PH is common in connective tissue diseases (CTD) and portends a poor prognosis. Although CTD-associated pulmonary arterial hypertension (CTD–APAH) is an important subgroup within Group 1 [1] pulmonary arterial hypertension, it is important to recognize that all groups of PH can occur in the setting of connective tissue disease (Table 9.1). Since interstitial lung disease (ILD) is also a common contributor to morbidity and mortality in the CTDs, this chapter will focus on the challenge of Group 3 pulmonary hypertension, which carries the worst prognosis.

PH and ILD are common in scleroderma/systemic sclerosis (SSc) [2, 3] and have equal weight in the most recent classification scheme for SSc. The survival of SSc patients with combined PH and ILD is particularly grim, with a fivefold increase in mortality compared to isolated SSc-associated PAH [2, 4]. Pulmonary involvement is also common in the other connective tissue diseases and an important cause of morbidity and mortality. Unfortunately, there is a striking paucity of data in the published literature across the other CTDs. Therefore, the key features seen in connective tissue disease-associated interstitial disease-related pulmonary hypertension

Table 9.1 Updated clinical classification of pulmonary hypertension 2013

1. *Pulmonary arterial hypertension (PAH)*
1.1. Idiopathic PAH
1.2. Heritable PAH
1.2.1. BMPR2
1.2.2. ALK, Endoglin, SMAD9, CAV1, KCNK3
1.2.3. Unknown
1.3. Drugs and Toxins induced
1.4. Associated with
1.4.1. Connective tissue disease
1.4.2. HIV
1.4.3. Portal hypertension
1.4.4. Congenital heart diseases
1.4.5. Schistosomiasis
1.5. Persistent pulmonary hypertension of newborn
1′ Pulmonary veno-occlusive disease/pulmonary capillary hemangiomatosis 1″ Persistent pulmonary hypertension of new born (PPHN)
2. *Pulmonary hypertension due to left heart disease*
2.1. Systolic dysfunction
2.2. Diastolic dysfunction
2.3. Valvular heart disease
2.4. Congenital/acquired/left heart inflow/outflow tract obstruction, congenital cardiomyopathies
3. *Pulmonary hypertension due to lung diseases and/or hypoxia*
3.1. Chronic obstructive pulmonary disease
3.2. Interstitial lung disease
3.3. Mixed restrictive and obstructive pulmonary disease
3.4. Sleep-disordered breathing
3.5. Alveolar hypoventilation disorders
3.6. Chronic exposure to high altitude
3.7. Developmental anomalies
4. *Chronic thromboembolic pulmonary hypertension (CTEPH)*
5. *Pulmonary hypertension with unclear multifactorial mechanisms*
5.1. Hematologic disorders, e.g., myeloproliferative diseases, chronic hemolytic anemia, splenectomy
5.2. Systemic disorders, e.g., sarcoidosis, Langerhans cell histiocytosis, lymphangioleiomyomatosis
5.3. Metabolic disorders, e.g., glycogen storage diseases, thyroid disorders
5.4. Others, e.g., fibrosing mediastinitis, chronic renal failure, segmental PH

Adapted from Simonneau et al. Updated clinical classification of pulmonary hypertension. *J Am Coll Cardiol*. 2013 Dec 24; 62(25 Suppl: D34–41)

(CTD–ILD–PH) highlighted in this chapter are mostly obtained from the evidence gathered in systemic sclerosis. Inevitably extrapolation of studies to other CTDs in regards to pathogenesis, clinical evaluation, and treatment is necessary despite inherent differences in these conditions [5].

Interstitial Lung Disease in the CTDs

ILD is a heterogeneous group of disorders characterized by interstitial inflammation and/or fibrosis, leading to restrictive pulmonary physiology and impaired gas exchange. Most parenchymal abnormalities are easily appreciated on high-resolution computed tomography (HRCT) chest, characterized by reticulation, ground-glass opacities, traction bronchiectasis, and honeycombing [6]. ILD is more commonly seen in SSc, rheumatoid arthritis (RA), polymyositis/dermatomyositis (PM/DM), mixed connective tissue disorder (MCTD), and less frequently in systemic lupus erythematosus (SLE) or Sjogren's syndrome (SS). ILD has a variable relationship with the extrapulmonary manifestations of the CTDs and can be a presenting manifestation in all forms of CTD, with classifiable CTD usually occurring within several years. However, it can also have a "forme fruste" presentation, often known as lung dominant CTD or autoimmune featured ILD akin to the rheumatologic diagnosis of "undifferentiated connective tissue disease."

Nonspecific interstitial pneumonia (NSIP) is the most common histopathologic pattern seen in the CTDs with the exception of rheumatoid arthritis, which is more commonly associated with usual interstitial pneumonia (UIP). Other histologic clues for a CTD-associated ILD (CTD–ILD) include dense perivascular collagen, extensive pleuritis, lymphoid aggregates with germinal centers, prominent plasmacytic infiltration, and fewer fibroblastic foci [7, 8]. Lymphocytic interstitial pneumonia (LIP), organizing pneumonia (OP), diffuse alveolar damage (DAD), and desquamative interstitial pneumonia (DIP) have also been described in the CTDs [4].

The risk factors for development of ILD in different CTDs are presented in Table 9.2. The survival in CTD–ILD is considered better than in idiopathic pulmonary fibrosis and is dictated by the underlying histopathology and extent of disease with patients having organizing pneumonia or limited extent (<20% of involvement on HRCT) NSIP having the best prognosis and patients with extensive extent of NSIP, UIP, or DAD having the worse prognosis [9].

CTD-Associated Pulmonary Hypertension

Pulmonary hypertension is associated with all the connective tissue diseases, most frequently in SSc. Given the systemic nature of connective tissue diseases, CTD–PH may span WHO groups 1 through 4 and often is considered "multifactorial" with features of several groups. In addition, pulmonary veno-occlusive disease (PVOD) can be seen in CTD, which is characterized by the additional intimal

Table 9.2 Risk factors predisposing to ILD in CTD patients

Risk factors for severe ILD in SSC patients [48, 49]
• Male gender
• African American race
• Early disease stage (<5 years)
• Cardiac involvement
• Preexisting pulmonary fibrosis,
• Presence of dyspnea,
• Higher avascular scores on nailfold capillaroscopy,
• Esophageal dysfunction
• Anti-Scl-70 antibody (anti-topoisomerase)
Risk factors for ILD in SLE patients [50]
• Long-standing disease
• Presence of SS-A antibody
Risk factors for severe ILD in RA [51]
• Male gender,
• Late onset RA,
• History of tobacco use,
• Positive ANA and high titer rheumatoid factor
Risk factors for ILD in PM/DM [52]
• Female gender
• Arthralgias/polyarthritis
• Presence of antisynthetase antibodies (e.g., Jo-1), and anti-Ro/SSA antibody

proliferation and fibrosis of the intrapulmonary veins and venules. The development of PH is a well-recognized complication of interstitial lung diseases and the presence of high titers of certain autoantibodies make the CTD patients susceptible to increased risk of developing ILD–PH [3, 10–14] (Table 9.3).

The exact prevalence of ILD-associated PH (ILD–PH) in connective tissue diseases is not known and likely varies greatly according to underlying CTD and data regarding CTD–ILD–PH are sparse; most observations are extrapolated from the evidence obtained from SSc patients. In a single-center analysis of 619 SSc patients, 22.5% had isolated ILD, 19.2% had isolated PH, and 18.1% had combined ILD and PH [15]. In a survey of community-based rheumatology clinics, patients with SSc and ILD tended to have higher pulmonary artery pressure than those without ILD [10]. In another retrospective case series [10] of scleroderma-ILD, the prevalence of pulmonary hypertension was 45% and of these, 25% of SSc patients with ILD had a mean pulmonary artery pressure (mPAP) ≥35 mm Hg suggesting the possibility of coexisting pulmonary arterial hypertension since the mPAP in the setting of ILD is generally ≤35 mm Hg. The presence of an elevated mPAP was associated with a lower survival rate [10]. Data from the PHAROS registry revealed that ILD–PH patients in SSc are more likely to be female and Caucasian with an average age at presentation of 50 years. Other risk for actors for the development of ILD–PH in SSc includes late onset SSc, disease duration of more than 10 years, presence of

Table 9.3 Higher titers of certain autoantibodies lead to development of ILD-associated PH in CTD

High titers of autoantibodies frequently present with ILD-associated PH in CTD patients
• SSc-anti Scl70 antibody, Nucleolar speckled ANA (U3RNP), Topoisomerase antibody
• SLE-anticardiolipin antibody without evidence of thromboembolism, anti-sm antibody
• MCTD-U1RNP antibody

telangiectasias, and severe Raynaud phenomenon [15]. At baseline, these patients are frequently a more advanced WHO functional class than isolated PAH with similar hemodynamics. They often have diffuse cutaneous form of scleroderma, unlike isolated PAH, which is more commonly seen in limited cutaneous SSc [16, 17].

In a series of SLE patients with PH, 8.3% had associated ILD and 20% had a combination of pulmonary embolism, left heart disease along with ILD [11]. Patients presenting with ILD–PH in SLE tended to have a longer duration illness than in those with just PAH. In MCTD patients, progressive ILD tends to be more frequently associated with PH and these patients generally have predominant manifestations of SSc. PH in RA is most commonly due to ILD, in which case prognosis is grim. In a series of 146 RA patients, 6% had PH, which was thought to be secondary to significant ILD [18]. PH in RA-associated ILD typically develops after a prolonged course of illness, suggesting a protracted subclinical inflammation, possibly similar to the mechanism accounting for the high cardiovascular death seen in these patients.

Etiopathogenesis

The concept regarding etiopathogenesis of ILD–PH has evolved in recent times. Histologically, in CTD–ILD–PH, the pulmonary parenchymal disease leads to isolated medial hypertrophy in the precapillary pulmonary arterial bed with or without concurrent intimal fibrosis. Since the distal pulmonary vasculature resides inside the interstitium, the underlying pathologic process that characterizes ILD would also affect these pulmonary vessels in most cases. The potential "unifying pathogenic mechanism" of developing interstitial fibrosis and pulmonary vascular remodeling include oxidant–antioxidant imbalance, specifically a lack of glutathione, which promotes fibrogenesis and inhibits vasodilation. The oxygen-free radicals and lack of antioxidants are attributed to apoptosis of alveolar cells and fibroblast proliferation. The inflammatory injury also leads to damage of epithelial cells and basement membranes, leading to fibrin exudation, fibroblast activation, and proliferation. Tumor growth factor (TGF-β), platelet-derived growth factor (PDGF), insulin-like growth factor 1 (IGF 1), and connective-tissue growth factor (CTGF) also play an important role in this respect. For example, in SSc-associated ILD–PH, gene polymorphism of CTGF and autoantibodies to PDGF have been described [56].

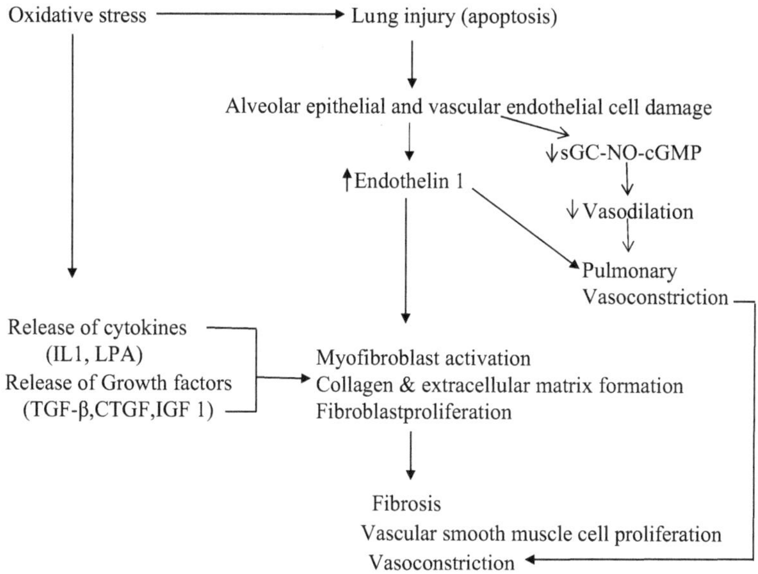

Fig. 9.1 Unifying etiopathogenic mechanism of development of ILD and pulmonary hypertension. *IL* interleukin, *LPA* Lipopolysaccharide, *TGF* transforming growth factor, *CTGF* connective tissue growth factor, *IGF* Insulin like growth factor, *sGC* soluble guanylate cyclase, *NO* nitric oxide, *cGMP* cyclic guanylate monophosphate

The unbalanced oxidative stress also leads to inactivation of soluble guanylyl cyclase (sGC), and the inhibition of its potent vasodilatory and antifibroproliferative effects via the sGC–NO–cGMP pathway [14, 19, 20]. Another common pathway to fibrosis and PH is endothelin 1 (ET-1). Endothelin-1 is not only a potent pulmonary vasoconstrictor but also a growth factor for endothelial cells and myofibroblasts. In experimental models, overexpression of ET1 has been noted in pulmonary fibrosis in addition to pulmonary hypertension. The ET-1 type-A receptor has been found to induce TGF-β1 and subsequent fibrosis. This "unifying mechanism" cascade leading to development of pulmonary fibrosis and pulmonary hypertension is illustrated in Fig. 9.1.

Clinical Manifestations

The clinical features of CTD–ILD–PH are nonspecific including progressive dyspnea, oxygen desaturation, fatigue, and functional limitations, which are often worse because of the combination of PH and ILD; often in excess of what would be expected from pulmonary function testing or parenchymal abnormalities. In advance stages, patients may present with symptoms of presyncope or syncope, chest pain, and peripheral edema due to cor pulmonale.

The physical examination has features of both pulmonary hypertension and interstitial lung disease. A loud P2 due to increased pulmonary artery pressure and a right ventricular heave suggesting right ventricular hypertrophy may be appreciated. Additionally, there may be an apical mid-diastolic rumble and a left parasternal holosystolic murmur, both increasing in inspiration due to a dilated pulmonary artery and tricuspid regurgitation, respectively. With advanced PH, patients may develop signs of right heart failure including elevated jugular venous pressure with prominent V waves with rapid y descent, right-sided S3 and/or S4, tender pulsatile hepatomegaly, ascites, and peripheral edema. In addition, frequently patients have a resting tachycardia and cardiac cachexia [10]. The presence of end-inspiratory crackles is associated with the presence of interstitial lung disease.

A complete detailed physical may

suggest the presence of an underlying CTD. For example, the presence of telangiectasias, digital ulcerations/pits, calcinosis, sclerodactyly, and/or more proximal skin thickening suggests a diagnosis of scleroderma. The presence of a rash, alopecia, keratoconjunctivitis sicca, arthritis, and/or proximal muscle weakness are other clues indicating the presence of an underlying connective tissue disease.

Diagnostic Strategy

Despite a high prevalence of PH complicating ILD in the CTD patients, diagnosis often gets delayed due to the inherent difficulty in detecting PH in the context of ILD. The clinical symptoms such as dyspnea, fatigue, and poor exercise tolerance are nonspecific, so the detection of PH in ILD patients relies on a high index of suspicion. Profound exercise desaturation during 6 min walk testing (6MWT) is a hallmark for the presence of PH in ILD patients. Nonetheless, concomitant musculoskeletal involvement, particularly pain, confounds the utility of 6MWT in CTD [21].

A restrictive ventilatory defect can also be seen in both PH and ILD, although the defect is typically mild in isolated PAH and more substantial in interstitial lung disease. A low diffusion capacity (DLco) may be seen in either PH or ILD. In SSc, a low DLco <40% is a highly sensitive screen for the presence of PH and a FVC/DLco ratio >1.6 strongly suggests the presence of PH in a background of interstitial fibrosis. Interestingly, the absolute DLco value does not correlate with the severity of PH in these patients [10, 14, 16].

The chest X-ray in CTD–ILD–PH may demonstrate features of pulmonary hypertension including central pulmonary artery dilation with peripheral pruning and dilated right-sided chambers in addition to reticulation and infiltrates due to ILD (Fig. 9.2) [22]. High-resolution chest computed tomography (HRCT) has the ability of simultaneously assessing the degree of parenchymal lung disease and has been used to predict the presence of concomitant pulmonary hypertension. In a retrospective study analyzing the relationship between PH and ILD, a mean pulmonary artery diameter (MPAD) greater than 2.9 cm had a sensitivity of 87% and specificity of 89% in predicting the presence of PH [23]. Similar results have been

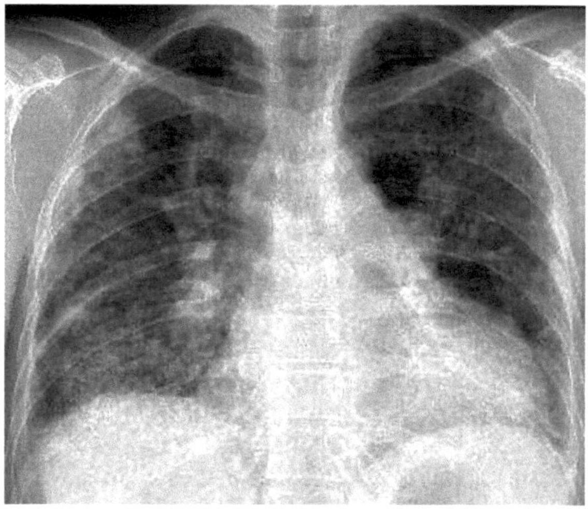

Fig. 9.2 Chest X-ray of a systemic sclerosis patient showing reticulo-nodular opacities in keeping with interstitial lung disease. It also demonstrates enlarged cardiac silhouette prominent central pulmonary vasculature, consistent with pulmonary hypertension

shown in patients with patients with SSc with combined ILD–PH, although results were attenuated by a low % forced vital capacity [24]. A ratio of main PA to ascending aorta diameter greater than one (MPA/AA >1) correlates strongly with presence mPAP >20 mm of Hg [25]. Interestingly, these radiographic correlations for presence of PH have not been reproduced in other studies in the context of ILD [26, 27].

Cardiac MRI variables such as ventricular area and diameter ratios, right ventricular mass, ventricular mass index (VMI), size of pulmonary artery, and pulmonary artery/aorta ratio (PA/Ao) have greater diagnostic and prognostic utility in CTD patients with suspected PH, compared to HRCT. However, it is an expensive tool and its clinical value in assessing CTD–ILD–PH is yet to be determined [28].

The eletrocardiogram (ECG) may demonstrate right atrial enlargement, right ventricular hypertrophy, and right axis deviation as well as rhythm abnormalities, most commonly supraventricular in origin (Fig. 9.3). A low voltage ECG may be seen in the setting of a pericardial effusion, which is not uncommon in patients with CTD. Although ECG is frequently abnormal, it is not sensitive or specific enough as a screening tool.

Although the transthoracic echocardiogram is still the best screening tool to detect PH associated with CTD–ILD [29], the measurement of the systolic pulmonary artery pressure (SPAP) in patients with advanced lung diseases may be misleading [30, 53]. PH is likely if the tricuspid regurgitant (TR) jet velocity is >3.4 m/s and/or the systolic pulmonary artery pressure (SPAP) is >50 mm of Hg. PH may also be possible if the TR jet velocity is 2.8–3.4 m/s and systolic SPAP >36 mm of Hg if there are other associated features such as increased dimensions of right heart chambers, increased right ventricular (RV) wall thickness, RV hypokinesis, dyskinesia of the interventricular septum, and/or a dilated main pulmonary artery [29]. In general, the sensitivity and specificity of Doppler-estimated SPAP in predicting PH ranges from 0.79 to 1.0 and 0.6 to 0.98, respectively [10]. In a retrospective study, right ventricular dilatation on echocardiogram predicted early mortality patients with

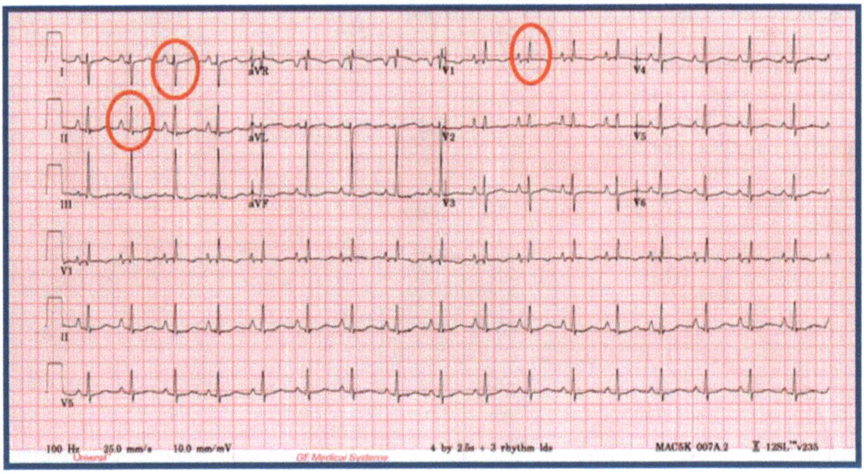

Fig. 9.3 EKG demonstrating cor pulmonale due to pulmonary hypertension. It shows tall peaked P-wave in lead II, consistent with right atrial enlargement and positive tall QRS deflection in lead V1 due to right ventricular hypertrophy

ILD. Moreover, SSc patients with PH often have disproportionately severe RV dysfunction; in fact severe RV depression may even be seen without associated PH [31]. Although echocardiogram can aid in predicting PH in ILD patients, it should not be solely relied upon. In ILD patients, a composite index of CT scan measured MPAD and SPAP on echocardiogram predicts PH better than each parameter alone [32].

Serum biomarkers are also useful in determining and prognosticating PH in ILD patients. An elevated B-type natriuretic peptide (BNP) and N-terminal pro-BNP (NT pro BNP) have been found to be an accurate predictor for the presence of PH in ILD. An NT pro-BNP level >240 pg/ml has a 90% specificity for detecting PH in SSc patients, and serial changes in NT pro-BNP also correlate with survival [33]. However, it should not be viewed in isolation as pro-BNP may remain elevated in other causes of CTD-related PH such as cardiac dysfunctions or in patients with renal insufficiency.

The gold standard for the diagnosis of pulmonary hypertension remains the right heart catheterization (RHC) and is useful in excluding PH due to elevated left-sided filling pressure (Group 2 PH), which is also commonly seen in CTD. The RHC can also be used prognostically. In patients with diffuse fibrotic lung diseases, early mortality is strongly linked to an elevated pulmonary vascular resistance (PVR) [30].

Prognosis

Although most of the published cohorts of CTD–PH involved SSc patients, limited data suggests similar outcomes in other CTDs. The presence of PH is an important predictor of mortality in CTD patients. This adverse prognosis is further compounded by coexisting ILD. Even in the modern treatment era, the outcome in CTD–ILD–PH is depressingly low. In a retrospective analysis of SSc patients who developed ILD–PH, the 1-, 2-, and 3-year mortality was 29%, 61%, and 79%, respectively, in spite of PH-specific therapy [34]. The predictors of adverse outcome included a low arterial oxygen tension and poor kidney function. A RHC-based study in SSc patients has reported that the 3-year survival with isolated PAH is 45% whereas for ILD–PH, it is only 28%. Little is known regarding the survival of ILD–PH in other CTDs. Mitto and coworker noted median survival of 34 months in a case series of patients with CTD–ILD–PH, although the majority of his patients were SSc [2]. Interestingly, in this series, the SSc patients had a worse survival than the other CTD cohorts. Age greater than70 years, male gender, NYHA functional class 4, severely reduced DLco (<39%), reduced 6MWD, impaired renal function, presence of pericardial effusion, and a low mixed venous oxygen saturation are risk factors for a poor prognosis in SSc Group 3 PH [35–37, 54, 55].

Management

Although the survival of patients with CTD-associated PAH has improved in the modern treatment era, the response to PH specific therapy is disappointing in ILD-related PH. The major focus of treatment in ILD–PH is the management of the ILD with immunosuppression. Inflammation is also felt to play a vital part in the development of PH secondary to the CTDs; and small studies have suggested that immunosuppressive therapy with combined cyclophosphamide and corticosteroids is associated with clinical improvement in PH due to SLE, MCTD, and demonstrated by an improvement in WHO functional class, distance walked in 6MWD, as well as mPAP [38]. There are also case reports suggesting pulmonary arterial hypertension in SLE improves with rituximab therapy [39], and rituximab is currently under investigation for SSc-associated PAH [40] and is of interest for the treatment of SSc-associated ILD. Further research is needed to ascertain the exact role of immunosuppression in these subsets of patients given the paucity of data investigating the role of immunosuppression for combined ILD and PH in CTD patients.

In advanced lung diseases, chronic hypoxemia leads to vasoconstriction of the pulmonary vasculature, thus worsening PH. The use of supplemental oxygen to maintain an oxygen saturation above 90% is recommended. Lifestyle recommendations also have an important role in management of CTD–PH. Those include smoking cessation, counseling against pregnancy, reduced salt intake, immunization against influenza, and pneumococcal pneumonia. These patients are prone to suffer from anxiety and depression, so often need a psychosocial support. In CTD–PAH, exercise training, as an add-on to medical therapy, has been found to improve exercise capacity, quality of life, and 3-year survival rate [41, 42]. Studies are needed to assess similar efficacy of exercise training in CTD–ILD–PH. The role of anticoagulation in CTD–PH is unclear as patients may have an increased bleeding risk from intestinal telangiectasia. There are no data supporting anticoagulation in CTD–ILD–PH. Patients should be appropriately diuresed.

There was initial enthusiasm for the use of PAH-specific vasoactive medications in CTD–PH–ILD due to the common linkage in etiopathogenesis. In a retrospective analysis of 70 SSc ILD–PH patients, PH therapy with prostanoids, phosphodiesterase-5 inhibitors and endothelin receptor antagonists did not show any clear-cut benefit in terms of WHO functional class, 6MWD, and pulmonary hemodynamics [43]. Small clinical studies suggest that PAH-specific therapies may be associated with worsening hypoxemia due to V/Q mismatch. Nevertheless, inhaled iloprost and oral sildenafil have been found to decrease pulmonary vascular resistance without significantly reducing arterial oxygen tension in a small study [10]. In another small series of CTD–ILD–PH, both sildenafil and bosentan were well tolerated [2]. Intravenous or subcutaneous treprostinil has also been suggested to be efficacious in ILD-related PH for improving pulmonary hemodynamics and 6MWD [35]. However before treatment recommendations can be made, larger multicenter prospective randomized placebo-controlled trials in CTD–ILD–PH are required.

Lung Transplantation

Lung transplantation is being offered more frequently in CTD patients with ILD and/or PH, given the limited efficacy of conventional medical therapy. Since the inception of the lung allocation score (LAS), CTD–ILD patients receive additional points upon development of PH because of their worse prognosis. Many centers are reluctant to perform lung transplantation in CTD patients because of the concomitant involvement of other organs, particularly esophageal dysfunction that is believed to contribute to allograft dysfunction. Although other organ dysfunction is not an absolute contraindication for lung transplantation in CTD patients, it does portend a higher risk for posttransplant complications [36]. In SSc, transplant outcomes have been shown to be similar in carefully selected patients with ILD and/or PH, compared to patients with idiopathic pulmonary fibrosis and idiopathic PAH with a 72% and 55% 2-year and 5-year survival, respectively [37, 44]. Similar results have been reported in a small series of a heterogeneous population of connective tissue disorders undergoing lung transplantation [45].

Future Directions

The shared etiopathogenesis of pulmonary fibrosis and PH has led to management focus on addressing increased expression of growth factors. As a result, imatinib, a PDGF inhibitor, has been tested in experimental models and the subsequent results of Phase II trials are encouraging in this respect, although associated with increased adverse events [46]. Riociguat, a guanylate cyclase stimulator increasing production of NO, has a great potential for use in ILD-associated PH and is currently being investigated [47]. Research is also ongoing assessing the efficacy of the antifibrotic drugs, such as nintedanib, in SSc. These agents may be beneficial in treating both the underlying ILD as well as vascular remodeling due to fibroproliferation of the pulmonary vasculature.

Conclusion

PH is frequent in CTD–ILD, particularly in SSc and the presence of PH along with ILD leads to a fivefold increase in mortality. These patients generally have a suboptimal response to conventional PH therapies and robust data regarding the use of aggressive immunosuppressive therapy or PAH-specific therapy are lacking. Nevertheless, some patients may benefit from PAH-specific therapy and/or immunosuppressive therapies in order to control PH as well as ILD. However, because of the disappointingly poor prognosis, patients candidacy for lung transplantation should be evaluated.

Conflict of Interest Debabrata Bandyopadhyay: none

Tanmay S. Panchabhai: none

Kristin B. Highland is a consultant, has grants/contracts, and/or is on the speaker's bureau for: Actelion Pharmaceuticals, Bayer Healthcare, Boerhinger Ingelheim, Genentech, Gilead Sciences, Intermmune, Lung Biotechnology, and United Therapeutics.

References

1. Simonneau G, Gatzoulis MA, Adatia I, Celermajer D, Denton C, Ghofrani A, et al. Updated clinical classification of pulmonary hypertension. J Am Coll Cardiol. 2013;62(25 Suppl):D34–41.
2. Mittoo S, Jacob T, Craig A, Bshouty Z. Treatment of pulmonary hypertension in patients with connective tissue disease and interstitial lung disease. Can Respir J. 2010;17(6):282–6.
3. Gutsche M, Rosen GD, Swigris JJ. Connective tissue disease-associated interstitial lung disease: a review. Curr Respir Care Rep. 2012;1:224–32.
4. van den Hoogen F, Khanna D, Fransen J, Johnson SR, Baron M, Tyndall A, et al. 2013 classification criteria for systemic sclerosis: an American College of Rheumatology/European League against Rheumatism collaborative initiative. Arthritis Rheum. 2013;65(11):2737–47.
5. Wells AU, Denton CP. Interstitial lung disease in connective tissue disease—mechanisms and management. Nat Rev Rheumatol. 2014;10(12):728–39.
6. Ruano CA, Lucas RN, Leal CI, Lourenço J, Pinheiro S, Fernandes O, et al. Thoracic manifestations of connective tissue diseases. Curr Probl Diagn Radiol. 2015;44(1):47–59.
7. Fischer A, West SG, Swigris JJ, Brown KK, du Bois RM. Connective tissue disease-associated interstitial lung disease: a call for clarification. Chest. 2010;138(2):251–6.
8. Song JW, Do KH, Kim MY, Jang SJ, Colby TV, Kim DS. Pathologic and radiologic differences between idiopathic and collagen vascular disease-related usual interstitial pneumonia. Chest. 2009;136(1):23–30.

9. Kocheril SV, Appleton BE, Somers EC, Kazerooni EA, Flaherty KR, Martinez FJ, et al. Comparison of disease progression and mortality of connective tissue disease-related interstitial lung disease and idiopathic interstitial pneumonia. Arthritis Rheum. 2005;53(4):549–57.
10. Ryu JH, Krowka MJ, Pellikka PA, Swanson KL, McGoon MD. Pulmonary hypertension in patients with interstitial lung diseases. Mayo Clin Proc. 2007;82(3):342–50.
11. Pan TL, Thumboo J, Boey ML. Primary and secondary pulmonary hypertension in systemic lupus erythematosus. Lupus. 2000;9(5):338–42.
12. Nishimaki T, Aotsuka S, Kondo H, Yamamoto K, Takasaki Y, Sumiya M, et al. Immunological analysis of pulmonary hypertension in connective tissue diseases. J Rheumatol. 1999;26(11): 2357–62.
13. Lian F, Chen D, Wang Y, et al. Clinical features and independent predictors of pulmonary arterial hypertension in systemic lupus erythematosus. Rheumatol Int. 2012;32(6):1727–31.
14. Shlobin OA, Nathan SD. Pulmonary hypertension secondary to interstitial lung disease. Expert Rev Respir Med. 2011;5(2):179–89.
15. Chang B, Wigley FM, White B, Wise RA. Scleroderma patients with combined pulmonary hypertension and interstitial lung disease. J Rheumatol. 2003;30(11):2398–405.
16. Hinchcliff M, Fischer A, Schiopu E, Steen VD. PHAROS Investigators. Pulmonary Hypertension Assessment and Recognition of Outcomes in Scleroderma (PHAROS): baseline characteristics and description of study population. J Rheumatol. 2011;38(10):2172–9.
17. Chung L, Liu J, Parsons L, Hassoun PM, McGoon M, Badesch DB, et al. Characterization of connective tissue disease-associated pulmonary arterial hypertension from REVEAL: identifying systemic sclerosis as a unique phenotype. Chest. 2010;138(6):1383–94.
18. Dawson JK, Goodson NG, Graham DR, Lynch MP. Raised pulmonary artery pressures measured with Doppler echocardiography in rheumatoid arthritis patients. Rheumatology (Oxford). 2000;39(12):1320–5.
19. Farkas L, Kolb M. Pulmonary microcirculation in interstitial lung disease. Proc Am Thorac Soc. 2011;8(6):516–21.
20. Behr J, Ryu JH. Pulmonary hypertension in interstitial lung disease. Eur Respir J. 2008; 31(6):1357–67.
21. Garin MC, Highland KB, Silver RM, Strange C. Limitations to the 6-minute walk test in interstitial lung disease and pulmonary hypertension in scleroderma. J Rheumatol. 2009;36(2): 330–6.
22. McGoon MD, Kane GC. Pulmonary hypertension: diagnosis and management. Mayo Clin Proc. 2009;84(2):191–207.
23. Tan RT, Kuzo R, Goodman LR, Siegel R, Haasler GB, Presberg KW. Utility of CT scan evaluation for predicting pulmonary hypertension in patients with parenchymal lung disease. Medical College of Wisconsin Lung Transplant Group. Chest. 1998;113(5):1250–6.
24. McCall RK, Ravenel JG, Nietert PJ, Granath A, Silver RM. Relationship of main pulmonary artery diameter to pulmonary arterial pressure in scleroderma patients with and without interstitial fibrosis. J Comput Assist Tomogr. 2014;38:163–8.
25. Ng CS, Wells AU, Padley SP. A CT sign of chronic pulmonary arterial hypertension: the ratio of main pulmonary artery to aortic diameter. J Thorac Imaging. 1999;14(4):270–8.
26. Devaraj A, Wells AU, Meister MG, et al. The effect of diffuse pulmonary fibrosis on the reliability of CT signs of pulmonary hypertension. Radiology. 2008;249:1042–9.
27. Zisman DA, Karlamangla AS, Ross DJ, Keane MP, Belperio JA, Saggar R, et al. High-resolution chest CT findings do not predict the presence of pulmonary hypertension in advanced idiopathic pulmonary fibrosis. Chest. 2007;132(3):773–9.
28. Rajaram S, Swift AJ, Capener D, Elliot CA, Condliffe R, Davies C, et al. Comparison of the diagnostic utility of cardiac magnetic resonance imaging, computed tomography, and echocardiography in assessment of suspected pulmonary arterial hypertension in patients with connective tissue disease. J Rheumatol. 2012;39(6):1265–74.
29. Galiè N, Hoeper MM, Humbert M, Torbicki A, Vachiery JL, Barbera JA, et al. ESC Committee for Practice Guidelines (CPG). Guidelines for the diagnosis and treatment of pulmonary

hypertension: the task force for the diagnosis and treatment of pulmonary hypertension of the European Society of Cardiology (ESC) and the European Respiratory Society (ERS), endorsed by the International Society of Heart and Lung Transplantation (ISHLT). Eur Heart J. 2009;30(20):2493–537.
30. Corte TJ, Wort SJ, Gatzoulis MA, Macdonald P, Hansell DM, Wells AU. Pulmonary vascular resistance predicts early mortality in patients with diffuse fibrotic lung disease and suspected pulmonary hypertension. Thorax. 2009;64(10):883–8.
31. Hsiao SH, Lee CY, Chang SM, Lin SK, Liu CP. Right heart function in scleroderma: insights from myocardial Doppler tissue imaging. J Am Soc Echocardiogr. 2006;19(5):507–14.
32. Devaraj A, Wells AU, Meister MG, Corte TJ, Wort SJ, Hansell DM. Detection of pulmonary hypertension with multidetector CT and echocardiography alone and in combination. Radiology. 2010;254(2):609–16.
33. Chaisson NF, Hassoun PM. Systemic sclerosis-associated pulmonary arterial hypertension. Chest. 2013;144(4):1346–56.
34. Le Pavec J, Girgis RE, Lechtzin N, Mathai SC, Launay D, Hummers LK, et al. Systemic sclerosis-related pulmonary hypertension associated with interstitial lung disease: impact of pulmonary arterial hypertension therapies. Arthritis Rheum. 2011;63(8):2456–64.
35. Saggar R, Belperio JA, Shapiro SS, Weight SS, Sager JS, Derhovanessian A, et al. A single center, prospective, open label, pilot study evaluating the safety and efficacy of IV/SQ treprostinil in the treatment of pulmonary arterial hypertension associated with advanced interstitial lung disease. Presented at American Thoracic Symposium; 2010 May 14–19; New Orleans, LA. Meeting Abstract. A5261.
36. Takagishi T, Ostrowski R, Alex C, Rychlik K, Pelletiere K, Tehrani R. Survival and extrapulmonary course of connective tissue disease after lung transplantation. J Clin Rheumatol. 2010;18:283–9.
37. Shitrit D, Amitai A, Peled N, Raviv Y, Medalion B, Saute M, et al. Lung transplantation in patients with scleroderma: case series, review of the literature, and criteria for transplantation. Clin Transplant. 2009;23:178–83.
38. Sanchez O, Sitbon O, Jaïs X, Simonneau G, Humbert M. Immunosuppressive therapy in connective tissue diseases-associated pulmonary arterial hypertension. Chest. 2006;130(1):182–9.
39. Hennigan S, Channick RN, Silverman GJ. Rituximab treatment of pulmonary arterial hypertension associated with systemic lupus erythematosus: a case report. Lupus. 2008;17(8):754–6.
40. Rituximab for treatment of systemic sclerosis associated pulmonary arterial hypertension. https://clinicaltrials.gov/ct2/show/NCT01086540. Published March 11, 2010. Updated May 11, 2015. Accessed 1 July 2015.
41. Grünig E, Maier F, Ehlken N, Fischer C, Lichtblau M, Blank N, et al. Exercise training in pulmonary arterial hypertension associated with connective tissue diseases. Arthritis Res Ther. 2012;14(3):R148.
42. Task Force for Diagnosis and Treatment of Pulmonary Hypertension of European Society of Cardiology (ESC), European Respiratory Society (ERS), International Society of Heart and Lung Transplantation (ISHLT), Galiè N, Hoeper MM, Humbert M, et al. Guidelines for the diagnosis and treatment of pulmonary hypertension. Eur Respir J. 2009;34(6):1219–63.
43. Bussone G, Mouthon L. Interstitial lung disease in systemic sclerosis. Autoimmun Rev. 2011;10(5):248–55.
44. Schachna L, Medsger Jr TA, Dauber JH, Wigley FM, Braunstein NA, White B, et al. Lung transplantation in scleroderma compared with idiopathic pulmonary fibrosis and idiopathic pulmonary arterial hypertension. Arthritis Rheum. 2006;54:3954–61.
45. Hajari AS, Willie KM, de Andrade JAM, Harrington KF. Lung transplant outcomes in connective tissue disorders. Chest. 2009;136:17S.
46. Berghausen E, ten Freyhaus H, Rosenkranz S. Targeting of platelet-derived growth factor signaling in pulmonary arterial hypertension. Handb Exp Pharmacol. 2013;218:381–408.

47. Hoeper MM, Halank M, Wilkens H, Günther A, Weimann G, Gebert I, et al. Riociguat for interstitial lung disease and pulmonary hypertension: a pilot trial. Eur Respir J. 2013;41(4): 853–60.
48. Bredemeier M, Xavier RM, Capobianco KG, Restelli VG, Rohde LE, Pinotti AF, et al. Nailfold capillary microscopy can suggest pulmonary disease activity in systemic sclerosis. J Rheumatol. 2004;31(2):286–94.
49. Jacobsen S, Ullman S, Shen GQ, Wiik A, Halberg P. Influence of clinicalfeatures, serum antinuclear antibodies, and lung function on survival of patients with systemic sclerosis. J Rheumatol. 2001;28(11):2454–9.
50. Alamoudi OS, Attar SM. Pulmonary manifestations in systemic lupus erythematosus: association with disease activity. Respirology. 2015;20(3):474–80.
51. Cavagna L, Monti S, Grosso V, Boffini N, Scorletti E, Crepaldi G, et al. The multifaceted aspects of interstitial lung disease in rheumatoid arthritis. Biomed Res Int. 2013;2013:759760.
52. Hirakata M, Nagai S. Interstitial lung disease in polymyositis and dermatomyositis. Curr Opin Rheumatol. 2000;12:501–8.
53. Arcasoy SM, Christie JD, Ferrari VA, Sutton MS, Zisman DA, Blumenthal NP, et al. Echocardiographic assessment of pulmonary hypertension in patients with advanced lung disease. Am J Respir Crit Care Med. 2003;167(5):735–40.
54. Mathai SC, Hummers LK, Champion HC, Wigley FM, Zaiman A, Hassoun PM, et al. Survival in pulmonary hypertension associated with the scleroderma spectrum of diseases: impact of interstitial lung disease. Arthritis Rheum. 2009;60(2):569–77.
55. Ngian GS, Stevens W, Prior D, Gabbay E, Roddy J, Tran A, et al. Predictors of mortality in connective tissue disease-associated pulmonary arterial hypertension: a cohort study. Arthritis Res Ther. 2012;14(5):R213.
56. Shahane A. Pulmonary hypertension in rheumatic diseases: epidemiology and pathogenesis. Rheumatol Int. 2013;33(7):1655–67.

Chapter 10
Pulmonary Hypertension in Rare Parenchymal Lung Diseases

Oksana A. Shlobin and Steven D. Nathan

Introduction

This chapter summarizes data published on pulmonary hypertension (PH) in rare parenchymal lung diseases including Pulmonary Langerhan's Histiocytosis, Lymphangioleiomyomatosis, Neurofibromatosis 1, Cystic Fibrosis, and several others. These diseases have widely differing etiologies and pulmonary pathophysiology changes; however, all of them may be complicated by the development of PH. These conditions often share similar mechanisms responsible for the development of PH, but in some, there are also unique elements that may be contributory. Figure 10.1 summarizes the various mechanisms that may account for the development of PH.

PH in Pulmonary Langerhans's Histiocytosis (PLCH-PH)

Pulmonary Langerhans's cell histiocytosis (PLCH) (also known as histiocytosis X and previously called Eosinophilic Granuloma (EG)) is an uncommon lung disease which affects primarily young adults, almost exclusively with a history of current or prior cigarette smoking [1]. Rarely, patients with PLCH have systemic manifestations (Langerhan's cell histiocytosis) with involvement of the skin, lymph nodes, as

O.A. Shlobin, MD (✉) • S.D. Nathan, MD
Inova Fairfax Advanced Lung Disease and Transplant Program, Inova Fairfax Hospital, 3300 Gallows Road, Falls Church, VA 22042, USA
e-mail: oksana.shlobin@inova.org; steven.nathan@inova.org

R.P. Baughman et al. (eds.), *Pulmonary Hypertension and Interstitial Lung Disease*, DOI 10.1007/978-3-319-49918-5_10

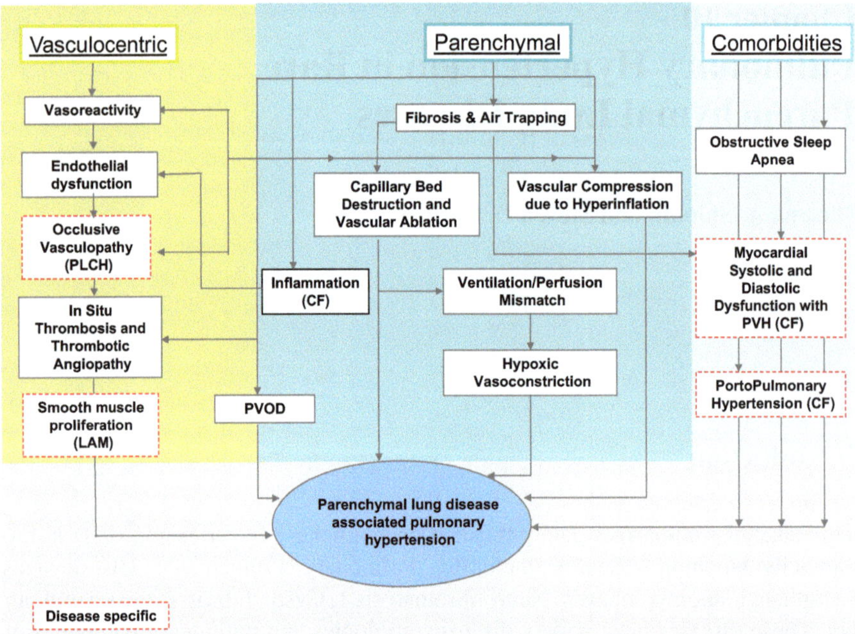

Fig. 10.1 Pathogenesis of parenchymal lung disease-associated PH. *CF* cystic fibrosis, *PVOD* pulmonary veno-occlusive disease, *LAM* Lymphangioleiomyomatosis, *PLCH* pulmonary Langerhans's cell histiocytosis

well as the liver, spleen, bone marrow, thymus, and the central nervous system [1]. Systemic disease is not associated with history of smoking.

The true incidence of the disease is unknown. In adults, the incidence is estimated to be one to two cases per million adults. A male predominance has been described in some case series, while the incidence appears to be higher in whites of northern European descent than in blacks [2].

The true incidence and prevalence of PLCH are unknown. In a 5-year prospective study in 20 pulmonology centers in Belgium, 3% of 360 patients with interstitial pneumonia had LCH [3]. A survey of discharge diagnoses in large hospitals in Japan over a 1-year period found 160 cases of PLCH, with the crude prevalence of the disease estimated at 0.27 and 0.07 per 100,000 in males and females, respectively [4]. Although not comprehensive and with inherent bias, these data confirm that PLCH is relatively rare. The prevalence of PLCH is, however, probably underestimated because some patients exhibit no symptoms or experience spontaneous remission, and histological findings are nonspecific in the advanced forms. No occupational or geographic predisposition has been reported but tobacco smoke is thought to be a major etiologic factor.

The Langerhans cell, a differentiated cell of the monocyte–macrophage line, is the pathologic cell type of PLCH. It is characterized by pale staining cytoplasm, a large nucleus and nucleoli, and, on electron microscopy, classic pentalaminar cytoplasmic inclusions or Birbeck granules (X-bodies). Langerhans cells also demonstrate positive immunohistochemical staining for S100 protein (sensitive but not specific feature). Another characteristic is the strong presence of CD1 antigen on the cell surface, a feature not observed in other cells of histiocytic origin. Langerin, the most specific stain, is not routinely performed and not widely available. In the lung, early inflammatory lesions surround the smaller bronchioles and usually contain a mixture of eosinophils, lymphocytes, and neutrophils, with eosinophils not being a dominant cell type, thus making EG a misnomer [5].

Three pathologic features frequently seen along changes specific to pulmonary Langerhans cell histiocytosis include smoking-related changes:

a. Pseudo-desquamative interstitial pneumonia (DIP) which is characterized by the accumulation of alveolar macrophages in the pulmonary parenchyma between the typical lesions containing Langerhans cells.
b. Respiratory ("smokers") bronchiolitis which is characterized by pigmented macrophages filling the lumen of bronchioles and the surrounding alveolar spaces.
c. Intraluminal fibrosis which is characterized by alveolar obliteration and the development of intraluminal buds) [6, 7].

The disease course of PLCH is variable with approximately one quarter of the cases undergoing spontaneous regression, one half maintaining a stable disease state, and the remaining quarter developing progression to end-stage disease. This is characterized by chronic respiratory failure with irreversible airflow obstruction, hypoxemia, and less commonly hypercapnia [8, 9]. PH, as defined by right heart catheterization, is a common complication of end stage PLCH [10]. Most reports pertaining to PH in PLCH have been gleaned from cohorts of patients evaluated for lung transplantation [11] although the development of PH in patients with stable disease has also been described [12].

Pathologically, a vasculopathy comprised of lesions that affect small airways can involve both pulmonary arterioles and venules, including pulmonary veno-occlusive disease (PVOD)-like lesions [12]. Although the pathogenesis remains unclear, it is postulated to involve vascular remodeling with diffuse medial hypertrophy, intimal fibrosis, and/or proliferation of smooth muscle cells (Figs. 10.2 and 10.3). These pathologic changes may be due to or independent of parenchymal changes, secondary to the effects of chronic hypoxemia, and/or related to the abnormal production of inflammatory cytokines and growth factors (Interleukin-1, Interleukin-6, tumor growth factor beta, and platelet-derived growth factor (PDGF)) [13–15].

In advanced PLCH, right heart catheterization (RHC)-confirmed PH occurs with a reported prevalence of 92–100% [11, 16]. The majority of these patients (65–75%) have severe PH with a mean pulmonary arterial pressure (mPAP) over 35 mmHg. Therefore, the prevalence and severity of PLCH-PH seems to be higher than in other chronic respiratory diseases [15].

PH usually develops years following the diagnosis of PLCH; however, there are also instances of a simultaneous diagnosis of PLCH with PH [16]. A report from the largest published cohort from the French registry of PLCH patients showed that the patients were diagnosed with PH an average of 11 years post-PLCH diagnosis. In this registry, a total of 29 patients were described, 60% of whom were male with a

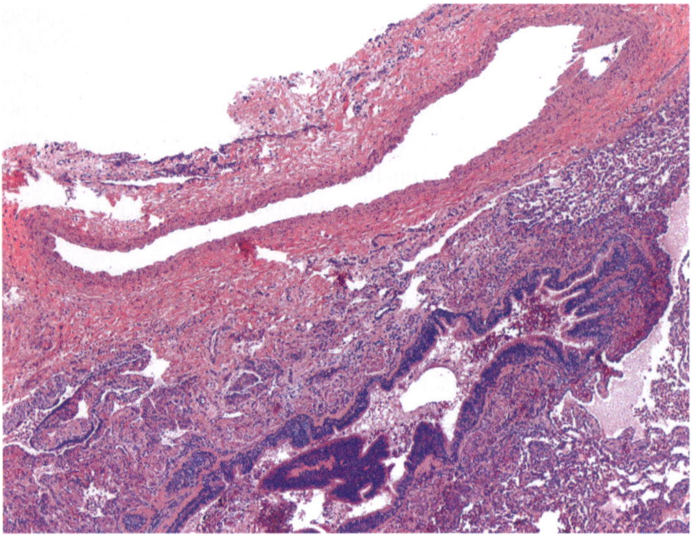

Fig. 10.2 This image shows a normal bronchiole and accompanying artery. Note that the diameter and caliber of the artery is similar to that of the airway, when normal (H&E, 40×)

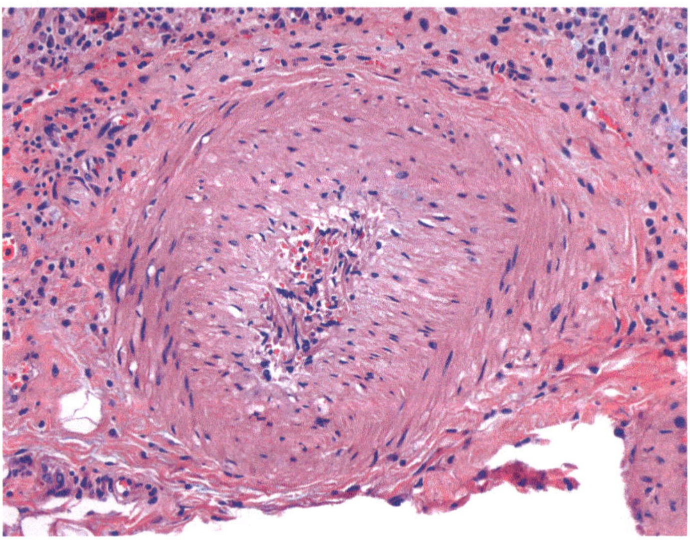

Fig. 10.3 This artery shows concentric fibrointimal thickening and significant medial hypertrophy, typical of hypertensive changes (H&E, 200×)

mean age of 43 years, and most had functional class II/III symptoms. Their mean six-minute walk test (6MWT) was 355 m while their hemodynamic profile included a mean right atrial pressure (RA) of 5 mmHg, mPAP of 45 mmHg, mean cardiac index (CI) of 3.2 L/min/m^2, and a mean pulmonary vascular resistance (PVR) of 6.9

Table 10.1 Response to PAH therapy in PLCH-PH patient cohort

Measurements	Baseline	Short-term follow up	Long-term follow up	*P* Value	*P* Value
WHO functional class I-II/III-IV, No.	1/11	6/6	4/6	.12	.37
6MWT, m	376 ± 96	403 ± 74	415 ± 90	.25	.20
Hemodynamics					
Mean BP, mmHg	102 ± 24	98 ± 15	90 ± 13	.57	.20
RAP, mmHg	8 ± 4	6 ± 4	8 ± 5	.18	.59
PCWP, mmHg	11 ± 4	10 ± 3	11 ± 3	.40	.71
mPAP, mmHg	56 ± 14	45 ± 12	43 ± 11	.03	.04
CO, L/min	5.5 ± 1.7	6.4 ± 1.7	6.9 ± 1.1	.08	<.01
Cardiac index, L/min/m^2	2.9 ± 0.8	3.4 ± 0.8	3.6 ± 0.5	.09	<.01
PVR, dyne/s/cm^5	701 ± 239	469 ± 210	348 ± 104	.01	<.01
Oxygen requirement in patients on oxygen at baseline, mean ± SD (No.), L/min	3.7 ± 2.1 [3]	2.0 ± 3.5 [3]	2.0 ± 3.4 [3]	.20	.20

Adapted from Le Pavec J, Lorillon G, Jaïs X, et al. Pulmonary Langerhans Cell Histiocytosis-Associated Pulmonary Hypertension Pulmonary Langerhans Cell Histiocytosis: Clinical Characteristics and Impact of Pulmonary Arterial Hypertension Therapies. Chest 2012; 142(5):1150–1157

wood units (Table 10.1). The patients had obstructive physiology with moderate-to-severe airflow obstruction, air trapping, and a severely reduced single breath diffusing capacity for carbon monoxide (DL_{CO}) [16].

Predictors of PH development in PLCH have not yet been described, as no formal comparison exists between patients with and without PH. In the French registry, a decrease in the DL_{CO}, along with a moderate reduction in the FEV1, appeared to be temporally related to the development of PH [16]. However, it does make intuitive sense that predictors of PH with demonstrated utility in other more common forms of diffuse parenchymal lung disease would have a role in predicting the presence of PH in PLCH. These predictors include a reduced 6MWT distance, desaturation, echocardiography (ECHO) findings, and elevated brain natriuretic peptide (BNP or pro-NT BNP), all of which could play a role in predicting the presence of PH in PLCH.

PH complicating the course of patients with PLCH appears to have significant ramifications. When PH is present, impairment in exercise capacity is likely primarily due to a vascular rather than a parenchymal limitation [9]. Survival in PLCH-PH remains poorly defined due to the small number of patients available for study. Outcomes of PLCH-PH (based on ECHO findings) patients suggest a median survival between 7.6 and 50 months [17, 18]. Not surprisingly, worsening of symptoms as measured by World Health Organization (WHO) functional class was found to be significantly associated with death in the French registry cohort ($p = .03$) [16].

The same registry reported 1-, 3-, and 5-year survivals of 96, 92, and 73%, respectively, although approximately half the patients received PAH-specific therapy which could have influenced these outcomes [16] (Table 10.1).

The treatment of PLCH-PH has not been standardized. There are theoretic concerns with the empiric treatment of PH in PLCH with PAH medications. Specifically, as there is a high incidence of pulmonary venular obstruction, there is the inherent risk of pulmonary edema when the right ventricle is unloaded. Also, there might be worsening in oxygenation as a result of increased ventilation/perfusion imbalance due to inhibition of hypoxic pulmonary vasoconstriction [19]. Therefore, the use of PAH-specific therapies has previously been thought to be hazardous [12]. Fourteen patients from the French Registry received PAH therapies, ten of whom were placed on an endothelin receptor antagonist (ERA), five on a phosphodiesterase 5 inhibitor (PDE5i), with 2 of 15 receiving upfront combination therapy. Five patients (35%) ultimately received a second PAH agent, either instead of or in combination with the initial drug. Follow-up assessment was available in 12 of the treated patients at a mean of 5.5 ± 2.5 months after baseline. WHO functional class improved by at least one in eight patients (67%), while five subjects (45%) demonstrated ≥10% increase in 6MWT, three (27%) of whom demonstrated ≥20% improvement. All 12 patients who underwent a follow-up RHC showed significant improvements in mPAP, PVR, and CI in comparison to their baseline measurements. This improvement in hemodynamics was sustained over time based on a third invasive evaluation performed 16 ± 4 months after baseline in ten patients (Table 10.1). These improvements were associated with a trend toward a better survival (p = .09) [16]. During a median observation period following the initial RHC of 35 months (range 2.7–130 months), five patients died and six underwent lung transplantation at a mean interval of 43 ± 30 months and 20 ± 15 months, respectively. In addition to this Registry data, there have been several other case reports attesting to the successful use of PAH specific therapy (bosentan and sildenafil) for PLCH-PH [20, 21].

PH in Lymphangioleiomyomatosis (PH-LAM)

Lymphangioleiomyomatosis (LAM) is a rare multisystem disease occurring almost exclusively in women of reproductive age. The term sporadic LAM is used for patients with pulmonary LAM not associated with tuberous sclerosis complex (TSC). TSC is characterized by germ line mutations, whereas the majority of LAM patients have biallelic mutations in the TSC1 or TSC2 genes [22].

The incidence and prevalence of pulmonary LAM are unknown. Based on data from the LAM registry, there are approximately 1300 known patients with LAM in North America [23]. Given the prevalence of TSC, however, it is estimated that at least 8000–10,000 women have cystic lung lesions consistent with LAM. Caucasians are afflicted much more commonly than other racial groups. LAM has rarely been reported in men, almost always in association with definite or probable TSC [23]. The pathogenesis is also unknown with some data suggesting a role for loss of

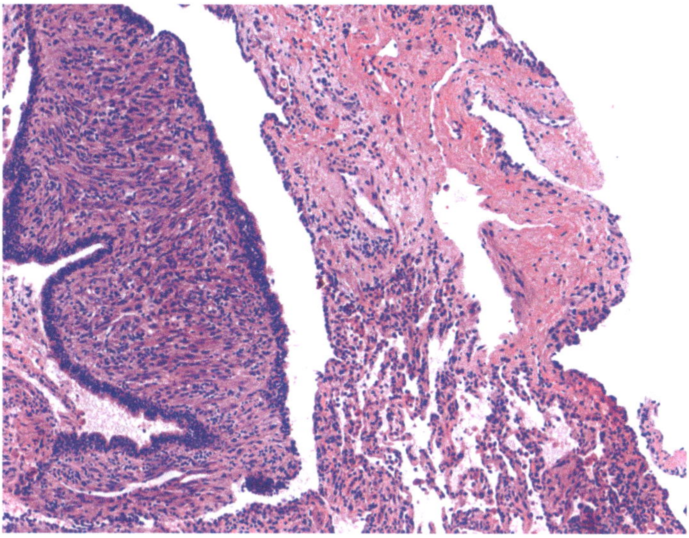

Fig. 10.4 In this example a LAM lesion is seen involving peribronchiolar lymphatics. The adjacent artery is normal (H&E, 100×)

tumor suppression functions of certain cellular proteins (e.g., hamartin, tuberin) or abnormalities in enzymes involved in the synthesis of catecholamines [24]. However, it is not clear how defects in these proteins result in LAM. LAM does not develop prior to puberty; it is extremely rarely postmenopause and is exceedingly rare in males. This predilection suggests that estrogen may have a pivotal role in disease progression, although probably not pathogenesis. Estrogen and progesterone receptors have been demonstrated in a subpopulation of the atypical smooth muscle (LAM) cells and appear to be downregulated by hormonal therapy [25].

Both sporadic and TSC-associated pulmonary LAM are characterized pathologically by interstitial collections of LAM cells and perivascular epithelioid cells around bronchovascular structures extending into the interstitium (Fig. 10.4). These result in tortuous and dilated lymphatics and venules as well as cyst formation. Hemosiderosis is common and is a consequence of clinically insignificant hemorrhage due to the rupture of dilated and tortuous venules [26].

Immunohistochemistry stains for melanocytic markers such as human melanoma black 45 (HMB-45), Melan-A, tyrosinase, microphthalmia transcription factor, and muscle markers such as smooth muscle actin, pan-muscle actin, muscle myosin, and calponin are typically positive [24]. In addition, immunohistochemical evaluation of lung tissue from LAM patients demonstrates immunoreactivity of LAM cells for vascular endothelial growth factor-D (VEGF-D), which is a lymphangiogenic factor. This observation correlates with several reports of elevated serum VEGF-D levels in LAM patients with lymphatic involvement [27].

Radiographically, pulmonary involvement typically manifests as diffuse thin-walled cysts, ranging from 0.1 cm to several centimeters in diameter [28]. The thoracic duct is frequently thickened and dilated. Clinically, most patients present with progressive dyspnea on exertion. Spontaneous pneumothorax, chylothorax, and PH are other pulmonary manifestations. Extrathoracic involvement includes lymphangioleiomyomas (benign neoplasms of lymphatic vessels that appear as cystic masses in the mediastinum, retroperitoneum, or pelvis), chyloperitoneum, renal angiomyolipomas, and meningiomas.

There is a paucity of data on PH complicating LAM. It is thought to be rare, with a reported prevalence of 7% in LAM patients across a wide spectrum of disease [29]. In with more advanced disease, specifically those LAM patients being evaluated for lung transplantation, the prevalence has been reported as high as 45–100% [30, 31], suggesting that the prevalence increases with worsening of the underlying disease process. In the French series [29], a comparison of those patients with and without PH revealed no difference between the two groups in age, menopause status, smoking history, imaging, occurrence of renal tumors, pneumo and/or chylothoraces, or association with tuberous sclerosis complex. However, study subjects with PH had more pronounced airflow obstruction, lower DL_{CO}, and a shorter distance and more desaturation on 6MWT. There was no correlation with physiological disease severity and PH was therefore also seen in patients with preserved lung volumes. PH was mild to moderate (mean mPAP ~32 mmHg) in severity and generally occurred with a preserved cardiac output (5.4 ± 1.9 L/min) without evidence of right heart failure.

The pathogenesis of PH in LAM is not completely understood. As in other advanced lung diseases, chronic hypoxia with pulmonary hypoxic vasoconstriction may play a role. Interestingly, in a study of six patients, no correlation between hemodynamic parameters and the partial pressure of oxygen was demonstrated [32], most likely due to the very small cohort studied. Vascular bed obliteration due to parenchymal destruction and vascular compression from obstructive physiology may also occur. On the cellular level, involvement of the PA walls by characteristic HMB-45 positive cells may contribute to the pathogenesis, potentially via activation of the mammalian target of rapamycin (mTOR) signaling [33].

The presence of PH has significant clinical implications for LAM patients. In one study, the estimated pulmonary artery systolic pressure (sPAP) during peak exercise assessed by TTE had a negative correlation with oxygen saturation. Moreover, increases in sPAP were noted during low-level exercises fairly commonly [34]. In the French series [29], patients with PH had significantly more dyspnea, day-to-day limitations, and were all categorized as NYHA functional class 3 or 4. Almost a quarter of the patients died or underwent lung transplantation within 2 years of PH diagnosis; indeed, the transplant-free probability of survival was 87% at 1 year, 78% at 2 years, and 56% at 3 years [29].

There is a paucity of data on the treatment of PH associated with LAM. In the six patient series earlier, all participants received oral PAH-specific therapy with a significant benefit seen in their hemodynamic profile as manifest by the mean mPAP decreasing from 33 ± 9 to 24 ± 10 mmHg with a decrease in the PVR from 481 ± 188 to 280 ± 79 dyn/w/cm^{-5} [29]. At this time, the treatment of PH in LAM cannot be routinely recommended and if considered should be undertaken at a tertiary PH referral center.

PH in Neurofibromatosis 1 (PH-NF1)

There are three major clinically and genetically distinct forms of neurofibromatosis: neurofibromatosis types 1 and 2 (NF1 and NF2) and schwannomatosis. Neurofibromatosis (NF1), or von Recklinghausen disease, is an autosomal dominant genetic disorder with an incidence of approximately 1 in 2600 to 1 in 3000 individuals, with half of the cases categorized as familial and the rest sporadic or so-called Segmental NF1. The de novo postzygotic mutations occur primarily in paternally derived chromosomes with the likelihood of de novo NF1 increasing with advanced paternal age [35].

NF1 develops as the result of mutations in the NF1 gene located at chromosome 17q11.2 with complete penetrance but highly variable expression. NF1 encodes neurofibromin which is expressed in many tissues, including the brain, kidney, spleen, and thymus. Neurofibromin is a guanosine triphosphate hydrolase (GTPase)-activating protein (GAP) and belongs to the ras p21 protein family that downregulate the cellular proto-oncogenes and are important determinants of cell growth and regulation as well as activators of a number of signaling pathways [36].

NF1 a multisystem disease characterized by café-au-lait spots, Lisch nodules (iris hamartomas), and neurofibromas with distinctive axillary and/or groin freckles on physical examination [35]. Very rarely, NF1 patients may develop PH, pulmonary artery stenosis, and interstitial lung disease. Interstitial lung disease is probably the most common manifestation and radiographically most often presents as cystic or bullous changes or a mosaic pattern of attenuation [37].

The pathogenesis of NF-1-associated PH is unknown. Pathologically, PAH-like plexiform lesions, intimal thickening and fibrosis, and hyperplasia of smooth muscle wall have all been described [38–40]. On a molecular level, it has been postulated that NF1 facilitates vascular remodeling via interactions with PDGF, Ras, mTOR, and extracellular signal-related kinase activities resulting in proliferative signaling and misguided angiogenesis [41, 42]. Unlike in some cases of familial PAH, no bone morphogenic protein receptor 2 (BMPR2) point mutations or large size allele rearrangements have been identified in several case studies [38, 40].

PH seems to develop late in the course of NF1, but the true prevalence is unknown. Most reported patients are >50 years of age and are predominantly female. In one series, a median delay from the time of diagnosis of 44 years was noted [39]. When PH is diagnosed, patients usually have moderate-to-severe disease with mildly decreased cardiac outputs and signs of right heart failure. Patients tend to be very symptomatic with NYHA class 3 symptoms and severely decreased exercise tolerance as demonstrated by a median 6MWT distance of only 180 m from one study. Lung volumes can be normal, obstructive, or restrictive in nature, but the DL_{CO} is always decreased out of proportion to other pulmonary function tests parameters [38]. Several case reports of NF1-PH treatment show very limited efficacy [38, 39].

PH in Cystic Fibrosis (PH-CF)

Cystic Fibrosis (CF) is a most common multisystem autosomal recessive progressive disease in Caucasian population, with a frequency of 1 in 2000–3000 live births in the United States. It is increasingly recognized in non-Caucasian population and occurs in approximately 1:9200 Hispanics, 1:10,900 Native Americans, 1:15,000 African Americans, and 1:30,000 Asian Americans, with prevalence estimates expected to increase with improved newborn screening and increasing recognition of nonclassic presentations of the disease [43]. According to the 2013 CF Foundation Registry Report published in 2014, the median survival for CF patients in the United States is 40.7 years [44], a significant increase over the last two decades.

CF is caused by mutations in a single large gene located on chromosome 7 that encodes the CF transmembrane conductance regulator (CFTR) protein, with clinical disease development predicated by disease-causing mutations in both copies of the CFTR gene [45]. CFTR functions as a regulated chloride channel, which in turn may regulate the activity of other chloride and sodium channels at the cell surface. To date, the CF Mutation Database lists more than 1900 different mutations with disease-causing potential, with delta F508 (being the most common mutation [46]).

Mutations of the CFTR are divided into five different classes: defective protein production (Class I), defective protein processing (Class II), defective regulation (Class III), defective conduction (Class IV), and reduced amounts of functional CFTR protein (Class V). Class I–III mutations are thought to cause more severe disease than the others, although genotype–phenotype correlations are weaker for pulmonary manifestations compared to pancreatic insufficiency phenotypes [46, 47]. Delta F508 is a Class II mutation and accounts for 70% of disease-causing alleles in the United States. Over 50% of CF patients are homozygous and 90% are heterozygous for delta F508. Finally, in up to 20% of patients, inconsistency in phenotypic expression of the disease is thought to be in part a result of action of gene modifiers (such as transforming growth factor-beta 1 and mannose-binding lectin) that are not directly related to the CFTR gene but nevertheless affect the severity of clinical disease manifestations [48].

Traditionally, patients with the typical form of CF were described as having "classic" CF with clinical disease in one or more organ systems, an elevated sweat chloride test, and lungs being the most commonly affected organ. Approximately 20% of CF patients have the "nonclassic" phenotype and fulfill the diagnostic criteria of CF but have normal or intermediate sweat chloride tests [49]. Presently, their diagnosis is most often confirmed by gene sequencing. It is increasingly recognized that there is a wide spectrum of disease severity in CF. Patients with a nonclassic clinical phenotype tend to be diagnosed later, usually have less severe pulmonary disease, no gastrointestinal involvement, and genetically, a higher frequency of unusual CFTR mutations [50].

Pulmonary manifestations of adult CF develop due to thickened and viscous airway secretions as a consequence of the abnormal transport of chloride and sodium across the respiratory epithelium. This results in chronic bronchiectasis and colonization of the airways by a variety of pathogens, most commonly *Pseudomonas aeruginosa* and *Staphylococcus aureus.* Clinically, patients typically present with a chronic productive cough and progressive dyspnea. Radiographically, hyperinflation and bronchiectasis are seen, while PFTs show progressive obstructive physiology with concomitant hyperinflation. Pulmonary function abnormalities may be detectable even in the absence of clinical symptoms. The severity of the disease tends to be variable due to differences in CFTR genotypes interacting with various individual factors. For those with a more aggressive phenotype, the disease progresses to severe obstruction, hypercapneic and hypoxic respiratory failure invariably ensues [51, 52].

Over the last decade, the treatment of the pulmonary manifestations of CF has undergone a period of rapid evolution, characterized by several innovations that have collectively resulted in an improved quality of life and increased longevity [53]. These advances include targeted treatment with IV and cycled inhaled antibiotics, chronic azithromycin use for its inflammatory properties in patients colonized with *Pseudomonas*, aggressive airway clearance with inhaled hypertonic saline, DNase, and most recently CFTR modulators [54, 55].

Pulmonary Hypertension in association with cystic fibrosis (CF) is categorized under Group III PH according to the fifth World PH Symposium classification, under the subgroup of "Other pulmonary diseases with mixed restrictive and obstructive patterns." As CF progresses, many patients succumb due to hypercapneic and/or hypoxemic respiratory failure [56], with PH a common accompanying factor. The prevalence of PH-CF depends on the age of the recipient, possibly gender, severity of the lung disease, as well as the methodology and definition used for the diagnosis [56–59]. In the adult CF population, most existing data is from patients with severe underlying parenchymal disease who are often on the transplant waiting list. This might explain the seemingly high reported prevalence range of 25–91% [60, 61].

The pathophysiology of PH in CF has not been fully elucidated. As in other interstitial lung diseases, chronic alveolar hypoxemia due to lung destruction, ventilation/perfusion mismatch, right to left shunt, progressive destruction of pulmonary vascular bed, air trapping with vessel compression, and/or persistent increase in cardiac output are all thought to play a role [62–66]. As a consequence of the dysfunctional CFTR, chronic respiratory tract infections, as well as the accompanying local and systemic inflammatory-immune response result in greater systemic inflammation which in turn has been demonstrated to cause vascular endothelial dysfunction [65]. Human vascular endothelium itself also expresses the CFTR protein channel [67]. Therefore, it is conceivable that dysfunctional ion regulation could result in compromised control of calcium concentrations in the smooth muscle resulting in a decrease in systemic NO production and lower NO bioavailability locally [65]. Other contributing factors include CF-related porto-pulmonary hypertension, obstructive sleep apnea (OSA), hypothyroidism, heart failure with preserved ejection fraction, as well as an increased incidence of venous thromboembolic events [57, 68, 69]. Histologically, intimal proliferation, subintimal fibrosis, and muscularization of pulmonary arterioles have all been described (Figs. 10.5 and 10.6).

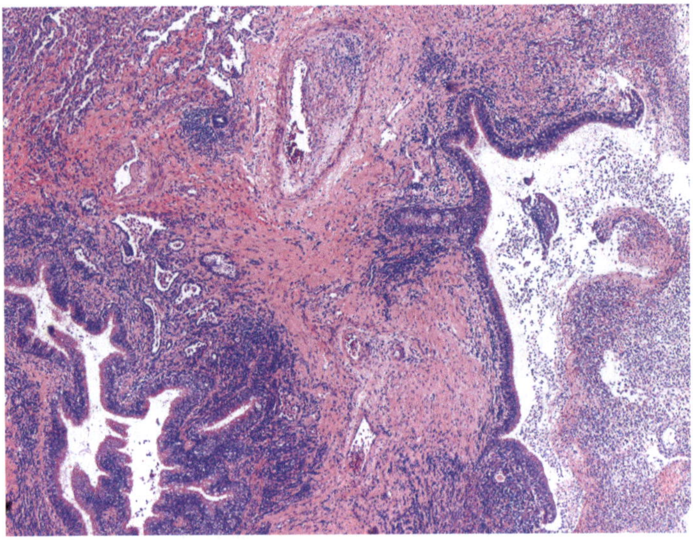

Fig. 10.5 There is bronchiolectasis with mucostasis, consistent with cystic fibrosis. The accompanying artery (*top center*) is abnormal and shows eccentrically thickened fibrointimal cushion with mild inflammation (H&E, 40×)

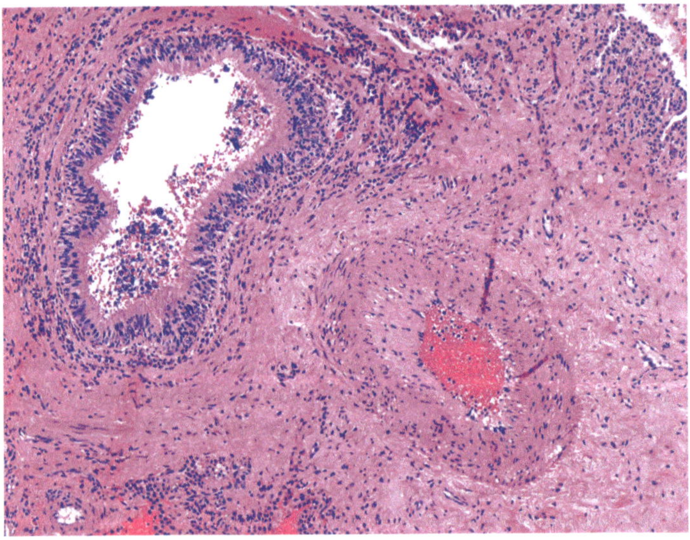

Fig. 10.6 This artery shows mild medial hypertrophy and fibrointimal thickening. The adjacent bronchiole is inflamed, although mucostasis is not evident (H&E, 100×)

Several prospective studies have investigated the function of the right ventricle (RV) in pediatric patients with CF [70, 71]. Interestingly, the presence of RV dysfunction in patients with no or mild obstructive disease without the presence of PH has been reported. The reasons for this finding are still unclear, as usually the development of PH precedes RV dysfunction. It has been postulated that chronic airway inflammation, direct involvement of the heart by the disease itself, and upregulation of neurohormones may be responsible for this finding. In addition, a small study examining exercise hemodynamics in a cohort of CF patients with moderate obstructive disease (FEV1 of 43 ± 11%) reported a significant increase in mPAP with stationary bicycle exertion. Although baseline characteristic showed only mildly elevated PAPs at rest (mean mPAP of 27.8 ± 4.9 and PVR 3.15 ± 0.3), they appeared to be increase significantly with activity (mean mPAP 47.2 ± 5.4 and PVR 12.8 ± 0.6) in 75% of the cohort [66].

To date, no large studies have examined the hemodynamic characteristics of CF patients with concomitant PH across the spectrum of underlying disease severity. An ECHO cohort of 109 adult CF patients showed that ~38% of patients had a trans-tricuspid pressure gradient above 30 mmHg. Patients with severe obstructive disease had the highest prevalence of ECHO-derived PH. The presence of PH also correlated with rest, exercise, and nocturnal need for supplemental oxygen. In a multiple step-wise regression model, the forced expiratory volume at 1 s and partial pressure of oxygen were the only two variables demonstrated to correlate with the presence of PH [72]. Radiographic parenchymal disease severity assessed by the modified Brody score does not correlate to CT scan signs of pulmonary hypertension in CF patients [73]. However, it has been shown in other disease that CT scan evidence of PH is only loosely correlated with RHC data. Indeed, in CF no study as yet has correlated radiographic extent of parenchymal disease to RHC-derived hemodynamic data.

The majority of the published studies that have examined the effect of PH in CF are based on retrospective analyses of large databases or patient cohorts being evaluated for lung transplant. Most studies conclude that the presence of PH has a negative impact on survival; notably different hemodynamic variables and cut points have been employed in these studies including various levels of the mPAP, the systolic PAP and PVR. The largest study to date was based on a retrospective evaluation of a UNOS cohort of 2781 CF patients listed for transplant. A multivariate Cox analysis identified that there was a significant risk of death associated with both mild (mPAP ≥25 mmHg, hazard ratio (HR) of 1.757; 95% confidence interval (CI) 1.367–2.258)) and severe PH (mPAP ≥35 mmHg, HR 2.284; 95% CI 1.596–3.268) [59]. Another analysis of a cohort of 179 CF lung transplant candidates at a single center demonstrated that the presence of any PH in 7.8% of the cohort was associated with worse survival while on the transplant list. A receiver operating characteristic curve demonstrated that sensitivities and specificities for predicting 1-year mortality differed based on the cut-off point of the mPAP (≥25 mmHg 70.2% and 69.7%, respectively, ≥35 mmHg 17.5 and 97%, respectively) [74]. As in other parenchymal diseases, it is not entirely clear whether PH is a marker of advanced disease or a driver of the outcomes. It is arguably likely that severe PH or PH with resultant right ventricular dysfunction is what ultimately affects mortality. Indeed, one study demonstrated that the presence of RV dysfunction, rather than PH, was more common in CF patients who died (51%) compared to those who survived (21%) while awaiting lung transplantation [75].

By virtue of their young age and natural disease progression, many CF patients ultimately advance to the point of requiring lung transplantation. A recent study of 831 CF patients from the UNOS database assessed the impact of pretransplant PH on posttransplant outcomes, and demonstrated that neither the presence nor severity of pretransplant PH negatively affected posttransplant survival [58].

Although there is data supporting that the presence of PH is associated with worse outcomes in CF, no placebo-controlled trials have been conducted to determine if the treatment of PH improves either morbidity or mortality. As with other parenchymal diseases, if PH is a reflection of underlying disease severity, its treatment might not necessarily improve outcomes. However, if PH is a driver of mortality, its treatment may prove beneficial. The potential deleterious effects of treating PH in the setting of CF, such as increased ventilation–perfusion mismatching with worsened hypoxemia, have been raised as a possibility. There is a paucity of data with only several case reports and one small case series describing the safe administration and functional improvement in PH CF patients treated with PDE5 inhibitors ±bosentan and inhaled iloprost [76–78]. In one case report, with PH only assessed by ECHO (RVSP of 41 mmHg at rest and 74 mmHg with exercise at baseline), following 4 months of treatment with low-dose sildenafil, the 6MWT distance increased from a baseline of 488–671 m, and the RVSP decreased to 28 mmHg at rest and 55 mmHg with activity [76]. Another case report described both functional and hemodynamic improvement after a 4-month treatment course with inhaled iloprost. Pulmonary vascular resistance and cardiac output both improved by 23 and 38%, respectively, and WHO functional class changed from 3 to 2 [77]. A case series of three patients evaluated the safety of oral vasodilator therapy with RHC-proven PH (two treated with PDE5 inhibitors and one with combination sildenafil and bosentan) and demonstrated no worsening in oxygenation in any of the patients [78].

Rare Reports of PH in Rare Diseases with ILD Manifestations

Occasional cases of PH have been reported in the literature in diseases such as anti-neutrophil cytoplasmic antibodies (ANCA)-associated systemic vasculitis with parenchymal involvement [79, 80], systemic primary amyloidosis without cardiac but with pulmonary involvement [81, 82], asbestosis-related lung disease [83], silicosis [84], and coal worker's pneumoconiosis [85]. Most papers describe either single cases or small case series employing different methods for diagnosis. It is therefore difficult to draw any conclusions on causal relationship and the true incidence of PH in the earlier diseases.

Two papers describe a total of five patients with ANCA-associated vasculitis (one with microscopic polyangiitis and the rest with Wegener's). All patients presented with hemodynamically severe disease and right heart failure [79]. Several improved with Wegener's specific therapy, while one patient was treated with intravenous epoprostenol and improved significantly. It has been speculated that the development of PH may be caused by small vessel vasculitis with subsequent endovascular fibrosis and microvascular in situ thrombosis.

A single center case series of five patients with systemic amyloidosis-associated interstitial lung disease and concomitant PH diagnosed either by RHC or ECHO reported a mortality of 100%. However, none of the patients were treated with a PAH medication and all were reported to have died from cardiac causes [81]. The authors postulated that microvascular obstruction and resultant endothelial dysfunction due to amyloid deposits in the pulmonary tree resulted in the development of PH. Whatever the pathogenesis of PH in the context of amyloidosis, this obviously portends a very poor prognosis.

One retrospective chart review of 48 patients with coal workers' pneumoconiosis examined the relationship between radiological abnormalities, pulmonary function tests, and PH. In this study, PH was defined by a RHC-derived mPAP of >20 mmHg and found that it could be present even in radiographically apparent but clinically asymptomatic disease. The author reported that spirometric abnormalities correlated with the radiographic appearance of emphysema, while the presence of PH was directly related to the extent of pneumoconiotic nodules. Presumably these nodules may result in obliteration of the vascular bed which may explain this correlation [85].

Conclusion

As with most other forms of diffuse parenchymal lung disease, the development of PH appears to portend a poor prognosis in all of the described conditions. Whether the presence of PH has a causal relationship with mortality or simply represents a marker of disease severity remains unclear. Patients with underlying parenchymal lung disease with concomitant PH remain an intriguing population with regards to their treatment and no clear guidelines exist on if and when to implement therapy. Randomized controlled trials are needed in an effort to better identify subgroups that would benefit from treatment, however such studies are extremely difficult to conduct given the very small afflicted patient populations. If treatment of PH is being considered in any of these patient populations, then it is best undertaken in the context of a tertiary referral center with expertise in PH.

References

1. Baumgartner I, von Hochstetter A, Baumert B, Luetolf U, Follath F. Langerhans' cell histiocytosis in adults. Med Pediatr Oncol. 1993;28(1):9–14.
2. Aricò M, Girschikofsky M, Généreau T, Klersy C, McClain K, Grois N, et al. Langerhans cell histiocytosis in adults. Report from the International Registry of the Histiocyte Society. Eur J Cancer. 2003;39(16):2341–8.

3. Thomeer M, Demedts M, Vandeurzen K. Registration of interstitial lung diseases by 20 centres of respiratory medicine in Flanders. Acta Clin Belg. 2001;56:163–72.
4. Watanabe R, Tatsumi K, Hashimoto S, Tamakoshi A, Kuriyama T. Clinico-epidemiological features of pulmonary histiocytosis X. Int Med. 2001;40:998–1003.
5. Basset F, Corrin B, Spencer H, Lacronique J, Roth C, Soler P, et al. Pulmonary histiocytosis X. Am Rev Respir Dis. 1978;118(5):811–20.
6. Travis WD, Borok Z, Roum JH, Zhang J, Feuerstein I, Ferrans VJ, et al. Pulmonary Langerhans cell granulomatosis (histiocytosis X). A clinicopathologic study of 48 cases. Am J Surg Pathol. 1993;17(10):971–86.
7. Fukuda Y, Basset F, Soler P, Ferrans VJ, Masugi Y, Crystal RG. Intraluminal fibrosis and elastic fiber degradation lead to lung remodeling in pulmonary Langerhans cell granulomatosis (histiocytosis X). Am J Pathol. 1990;7(2):415–24.
8. Tazi A. Aduly pulmonary Langerhan's cell histiocytosis. Eur Respir J. 2006;27(6):1272–85.
9. Crausman RS, Jennings CA, Tuder RM, Ackerson LM, Irvin CG, King Jr TE, et al. Pulmonary histiocytosis X: pumonary function and exercise phatophysiology. Am J Respir Crit Care Med. 1996;153(1):426–35.
10. Vassalo R, Ryu JH, Schroeder DR, Decker PA, Limper AH. Clinical outcomes of pulmonary Langerhans' cell histiocytosis in adults. N Engl J Med. 2002;346(7):484–90.
11. Dauriat G, Mal H, Thabut G, Mornex JF, Bertocchi M, Tronc F, et al. Lung transplantation for pulmonary Langerhan's cell histiocytosis: a multicenter analsys. Transplantation. 2006;81: 746–50.
12. Fartoukh M, Humbert M, Capron F, Maître S, Parent F, Le Gall C, et al. Severe pulmonary hypertension in histiocytosis X. J Respir Crit Care. 2000;161:216–23.
13. Nathan SD, Hassoun P. Pulmonsty hypertension due to lung disease and/or hypoxemia. Clin Chest Med. 2013;34:695–705.
14. Sundar KM, Gosselin MV, Chung HL, Cahill BC, et al. Pulmonary Langerhan's cell histiocytosis: emerging concepts in pathobiology, radiology, and clinical evolution of the disease. Chest. 2003;123:1673–83.
15. Lahm T, Chakinala M. World Health Organization Group 5 Pulmonary HYpertension. Clin Chest Med. 2014;34:753–78.
16. Le Pavec J, Lorillon G, Jaïs X, Tcherakian C, Feuillet S, Dorfmüller P, et al. Pumonnary Langerhans cell histiocytosis-asscociated pulmonary hypertension: clinical characteristics and impact of pulmonary arterial hypertension therapies. Chest. 2012;142(5):1150–7.
17. Harari S, Brenot F, Barberis M, Simmoneau G. Advanced pulmonary histiocytosis X is associated with severe pulmonary hypertension. Chest. 1997;111(4):1142–4.
18. Chaowalit N, Pellikka PA, Decker PA, Aubry MC, Krowka MJ, Ryu JH, et al. Echocardiographic and clinical characteristics of pulmonary hypertension complicating pulmonary Langerhands cell histiocytosis. Mayo Clin Proc. 2004;111(4):1269–75.
19. Simmonneau G, Escourrou P, Duroux P, Lockhart A. Inhibition of hypoxic vasocontriction by nifedipine. N Engl J Med. 1981;304(26):1582–5.
20. Fukuda Y, Miura S, Fujimi K, Yano M, Nishikawa H, Yanagisawa J, et al. Effects of treatment with a combination of cardiac rehabilitaion and bosentan in patients with pulmonary Lagerhans cell histiocytosis associated with pulmonary hypertension. Eur J Prev Cardiol. 2014;21(12):1481–3.
21. Kiakouama L, Cottin V, Etienne-Mastroïanni B, Khouatra C, Humbert M, Cordier JF, et al. Severe pulmonary hypertension in histiocytosis X: long tern improvement iwth bosentan. Eur Respir J. 2010;36(1):202–11.
22. Kalassian KG, Doyle R, Kao P, Ruoss S, Raffin TA. Lymphangioleiomyomatosis: new insights. Am J Respir Crit Care Med. 1997;155(4):1183–6.
23. Moss J, Avila NA, Barnes PM, Litzenberger RA, Bechtle J, Brooks PG, et al. Prevalence and clinical characteristics of lymphangioleiomyomatosis (LAM) in patients with tuberous sclerosis complex. Am J Respir Crit Care Med. 2001;164(4):669–71.
24. Martignoni G, Pea M, Reghellin D, Gobbo S, Zamboni G, Chilosi M, et al. Molecular pathology of lymphangioleiomyomatosis and other perivascular epithelioid cell tumors. Arch Pathol Lab Med. 2010;124(1):33–40.

25. Matsui K, Takeda K, Yu ZX, Valencia J, Travis WD, Moss J, et al. Downregulation of estrogen and progesterone receptors in the abnormal smooth muscle cells in pulmonary lymphangioleiomyomatosis following therapy. An immunohistochemical study. Am J Respir Crit Care Med. 2000;161:1002–9.
26. McCormack FX, Travis WD, Colby TV, Henske EP, Moss J. Lymphangioleiomyomatosis: calling it what it is: a low-grade, destructive, metastasizing neoplasm. Am J Respir Crit Care Med. 2012;186(12):1210–2.
27. Glasgow CG, Avila NA, Lin JP, Stylianou MP, Moss J. Serum vascular endothelial growth factor-D levels in patients with lymphangioleiomyomatosis reflect lymphatic involvement. Chest. 2009;135(5):1293–300.
28. Johnson SR. Lymphangioleiomyomatosis. Eur Respir J. 2006;27:1056–65.
29. Cottin V, Harari S, Humbert M, Mal H, Dorfmüller P, Jaïs X, et al. Pulmonary hypertenison in lymphangioleiomyomatosis: charecteristics in 20 patients. Eur Respir J. 2012;40:630–40.
30. Reynaud-Gaubert M, Mornex JF, Mal H, Treilhaud M, Dromer C, Quétant S, et al. Lung transplantation for lymphangioleiomyomatosis: the French experience. Transplantation. 2008;86:515–20.
31. Ansótegui Barrera E, Mancheño Franch N, Peñalver Cuesta JC, Vera-Sempere F, Padilla Alarcón J, et al. Sporadic lymphangioleiomyomatosis and pulmonary hypertension. Clinical and pathological study in patients undergoing lung transplantation. Med Clin. 2012;138(13):570–3.
32. Carrington CB, Cugell DW, Gaensler EA, Marks A, Redding RA, Schaaf JT, et al. Lymphangioleiomyomatosis. Physiologic-pathologic-radiologic correlations. Am Rev Respir Dis. 1977;116:977–95.
33. Krymskaya VP, Snow J, Cesarone G, Khavin I, Goncharov DA, Lim PN, et al. mTOR is required for pulmonary arterial vascular smooth muscle proliferaton under chronic hypoxia. FASEB J. 2011;25:1922–33.
34. AM T-DS, Stylianou MP, Hedin CJ, Kristof AS, Avila NA, Rabel A, et al. Maximal oxygen uptake and severity of disease in lymphangioleiomyomatosis. Am J Respir Crit Care Med. 2003;168:1427–31.
35. Reynolds RM, Browning GG, Nawroz I, Campbell IW, et al. Von Recklinghausen's neurofibromatosis: neurofibromatosis type 1. Lancet. 2003;361:1552–4.
36. Gutmann DH, Blakeley JO, Korf BR, Packer RJ. Optimizing biologically targeted clinical trials for neurofibromatosis. Expert Opin Investig Drugs. 2013;22(4):443–62.
37. Zamora AC, Collard HR, Wolters PJ, Webb WR, King TE, et al. Neurofibromatosis-associated lung disease: a case series and literature review. Eur Respir J. 2007;29:210–4.
38. Montani D, Coulet F, Girerd B, Eyries M, Bergot E, Mal H, et al. Pulmonary hypertension in patients with neurofibromatosis type I. Medicine. 2011;90:201–11.
39. Aoki Y, Kodama M, Mezaki T, Ogawa R, Sato M, Okabe M, et al. Von Recklinghausen disease complicated by pulmonary hypertension. Chest. 2001;119:1606–8.
40. Stewart DR, Cogan JD, Kramer MR, Miller Jr WT, Christiansen LE, Pauciulo MW, et al. Is pulmonary arterial hypertension in neurofibromatosis type 1 secondary to a plexogenic arteriopathy? Chest. 2007;132:798–808.
41. Xu J, Ismat FA, Wang T, Yang J, Epstein JA, et al. NF1 regulates a ras dependent vascular smooth muscle proliferative injury response. Circulation. 2007;116:2148–56.
42. Munchhof AM, Li F, White HA, Mead LE, Krier TR, Fenoglio A, et al. Neurofibromatosis-associated growth factors activate a distinct signaling network to alter the funcion of neurofibromin-deficient endothelial cells. Hum Mol Genet. 2006;15:1858–69.
43. Ratjen F, Doring G. Cystic fibrosis. Lancet. 2003;361:681–9.
44. Cystic Fibrosis Foundation Patient Registry. 2013 Annual Data Report. 2014. http://www.cff.org/UploadedFiles/research/ClinicalResearch/PatientRegistryReport/2013_CFF_Annual_Data_Report_to_the_Center_Directors.pdf. Accessed 13 Feb 2015.
45. Drumm ML, Collins FS. Molecular biology of cystic fibrosis. Mol Genet Med. 1993;3:33–68.
46. The Cystic Fibrosis Consortium. Correlation between genotype and phenotype in patients with cystic fibrosis. N Engl J Med. 1993;329:1308–13.
47. de Gracia J, Mata F, Alvarez A, Casals T, Gatner S, Vendrell M, et al. Genotype-phenotype correlation for pulmonary function in cystic fibrosis. Thorax. 2005;60:558–63.

48. Drumm ML, Konstan MW, Schluchter MD, Handler A, Pace R, Zou F, et al. Genetic modifiers of lung disease in cystic fibrosis. N Engl J Med. 2005;353:1443–53.
49. Boyle MP. Nonclassic cystic fibrosis and CFTR-related disease. Curr Opin Pulm Med. 2009;9:498–503.
50. Keating CL, Liu X, Dimango EA. Classic respiratory disease but atypical diagnostic testing distinguishes adult presentation of cystic fibrosis. Chest. 2010;127:1157–63.
51. Gilljam M, Ellis L, Corey M, Zielenski J, Durie P, Tullis DE, et al. Clinical manifestations of cystic fibrosis among patients with diagnosis in adulthood. Chest. 2004;126:1215–24.
52. Rowe SM, Miller S, Sorscher EJ. Cystic fibrosis. N Engl J Med. 2005;352:1992–2001.
53. George PM, Banya W, Pareek N, Bilton D, Cullinan P, Hodson ME, et al. Improved survival in low lung function in cystic fibrosis: cohort study from 1990 and 2007. BMJ. 2011;342:d1008.
54. Hoffman LR, Ramsey BW. Cystic fibrosis therapeutics: the road ahead. Chest. 2013;143:207–13.
55. Ashlock MA, Olson ER. Therapeutic development for cystic fibrosis: a successful model for a multisystem genetic disease. Annu Rev Med. 2011;62:107–25.
56. Tonelli AR, Fernandez-Bussy S, Lodhi S. Prevalence of pulmonary hypertension in end-stage cystic fibrosis and correlation with mortality. Heart Lung Transplant. 2010;29:865–72.
57. Tonelli AR. Pulmonary hypertension survival effects and treatment options in cystic fibrosis. Curr Opin Dent. 2013;19:652–61.
58. Hayes Jr D, Higgins RS, Kirkby S, KS MC, Wehr AM, Lehman AM, et al. Impact of pulmonary hypertension on survival in patients with cystic firbrosis undergoing lung transplantation: an analysis of the UNOS registry. J Cyst Fibros. 2014;13:416–23.
59. Hayes Jr D, Tobias JD, Mansour HM, Kirkby S, KS MC, Daniels CJ, et al. Pulmonary hypertension in cystic fibrosis wtih advaced lung disease. Am J Respir Crit Care Med. 2014;190(8):898–905.
60. Belle-van Meerkerk G, Cramer MJ, Kwakkel-van Erp JM, Nugroho MA, Tahri S, de Valk HW, et al. Pulmonary hypertension is a mild comorbidity in end-stage cystic fibrosis patients. J Heart Lung Transplant. 2013;32:609–14.
61. Venuta F, Rendina EA, Rocca GD, De Giacomo T, Pugliese F, Ciccone AM, et al. Pulmonary hemodynamics contribute to indicate priority for lung transplantation in patients with cystic fibrosis. J Thorac Cardiovasc Surg. 2000;119:682–9.
62. Fraser KL, Tullis DE, Sasson Z, Hyland RH, Thornley KS, Hanly PJ, et al. Pulmonary hypertension and cardiac function in adult cystic fibrosis. Chest. 1999;115:1321–8.
63. Hopkins N, McLoughlin P. The structural basis of pulmonary hypertension in chronic lung disease: remodeling, rarefaction or angiogenesis? J Anat. 2002;201:335–48.
64. Fauroux B, Hart N, Belfar S, Boulé M, Tillous-Borde I, Bonnet D, et al. Burkholderia cepacia is associated with pulmonary hypertension and increased mortality among cystic fibrosis patients. J Clin Microbiol. 2004;42:5537–41.
65. Poore S, Berry B, Eidson D, KT MK, Harris RA, et al. Evidence of vascular endothelial dysfunction in young patients with cystic fibrosis. Chest. 2013;143:939–45.
66. Hayes Jr D, Daniels CJ, Kirkby S, Kopp BT, Nicholson KL, Nance AE, et al. Polysomnographic differences assoaited with pulmonary hypertension in patients with advanced lung disease due to cystic fibrosis. Lung. 2014;192:413–9.
67. Tousson A, Van Tine BA, Naren AP, Shaw GM, Schwiebert LM. Characterization of CFTR expression and chloride channel activity in human endothelia. Am J Physiol. 1998;275(6 Pt 1):C1555–64.
68. De Luca F, Trimarchi F, Sferlazzas C, Benvenga S, Costante G, Mami C, et al. Thyroid function in children with cystic fibrosis. Eur J Pediatr. 1982;138:327–30.
69. Takemoto CK. Venous thromboembolism in cystic fibrosis. Pediatr Pulmonol. 2012;47:105–12.
70. Ozcelik N, Shell R, Holtzlander M, Cua C. Decreased right ventricular function in healty pediatric patients wtih cystic fibrosis versus noncystic patients. Pediatr Cardiol. 2013;34:159–64.
71. Baño-Rodrigo A, Salcedo-Posadas A, Villa-Asensi JR, Tamariz-Martel A, Lopez-Neyra A, Blanco-Iglesias E, et al. Right ventricular dysfunction in adolescents with mild cystic fibrosis. J Cyst Fibros. 2012;11:274–80.

72. Bright-Thomas R, Ray SG, Webb AK. Pulmonary artery pressure in cystic fibrosis adults: characteristics, clinical correlates and long-term follow up. J Cyst Fibros. 2012;11:532–8.
73. Simanovsky N, Gileles-Hilliel A, Frenkel R, Shosayov D, Hiller N. Correlation between computed tomography expression of pulmonary hypertension and severity of lung disease in cystic fibrosis patients. J Thorac Imaging. 2013;28(6):383–7.
74. Venuta F, Tonelli AR, Anile M, Diso D, De Giacomo T, Ruberto F, et al. Pulmonary hypertension is associated with higher mortality in cystic fibrosis patients awaiting lung transplantation. J Cardiovasc Surg (Torino). 2012;53:817–20.
75. Belkin RA, Henig NR, Singer LG, Chaparro C, Rubenstein RC, Xie SX, et al. Risk factors for death of patients with cystic fibrosis awaiting lung transplantation. Am J Respir Crit Care Med. 2006;173:659–66.
76. Montgomery GS, Sagel SD, Taylor AL, Abman SH. Effects of sildenafil on pulmonary hypertension and exercise tolerancce in severe cystic fibrosis-related lung disease. Pediatr Pulmonol. 2006;41:383–5.
77. Tissières P, Nicod L, Barazzone-Argiroffo C, Rimensberger PC, Beghetti M, et al. Aerosolized iloprost as a bridge to lung transplantation in a patient with cystic fibrosis and pulmonary hypertension. Ann Thorac Surg. 2004;78:e48–50.
78. Gorbett D, Hayes D, Daniels CJ, Smith JS. Pulmonary hypertension in advanced cystic fibrosis: pulmonary vasodilator therapy prior to lung transplantation. Am J Respir Crit Care. 2014;189:A4839.
79. Launay D, Souza R, Guillevin L, Hachulla E, Pouchot J, Simonneau G, et al. Pulmonary arterrial hypertension in ANCA-associated vasculitis. Sarcoidosis Vasc Diffuse Lung Dis. 2006;23:223–8.
80. Doyle DJ, Fanning NF, Silke CS, Salah S, Burke L, Molloy M, et al. Wegener's granulomatosis of the main pulmonary arteries: imaging findings. Clin Radiol. 2003;58:329–31.
81. Dingli D, Utz JP, Gertz MA. Pulmonary hypertension in patients with amyloidosis. Chest. 2001;120(5):1735–9.
82. Chapman AD, Brown PA, Kerr KM. Right heart failure as the domonant clinical picture in a case of primary amyloidosis affecting the pulmonary vasculature. Scott Med J. 1999;44:116–7.
83. Tomasini M, Chiappino G. Hemodynamics of pulmonary circulation in asbestosis: study of 16 cases. Ann J Ind Med. 1981;2(2):167–74.
84. Evers H, Liehs F, Harzbecker K, Wenzel D, Wilke A, Pielesch W, et al. Screening of pulmonary hypertension in chronic obstructibe pulmonary disease and silicosis by discriminant functions. Eur Respir J. 1992;5(4):444–51.
85. Akkoca Yildez O, Eris Gulbay B, Saryal S, Karabiyikoglu G. Evaluation of the relationship between radiological abnormalities and both pulmonary function and pulmonary hypertension in coal workers' pneumoconiosis. Respirology. 2007;12:420–6.

Index

R.P. Baughman et al. (eds.), *Pulmonary Hypertension and Interstitial Lung Disease*, DOI 10.1007/978-3-319-49918-5

MIX
Papier aus verantwortungsvollen Quellen
Paper from responsible sources
FSC® C105338
www.fsc.org

If you have any concerns about our products,
you can contact us on
ProductSafety@springernature.com

In case Publisher is established outside the EU,
the EU authorized representative is:
Springer Nature Customer Service Center GmbH
Europaplatz 3, 69115 Heidelberg, Germany

Printed by Libri Plureos GmbH
in Hamburg, Germany